Neurologic Emergencies

Editors

MICHAEL K. ABRAHAM
EVIE MARCOLINI

EMERGENCY MEDICINE CLINICS OF NORTH AMERICA

www.emed.theclinics.com

Consulting Editor
AMAL MATTU

February 2021 • Volume 39 • Number 1

ELSEVIER

1600 John F. Kennedy Boulevard • Suite 1800 • Philadelphia, Pennsylvania, 19103-2899

http://www.theclinics.com

EMERGENCY MEDICINE CLINICS OF NORTH AMERICA Volume 39, Number 1
February 2021 ISSN 0733-8627, ISBN-13: 978-0-323-76328-8

Editor: Joanna Collett
Developmental Editor: Casey Potter

Emergency Medicine Clinics of North America (ISSN 0733-8627) is published quarterly by Elsevier Inc., 360 Park Avenue South, New York, NY, 10010-1710. Months of issue are February, May, August, and November. Business and Editorial Offices: 1600 John F. Kennedy Boulevard, Suite 1800, Philadelphia, PA 19103-2899. Customer Service Office: 6277 Sea Harbor Drive, Orlando, FL 32887-4800. Periodicals postage paid at New York, NY, and additional mailing offices. Subscription prices are $100.00 per year (US students), $359.00 per year (US individuals), $926.00 per year (US institutions), $220.00 per year (international students), $462.00 per year (international individuals), $986.00 per year (international institutions), $100.00 per year (Canadian students), $423.00 per year (Canadian individuals), and $986.00 per year (Canadian institutions). International air speed delivery is included in all *Clinics'* subscription prices. All prices are subject to change without notice. **POSTMASTER:** Send address changes to *Emergency Medicine Clinics of North America*, Elsevier Periodicals Customer Service, 11830 Westline Industrial Drive, St. Louis, MO 63146. Customer Service (orders, claims, online, change of address): Elsevier Periodicals **Customer Service, 11830 Westline Industrial Drive, St. Louis, MO 63146. Tel: 1-800-654-2452 (U.S. and Canada); 314-453-7041 (outside U.S. and Canada). Fax: 314-453-5170. E-mail: journalscustomerservice-usa@elsevier.com (for print support); journalsonlinesupport-usa@elsevier.com (for online support)**.

Reprints. For copies of 100 or more of articles in this publication, please contact the Commercial Reprints Department, Elsevier Inc., 360 Park Avenue South, New York, NY 10010-1710. Tel.: 212-633-3874; Fax: 212-633-3820; E-mail: reprints@elsevier.com.

Emergency Medicine Clinics of North America is covered in *MEDLINE/PubMed (Index Medicus), Current Contents/Clinical Medicine, EMBASE/Excerpta Medica, BIOSIS, SciSearch, CINAHL, ISI/BIOMED,* and *Research Alert.*

Contributors

CONSULTING EDITOR

AMAL MATTU, MD, FAAEM, FACEP
Professor and Vice Chair of Academic Affairs, Department of Emergency Medicine, University of Maryland School of Medicine, Baltimore, Maryland

EDITORS

MICHAEL K. ABRAHAM, MD, MS
Adjunct Assistant Professor, Department of Emergency Medicine, University of Maryland School of Medicine, Baltimore, Maryland; Chair, Department of Emergency Medicine, University of Maryland, –Upper Chesapeake Health System, Bel Air, Maryland

EVIE MARCOLINI, MD
Associate Professor of Emergency Medicine and Neurology, Geisel School of Medicine at Dartmouth, Hanover, New Hampshire

AUTHORS

JORDAN BONOMO, MD, FCCM, FNCS
Departments of Emergency Medicine, Neurology and Rehabilitation Medicine, Neurosurgery, University of Cincinnati, Cincinnati, Ohio

JULIE BYKOWSKI, MD
Professor, Department of Radiology, UC San Diego Health, San Diego, California

KELSEY CACIC, MD
Department of Neurology and Rehabilitation Medicine, University of Cincinnati, Cincinnati, Ohio

RHONDA CADENA, MD
Associate Professor, Division of Neurocritical Care, Departments of Neurology, Neurosurgery, and Emergency Medicine, The University of North Carolina at Chapel Hill, Chapel Hill, North Carolina

MEGAN J. COBB, MD, DPT
Adjunct Clinical Instructor, Department of Emergency Medicine, University of Maryland School of Medicine, Maryland Emergency Medicine Network, Upper Chesapeake Emergency Medicine, Bel Air, Maryland

NICOLE M. DUBOSH, MD
Assistant Professor of Emergency Medicine, Harvard Medical School, Beth Israel Deaconess Medical Center, Boston, Massachusetts

KYLE M. DEWITT, PharmD
Pharmacist Clinician, Emergency Medicine, Department of Pharmacy, The University of Vermont Medical Center, Burlington, Vermont

JONATHAN A. EDLOW, MD
Professor of Medicine and Emergency Medicine, Harvard Medical School, Vice Chairman, Department of Emergency Medicine, Beth Israel Deaconess Medical Center, Boston, Massachusetts

SAMUEL M. GALVAGNO Jr, DO, PhD, FCCM
Professor, Medical Director, Multi Trauma Critical Care Unit, R Adams Cowley Shock Trauma Center, Program in Trauma, University of Maryland School of Medicine, Baltimore, Maryland

J. DAVID GATZ, MD
Assistant Professor of Emergency Medicine, University of Maryland School of Medicine, Baltimore, Maryland

KAREN GREENBERG, DO, FACOEP, FAAEM
Director, Neurologic Emergency Department, Global Neurosciences Institute, Crozer Chester Medical Center, Lawrenceville, New Jersey

KIERSTEN L. GURLEY, MD
Instructor of Emergency Medicine, Harvard Medical School, Assistant QI Director, Department of Emergency Medicine, Beth Israel Deaconess Medical Center, Boston, Massachusetts; Attending Physician, Anna Jaques Hospital, Newburyport, Massachusetts

ANNA KARPENKO, MD
Assistant Professor of Neurology and Neurocritical Care, Dartmouth Hitchcock Medical Center, Lebanon, New Hampshire

JOSHUA KEEGAN, MD
Assistant Professor of Emergency Medicine and Neurocritical Care, Dartmouth Hitchcock Medical Center, Lebanon, New Hampshire

DEENA KHAMEES, MD
Clinical Instructor, Emergency Medicine, University of Michigan Medical School, Ann Arbor, Michigan

DANYA KHOUJAH, MBBS, MEHP
Attending Physician, Emergency Medicine, MedStar Franklin Square Medical Center, Adjunct Volunteer Assistant Professor, Department of Emergency Medicine, University of Maryland School of Medicine, Baltimore, Maryland

STEPHEN Y. LIANG, MD, MPHS
Assistant Professor, Departments of Emergency Medicine and Internal Medicine, Division of Infectious Disease, Washington University School of Medicine, St Louis, Missouri

EVIE MARCOLINI, MD
Associate Professor of Emergency Medicine and Neurology, Geisel School of Medicine at Dartmouth, Hanover, New Hampshire

WILLIAM MEURER, MD
Associate Professor, Emergency Medicine, University of Michigan Medical School, Ann Arbor, Michigan

BLAKE A. PORTER, PharmD
Pharmacist Clinician, Emergency Medicine, Department of Pharmacy, The University of Vermont Medical Center, Burlington, Vermont

RYAN RAAM, MD
Assistant Professor of Clinical Emergency Medicine, Keck School of Medicine of USC, Assistant Program Director, LAC+USC Emergency Medicine Residency, Los Angeles, California

JESSE SHRIKI, DO, MS, FACEP
Fellow, Surgical Critical Care, R Adams Cowley Shock Trauma Center, Program in Trauma, University of Maryland School of Medicine, Baltimore, Maryland

MATTHEW S. SIKET, MD, MSc
Associate Professor, Division of Emergency Medicine, Departments of Surgery and Neurological Sciences, Larner College of Medicine at the University of Vermont, Burlington, Vermont

LUCAS SJEKLOCHA, MD
Emergency Medicine/Surgical Critical Care Fellow, R Adams Cowley Shock Trauma Center, Baltimore, Maryland

ROBERT J. STEPHENS, MD, MSCI
Resident Physician, Department of Emergency Medicine, Washington University School of Medicine, St Louis, Missouri

RAMIN R. TABATABAI, MD, MACM, FACEP
Associate Professor of Clinical Emergency Medicine, Keck School of Medicine of USC, Program Director, LAC+USC Emergency Medicine Residency, Los Angeles, California

BENJAMIN TOLCHIN, MD, MS
Assistant Professor, Department of Neurology, Yale School of Medicine, New Haven, Connecticut

Contents

Both blunt and penetrating trauma can cause injuries to the peripheral and central nervous systems. Emergency providers must maintain a high index of suspicion, especially in the setting of polytrauma. There are 2 major classifications of peripheral nerve injuries (PNIs). Some PNIs are classically associated with certain traumatic mechanisms. Most closed PNIs are managed conservatively, whereas sharp nerve transections require specialist consultation for urgent repair. Spinal cord injuries almost universally require computed tomography imaging; some require emergent magnetic resonance imaging. Providers should work to minimize secondary injury. Surgical specialists are needed for closed reduction, surgical decompression, or stabilization.

Neuroimaging should be obtained for all patients suspected of having acute ischemic stroke or transient ischemic attack. Noncontrast head computed tomography (CT) scans are used to exclude hemorrhage, evaluate for early brain injury, and exclude stroke mimics. CT angiography assists in identifying proximal vessel occlusions, dissection, or high-grade arterial stenoses. Additional imaging techniques have emerged to improve selection of patients likely to benefit from therapies. Artificial intelligence applications assist in acute stroke imaging assessment, identifying acute hemorrhage, and predicting risk of endovascular intervention in acute large vessel occlusion. Each should be considered an aid rather than stand-alone diagnostic tool.

The diagnosis and management of neurologic conditions are more complex at the extremes of age than in the average adult. In the pediatric population, neurologic emergencies are somewhat rare and some may require emergent consultation. In older adults, geriatric physiologic changes with increased comorbidities leads to atypical presentations and worsened outcomes. The unique considerations regarding emergency department presentation and

to epileptic seizures but are instead a common and highly disabling form of functional neurologic disorder, or conversion disorder. Consistent with the biopsychosocial model of mental illness, functional seizures are caused by biological, psychological, and social factors unrelated to epileptic discharges. People with functional seizures do not consciously fake their symptoms. Functional seizures can be differentiated from epileptic seizures through the clinical history, features of the seizures themselves, and electroencephalography findings. Psychotherapy is effective in treating functional seizures.

Emergency Neuropharmacology 133

Kyle M. DeWitt and Blake A. Porter

Management of acute neurologic disorders in the emergency department is multimodal and may require the use of medications to decrease morbidity and mortality secondary to neurologic injury. Clinicians should form an individualized treatment approach with regard to various patient specific factors. This review article focuses on the pharmacotherapy for common neurologic emergencies that present to the emergency department, including traumatic brain injury, central nervous system infections, status epilepticus, hypertensive emergencies, spinal cord injury, and neurogenic shock.

Diagnosis of Coma 155

Anna Karpenko and Joshua Keegan

The differential diagnosis for the comatose patient is includes structural abnormality, seizure, encephalitis, metabolic derangements, and toxicologic etiologies. Identifying and treating the underlying pathology in a timely manner is critical for the patient's outcome. We provide a structured approach to taking a history and performing a physical examination for this patient population. We discuss diagnostic testing and treatment methodologies for each of the common causes of coma. Our current understanding of the mechanisms of coma is insufficient to accurately predict the patient's clinical trajectory and more work needs to be done to investigate potential treatments for this often fatal disorder.

Approach to Acute Weakness 173

Deena Khamees and William Meurer

Weakness has a broad differential diagnosis. A paradigm for organizing possibilities is to consider what part of the nervous system is involved, ranging from brain, spinal cord, nerve roots, and peripheral nerves to the neuromuscular junction. The clinician can consider internal versus external causes. Some neurologic conditions have subtle presentations yet carry a risk of short-term decompensation if not recognized. It is helpful to consider whether an emergency department presentation of weakness is a new disease process or represents an exacerbation of an established condition. Emergency presentations of weakness are challenging, and one must carefully consider potential serious causes.

EMERGENCY MEDICINE CLINICS OF NORTH AMERICA

FORTHCOMING ISSUES

May 2021
Emergencies in the Older Adult
Robert Anderson, Phillip Magidson, and
Danya Khoujah, *Editors*

August 2021
Pediatric Emergency Medicine
Mimi Lu, Ilene Claudius and Chris Amato,
Editors

RECENT ISSUES

November 2020
Emergency Department Resuscitation
Michael E. Winters and Susan R. Wilcox,
Editors

August 2020
**Emergency Department Operations and
Administration**
Joshua W. Joseph and Benjamin A. Whie,
Editors

SERIES OF RELATED INTEREST

Orthopedic Clinics
https://www.orthopedic.theclinics.com/

THE CLINICS ARE NOW AVAILABLE ONLINE!
Access your subscription at:
www.theclinics.com

Foreword

Neurologic Emergencies

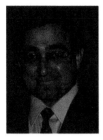

Amal Mattu, MD, FAAEM, FACEP
Consulting Editor

I'll bet that if you ask most emergency physicians about which organ system's emergencies cause them the most angst, it would be the neurologic system. Neurologic emergencies are the epitome of the proverbial "needle in a haystack." For example, the overwhelming majority of cases of headache, back pain, weakness, and dizziness turn out to be a haystack of benign causes. Our job in the emergency department is to find those rare needles...the subarachnoid hemorrhage, the spinal infection, the stroke, or the vertebral dissection. Further complicating our task is that misdiagnoses of many of these neurologic conditions can result in disastrous outcomes, including profound disability or death.

Disastrous outcomes certainly can occur in other organ systems as well, but we tend to be more comfortable in assessing those other conditions. Perhaps our discomfort with emergency neurology is due to inadequate training in neurologic conditions; or perhaps it is because the neurologic system cannot be seen, felt, or auscultated; or perhaps it is because the examination of the neurologic system is more complicated than other systems and the examination cannot simply be replaced with a blood test or radiograph. Regardless of the reason for our discomfort, we need to improve our skills in the diagnosis and management of patients presenting with neurologic emergencies.

I am, therefore, thrilled to welcome Drs Michael Abraham and Evie Marcolini to serve as Guest Editors of this issue of *Emergency Medicine Clinics of North America* focused on neurologic emergencies. Both of these educators have dedicated their careers to educating emergency physicians on the care of patients with neurologic emergencies. They have assembled an outstanding team to discuss a wide range of conditions, from the common to the catastrophic. Common presentations are addressed, including headaches, weakness, dizziness, trauma, and altered mental status, all the while focusing on separating out the catastrophic needles from the stacks of hay. Articles also focus on specific conditions, such as infections, seizures, coma, transient

Emerg Med Clin N Am 39 (2021) xiii–xiv
https://doi.org/10.1016/j.emc.2020.10.001
0733-8627/21/© 2020 Published by Elsevier Inc.

ischemic attack, and stroke. Presentations and conditions that are a bit more specific to extremes of age are addressed in a separate article as well. In addition, miscellaneous articles focusing on imaging techniques, neuropharmacology, sedation and intubation, and end-of-life care round out the issue.

This issue of *Emergency Medicine Clinics of North America* should be considered must-reading not only for us practicing emergency physicians but also for emergency medicine trainees and for any other health care providers who feel somewhat uncertain or inadequate about their ability to diagnose and manage the vast array of neurologic emergencies. Knowledge and practice of the concepts that are discussed in the following pages are certain to help pick out those needles in the haystack and save lives. Kudos to the Guest Editors and authors for providing us with this valuable addition to our specialty.

Amal Mattu, MD, FAAEM, FACEP
Department of Emergency Medicine
University of Maryland School of Medicine
110 South Paca Street
6th Floor, Suite 200
Baltimore, MD 21201, USA

E-mail address:
amattu@som.umaryland.edu

Preface

Neurologic Emergencies: 2020 Update

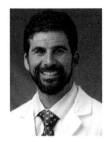 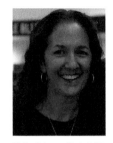

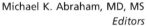

Michael K. Abraham, MD, MS   Evie Marcolini, MD
Editors

Emergency Medicine is a unique field in the house of medicine. We are expected to understand and assimilate the most pressing details of every specialty, often with limited resources and information, in a time-sensitive manner. This uniqueness is nowhere more exemplified than with emergency neurology. Neurology is a field of medicine both adored and feared by emergentologists. Most often this dichotomy can be attributed to the complexity, subtlety, and rapidly evolving nature of the field. *Emergency Medicine Clinics of North America* published a dedicated neurology issue in 2016. The fact that they have decided to publish another issue so quickly highlights the point that the field continues to evolve. While many of the articles in this issue are on topics similar to the 2016 issue, we have provided updates and new perspectives to mirror the evolving science. Topics covered in this issue will help to clarify some of the diagnostic challenges neurologic emergencies present for the Emergency Medicine clinician.

In this issue, we showcase experts in the field writing about neurologic emergencies that you see nearly every day in your practice, such as neurotrauma, headache, the dizzy patient, stroke, and neuroinfections, but all with important updates and new protocols. Some of the tools that you use will each have an article, such as neuroimaging, neuropharmacology, and sedation in the neurologically impaired patient. Finally, some of the more complex patient scenarios have articles to give you a useful framework with which to approach the patient, such as coma, functional seizures, neuromuscular diseases, neurologic emergencies at the extremes of age, and neuroethics.

Our goal for this issue is to demystify many of the complex and confusing subtleties of neurology and increase the comfort level for the emergency clinician taking care of these patients and teaching residents. We hope that you find this issue useful and as

Emerg Med Clin N Am 39 (2021) xv–xvi
https://doi.org/10.1016/j.emc.2020.09.015
0733-8627/21/© 2020 Published by Elsevier Inc.

emed.theclinics.com

interesting as it was for us to compile, and after reading it that you have a newfound comfort level with both the common and the complex neurologic emergencies.

Michael K. Abraham, MD, MS
Department of Emergency Medicine
University of Maryland School of Medicine
110 S. Paca Street, 6th Floor
Baltimore, MD 21201, USA

Evie Marcolini, MD
Emergency Medicine and Neurology
Geisel School of Medicine
Department of Emergency Medicine
1 Medical Center Drive
Lebanon, NH 03756, USA

E-mail addresses:
Mike.Abraham@gmail.com (M.K. Abraham)
Emarcolini@gmail.com (E. Marcolini)

Traumatic Injuries to the Spinal Cord and Peripheral Nervous System

Lucas Sjeklocha, MD[a], J. David Gatz, MD[b],*

KEYWORDS

- Peripheral nerve injury • Spinal cord injury • Trauma • Neurogenic shock
- Secondary injury

KEY POINTS

- Injuries to the peripheral nervous system and spinal cord regularly occur during blunt and penetrating trauma.
- Other life-threatening injuries should be prioritized in the setting of polytrauma before pursing definitive management of injuries to peripheral nerves or the spinal cord.
- Sharply transected peripheral nerve injuries should prompt consultation for immediate repair.
- Providers should have a low threshold for intubation during the acute management of spinal cord injuries because lower cervical and even thoracic injuries can result in insufficient airway protection or breathing.
- First-line management of neurogenic shock should be intravenous fluids followed by, if necessary, norepinephrine to maintain a mean arterial pressure of at least 85 mm Hg.

INTRODUCTION

All trauma, whether blunt or penetrating, has the potential to cause injury to the nervous system. This includes the brain and spinal cord of the central nervous system and the somatic and autonomic components of the peripheral nervous system (PNS). Traumatic injuries to the PNS are a significant source of morbidity. Peripheral nerve injury (PNI) can result in permanent disability and entail significant health care and patient costs. Acute costs associated with these injuries average nearly $6000 in the emergency department (ED) and $20,000 to $60,000 in inpatient expenses.[1–3] These costs do not consider the burden of decreased quality of life and long-term health care costs.

[a] R Adams Cowley Shock Trauma Center, 22 South Greene Street, Room S4D03, Baltimore, MD 21201, USA; [b] Department of Emergency Medicine, University of Maryland School of Medicine, 110 South Paca Street, 6th Floor, Suite 200, Baltimore, MD 21201, USA
* Corresponding author.
E-mail address: jgatz@som.umaryland.edu
Twitter: @DrDavidGatz (J.D.G.)

Emerg Med Clin N Am 39 (2021) 1–28
https://doi.org/10.1016/j.emc.2020.09.001
0733-8627/21/© 2020 Elsevier Inc. All rights reserved.

Spinal cord injuries (SCIs) similarly can cause significant permanent disability and even death. The financial cost to patients and society from SCIs is significant, accumulating average expenses in the United States between $375,000 and $1,150,000 in the first year alone, depending on severity of injury. Subsequent annual expenses average between $45,000 to $200,000.[4]

Emergency medicine providers play an essential role in the recognition and subsequent management of these patients. Presentations can be subtle and sometimes are missed, risking morbidity and even mortality for patients, and subjecting providers to high medicolegal liability. Prior malpractice suits involving missed cervical injuries in blunt trauma patients, for example, have resulted in multimillion-dollar awards.[5]

This article covers the pathophysiology, clinical assessment, and management of traumatic PNIs and SCIs. The primary population of this review is adult patients. Please see the article "Neurologic Emergencies at the Extremes of Age," by Khoujah and Cobb for further discussion of pediatric and geriatric populations.

PERIPHERAL NERVE INJURY
Epidemiology

Traumatic PNI represents a significant burden of disease. PNIs are thought to have an incidence of more than 350,000 per year in the United States.[6] Previous estimates using the National Inpatient Sample and National Emergency Department Sample show widely varying estimates of injuries based on diagnosis codes and likely underestimate the true burden of injury. The overall trend in injuries has been relatively stable, with upper extremity PNI more common than lower extremity PNI.[1,2] Among trauma patients evaluated at a level 1 trauma center, 2.8% were identified as having a PNI.[7] European trauma registry data showed PNIs associated with 3.3% of severe upper extremity trauma and 1.8% of severe lower extremity trauma.[8,9] PNIs may remain occult in severely injured patients given priorities of resuscitation and concomitant injuries that limit the examination. A previous case series of traumatic brain injury patients identified a 34% incidence of PNIs not recognized on initial evaluation.[10]

Males account for 80% of traumatic PNIs with a mean age of approximately 40 years in registry data.[8,9] Blunt mechanisms, including motor vehicle accidents and falls, account for the majority of injuries but disproportionately higher rates of PNIs are observed in penetrating trauma then compared to the overall trauma population.[9] In upper extremity trauma, the ulnar nerve is injured most commonly, followed by the radial and median nerves.[2] The peroneal nerve is the lower extremity nerve most commonly injured followed by the sciatic and tibial nerves.[1] Sports-related acute nerve injury represents less than 1% of all injuries but has been increasing.[11]

Key Anatomy and Pathophysiology

The terms, *peripheral nerve* and *PNS*, encompass nervous tissue and supporting structures between the central nervous system and target tissues or sensory areas. These include cranial nerves (except for the optic nerves) and the autonomic nervous system, in addition to motor and sensory branches originating in the spinal cord. Peripheral nerves have several specialized connective tissues: the endoneurium, the perineurium, and the epineurium (**Fig. 1**). These define the structure of the nerve and are critical for regeneration.[12]

Most PNIs can be attributed to a combination of mechanisms including traction or stretch, contusion, transection, and compression. Other mechanisms of traumatic injury include ischemia, burns, and electrical injuries. Nerves are vulnerable to different mechanisms along their length due to the changing composition of the nerves and

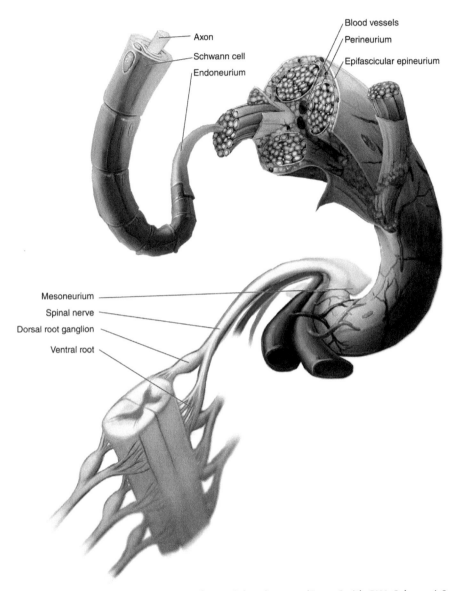

Fig. 1. Major anatomic components of a peripheral nerve. (*From* Smith BW, Sakamuri S, Spain DA, Joseph JR, Yang LJ, Wilson TJ. An update on the management of adult traumatic nerve injuries-replacing old paradigms: A review. J Trauma Acute Care Surg. 2019;86(2):299-306; with permission.)

regional anatomy. Nerve roots, for instance, lack both epineurium and perineurium and are relatively tethered to the spinal cord, making them vulnerable to traction and compression.[6] Proximity to bone makes nerves vulnerable to injury from fractures, whereas superficial nerves may be more easily contused or lacerated.

Nerve stretching can be part of normal function with changes in length as nerves cross over joints and at extremes of physiologic movement. Extremes of stretching overwhelm the ability of the connective tissue to compensate and result in injuries with associated hematomas and scarring.[13] Avulsion is an extreme stretch or traction injury causing mechanical failure and disruption of the nerve, often occurring at nerve roots and is associated with significant morbidity.

Compression can cause ischemic injury from direct or indirect pressure (eg, associated compartment syndrome). A classic example is compression of the radial nerve against the humerus as it travels in the radial groove, producing a Saturday night palsy. Hydrostatic forces from penetrating injury also can cause nerve injury or disruption. Crush injuries can occur directly or via entrapment from dislocation-relocation or associated fractures. Laceration or transection mechanisms can be divided into sharp and blunt.

Classification of Peripheral Nerve Injuries

In 1942, Seddon[14] proposed a classification scheme that is still in primary use today for grading nerve injuries based on severity of disruption to the nerve and supporting structures. Seddon divided injuries as neurapraxia, axonotmesis, and neurotmesis (**Fig. 2**). Sunderland[15] later expanded this to 5 degrees of injury (**Table 1**).

Presentation and Examination of Peripheral Nerve Injuries

Traumatic PNI initially is a clinical diagnosis and, because PNIs by themselves typically are not life threatening, other more dangerous and time-sensitive causes and associated injuries must be considered. In the trauma patient, prompt global assessment and resuscitation should be undertaken prior to detailed investigation for nerve injury. All sensory or motor abnormalities should be evaluated for alternative causes, especially central causes, such as intracranial hemorrhage and SCIs.[16] An evolving deficit should prompt evaluation for a dynamic process like progressive edema, hematoma formation, pseudoaneurysm formation, or shifting of fractures.

Evidence of nerve injury should prompt consideration of associated fractures, hematomas, compartment syndrome, and arterial injuries. Because nerves typically travel along the neurovascular bundles, and blood vessels are vulnerable to the same forces, approximately 13% of upper extremity PNIs from civilian trauma have an associated vascular injury.[9,17] Injuries associated with warfare and penetrating injury have an even higher association between PNIs and vascular injuries, with arterial injuries present in 48 of 119 patients in a case series of PNIs from the Balkan conflict.[18] Traumatic injuries typically present with maximal deficits.

It is critical to determine open versus closed injuries because this significantly alters management.[19–23] Exploration of an open wound and assessment of the wound mechanism can help identify an associated clinical nerve injury. A clean, sharp transection versus a blunt, ragged transection can affect the urgency of repair.[20,21,23] Providers should use motor grading and sensory testing to determine the severity and likely anatomic location(s) of injury (**Fig. 3** for sensory distribution of major peripheral nerves). Two-point discrimination is the preferred mode of testing for sensory injury with a recent case series of hand injuries, demonstrating 98.6% sensitivity for detecting nerve injury with a 2-point discrimination tool compared to 82.5% for dry gauze.[16,24] Tinel sign also may be present acutely at the area of injury with advancing location and increased pain present in regenerating injuries and developing neuromas, respectively.[25]

Providers should be prepared to recognize several classic PNIs of the upper (**Table 2**) and lower (**Table 3**) extremities.

A

Normal Nerve Schematic

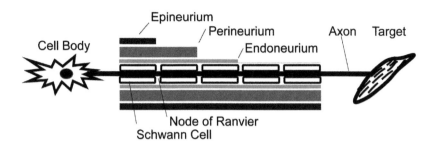

B

Nerve Injury Schematic

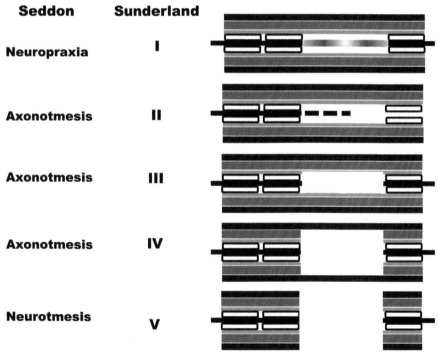

Fig. 2. (A) Intact peripheral nerve anatomy. (B) Anatomic schematic of PNI grades.

Diagnostic Evaluation of Peripheral Nerve Injuries

Clinical examination combined with potential surgical exploration, electromyography, and nerve conduction studies is important for overall assessment of PNIs. Additional diagnostics during acute presentations in the ED are largely supplements to the clinical examination and evaluate primarily for associated injuries and alternative causes.

Table 1
Seddon and Sunderland classification schemes of peripheral nerve injuries

Seddon	Sunderland	Clinical Correlate	Pathologic Correlate	Prognosis for Spontaneous Recovery	Surgical Intervention
Neurapraxia	1	Compression, ischemia	Demyelination	Good	Unnecessary
Axonotmesis	2	Ischemia, crush, percussion	Axon degeneration	Good to fair	Usually unnecessary
	3		Endoneural injury	Intermediate	May be required
	4		Perineural injury	Poor	May be required
Neurotmesis	5	Avulsion, transection	Epineural Injury	Poor	Required

From National Spinal Cord Injury Statistical Center. 2019 Annual Statistical Report for the Spinal Cord Injury. Model Systems. University of Alabama at Birmingham: Birmingham, Alabama; With permission.

X-ray and computed tomography evaluation

Peripheral nerves are not imaged by plain radiographs and are poorly imaged with computed tomography (CT). These images can evaluate for associated injuries. Individual nerve injuries may prompt specific radiographs to identify commonly associated fractures or dislocations (eg, hook of hamate fracture in distal ulnar nerve injury or evaluation for a Bankart or Hill-Sachs lesion suggestive of previous dislocation in axillary nerve dysfunction). Although CT is inadequate for direct evaluation of

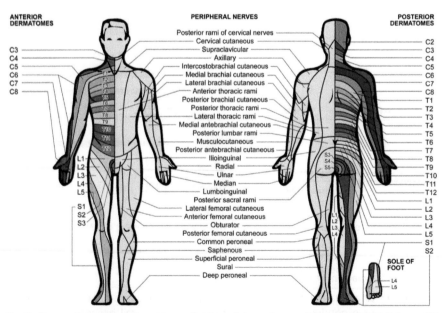

Fig. 3. Comparison of peripheral nerve fields and dermatomes. (*From* Smith BW, Sakamuri S, Spain DA, Joseph JR, Yang LJ, Wilson TJ. An update on the management of adult traumatic nerve injuries-replacing old paradigms: A review. *J Trauma Acute Care Surg.* 2019;86(2):299–306; with permission.)

Table 2
Classic peripheral nerve injuries of the upper extremities

Nerves	Example Mechanism(s)	Major Deficits	Pathologic Correlate
Brachial plexus	Stinger/burner Seatbelt injury	Variable; typically, C5-C6 or C8-T1, depending on direction of forces Autonomic deficits (eg, Horner syndrome) in C8-T1 lesions	Neuropraxia, nerve avulsion in severe trauma
Axillary	Shoulder dislocation Surgical neck fracture of humerus	Sensory: deltoid area Motor: shoulder flexion and abduction	Neuropraxia
Radial	Midshaft humerus fracture Saturday night palsy	Sensory: dorsal medial hand Motor: wrist extension, finger extension	Neuropraxia
Ulnar (proximal)	Elbow dislocation Medial epicondyle fracture cubital compression	Sensory: ulnar hand Motor: grip strength, fourth and fifth digits flexion (proximal)	Axonotmesis
Median	Supracondylar fracture of humerus Laceration (typically distal)	Sensory: palmar radial hand Motor: thumb opposition, second and third digits flexion	Variable
Long thoracic nerve	Penetrating chest, axilla, or supraclavicular trauma	Motor: scapular protraction (may significantly impair upper extremity function)	Neurotmesis

Table 3
Classic peripheral nerve injuries of the lower extremities

Nerves	Example Mechanism(s)	Major Deficits	Pathologic Correlate
Sciatic	Posterior hip dislocation Penetrating trauma	Sensory: posterior and lateral leg, dorsal and plantar foot Motor: knee flexion, ankle dorsiflexion and plantarflexion	Variable
Peroneal	Knee dislocation Fibular fracture Contusion	Sensory: dorsal foot Motor: ankle dorsiflexion and eversion	Variable
Inferior gluteal	Posterior hip dislocation	Sensory: none Motor: hip extension and extension of the flexed thigh	Variable
Tibial	Tibial fracture Knee dislocation	Sensory: plantar foot Motor: ankle plantarflexion	Variable

nerve injury, it has added utility for evaluating soft tissue lesions and vascular structures[25] CT myelography is sensitive and specific for brachial plexus injury and nerve root avulsion in later phases of injury.[26]

Magnetic resonance imaging

Magnetic resonance imaging (MRI), also called magnetic resonance neurography, is superior to CT for PNIs due to significantly improved contrast resolution, ability to assess nerve edema, and evolving use of sequences to assess nerve integrity.[25,27,28] The utility of MRI in the immediate or early evaluation of suspected injury is unclear, because there are no established guidelines and because of typically conservative overall management strategy of closed nerve injuries. Given the limitations of electrodiagnostic testing in the acute phase, there may be select cases of MRI that allow for earlier intervention.[29]

Ultrasonography

Ultrasonography, along with MRI, is the other preferred imaging technique for nerve injury. Ultrasound offers high spatial resolution, the ability to perform dynamic maneuvers, and comparatively low cost but with limited contrast resolution, limited ability to image deeper structures, and significant operator dependence.[28,30–32] Nerves are imaged best with a high-frequency linear array and have a characteristic echotexture due to bundles of nerve fibers or fascicles.

Superficial nerves are well visualized and can be traced along their course to evaluate for swelling, size, or echotexture changes (eg, loss of internal architecture) that may indicate neuropraxia, axonotmesis/neurotmesis, and disruption of nerve continuity.[30–32] These can be accentuated by dynamic maneuvers. Ultrasound is able to characterize much of the course of the most commonly injured nerves and can identify areas of nerve entrapment.[27,33,34]

The role of ultrasound in the ED is evolving but has been shown in some cases to be superior to MRI in evaluation of nerve lesions.[35] Ultrasound evaluation changes management in as many as 58% of cases, including decisions on immediate versus delayed surgery, identification of complete nerve disruption, detection of foreign bodies, and detection of multiple areas of injury.[36,37]

Electrodiagnostic testing

Electrodiagnostic testing is the interrogation of nerve function using electrical impulses and is widely used for evaluation of nerve function, including in traumatic injuries. This technique does not have a role in the acute setting because electromyography and nerve conduction studies cannot differentiate between neuropraxia, axonotmesis, and neurotmesis immediately after injury.[38,39] Neuropraxia and higher-grade injuries can be differentiated by 1 week postinjury. PNI features are variable between injury areas and type, and serial evaluations over time are used to help gauge recovery and plan interventions.

Management of Peripheral Nerve Injuries

Disposition and follow-up

Treatment can vary widely after initial evaluation of possible nerve injury because, depending on the type of injury, it may be supportive or surgical. Smith and colleagues outlined a proposed approach to management of nerve injury building on the approach of Grant and colleagues (**Fig. 4**).[20,23]

The rule of 3s can be helpful in considering the appropriate timing of follow-up and intervention in subspecialty care. Sharp nerve transections are best explored and repaired within 3 days. Open injuries that are ragged or contused may be best

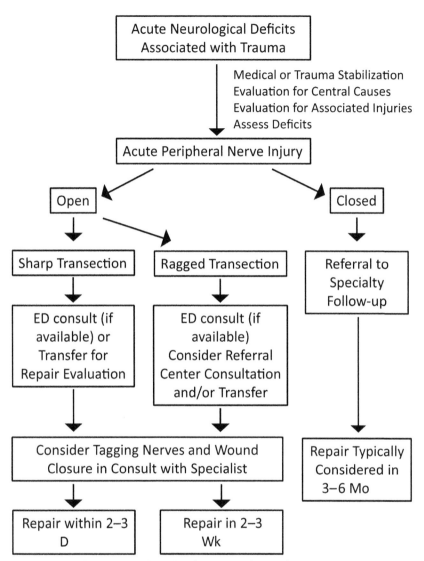

Fig. 4. Proposed treatment algorithm for PNIs. (*Adapted from* Smith BW, Sakamuri S, Spain DA, Joseph JR, Yang LJ, Wilson TJ. An update on the management of adult traumatic nerve injuries-replacing old paradigms: A review. *J Trauma Acute Care Surg.* 2019;86(2):299–306; with permission.)

explored for repair after 3 weeks to allow demarcation and healing of associated injuries as healthy nerve ends are needed for repair. Closed injuries typically are considered for surgery after 3 months postinjury.[16]

After stabilization and assessment, sharply transected PNIs should prompt consultation for immediate repair or transfer. Transections without cleanly incised ends for anastomosis should still prompt discussion with specialty care and should have urgent follow-up. Closed injuries also should have urgent referral to specialty care not only for possible surgery but also because such patients benefit from comprehensive rehabilitation services.

Wound Management

Wound management in the ED in part is driven by need for specialty care or transfer. Wounds should be decontaminated, explored, and assessed for foreign bodies, tetanus status updated, and pain addressed. Closure should be done in consultation with a specialist if the patient is not a candidate for immediate evaluation or transfer and if within the scope of the emergency provider's practice. Nerve ends can be tagged with suture to local structures to maintain nerve length, which facilitates better identification of nerves and preserves nerve length on re-exploration.

SPINAL CORD INJURY
Epidemiology

SCI affects approximately 300,000 individuals in the United States, with approximately 17,810 new cases occurring per year.[4] Like most trauma patients, these individuals tend to be younger and male. Overall, there is an almost 4:1 male predominance among new SCIs in the United States. Paralleling the aging population of the United States, the mean age of patients with acute traumatic SCI has risen gradually from 29 years to 43 years.[4] The most common age at the time of injury for the past several years is 19 years, and more than a quarter (25.61%) of all cases occur between the ages of 16 years and 22 years.[40] Non-Hispanic blacks make up approximately 24% of new cases despite representing approximately only 13% of the US population.[4]

The most common cause of SCIs varies with age and other factors, such as gender and race. Notably, the top 3 causes for both genders are the same: auto accidents, followed by falls and gunshot wounds (**Table 4**). Over the age of 45 years, falls become the leading cause of SCIs in the United States. The proportion of SCIs from vehicular accidents, acts of violence, and sports-related injuries have been declining from their peaks, while the proportion of SCIs from falls and medical/surgical complications have been increasing.[40]

Globally, approximately 750,000 traumatic SCIs occur each year.[41] Etiologies and consequences of SCIs vary in other countries. Higher-income countries tend to

Table 4
Ten most common causes of spinal cord injury by gender (all ages)

Rank	Cause of Spinal Cord Injuries Among Men (% of Total Cases)	Cause of Spinal Cord Injuries Among Women (% of Total Cases)
1	Auto accident (28.6)	Auto accident (46.6)
2	Fall (22.8)	Fall (23.1)
3	Gunshot wound (16.6)	Gunshot wound (9.3)
4	Motorcycle accident (7.1)	Medical/surgical complication (5.4)
5	Diving (6.5)	Diving (2.4)
6	Hit by falling/flying object (3.2)	Motorcycle accident (2.2)
7	Medical/surgical complication (2.3)	Pedestrian (2.0)
8	Bicycle (1.9)	Horseback riding (1.2)
9	Pedestrian (1.4)	Person-to-person contact (1.1)
10	Person-to-person contact (1.0)	Bicycle (1.0)

Data from National Spinal Cord Injury Statistical Center. 2019 Annual Statistical Report for the Spinal Cord Injury. Model Systems. University of Alabama at Birmingham: Birmingham, Alabama.

have older populations and see a bimodal distribution of traumatic SCIs, with peaks between the ages of 18 years and 32 years and at ages greater than 65 years. These older populations also see higher rates of tetraplegia with falls. Work-related falls in younger patients are more common in low-income countries.[42]

Although acute SCIs may involve any part of the spine, certain regions are more common. The needed flexibility of the cervical spine for flexion, extension, and rotation makes this region highly vulnerable to injury. The cervical spine is the most common site of injury in motor vehicle accidents and falls. Complete and incomplete tetraplegia consequently has made up approximately 60% of acute traumatic SCI cases since 2015.[4]

Key Anatomy and Pathophysiology

The spinal cord exits the foramen magnum and travels the length of the spine to the conus medullaris. The anterior-posterior diameter remains relatively constant, with transverse enlargements occurring in cervical and lumbar spine, around C5 and L3, respectively.[43] The bony boundaries of the spinal canal are relatively wide in the upper cervical spine, which can help protect the spinal cord from potentially devasting injuries in this area. The relative area of the cervical canal compared to the cord gets progressively smaller, increasing the chance of SCI in the lower cervical spine.[44]

The spinal cord contains several important paired nerve tracts:

- Corticospinal tracts—located both anteriorly/medially and posteriorly/laterally. These are the major descending motor pathways.
- Spinothalamic tracts—located anteriorly/laterally. These ascending pathways communicate light touch, temperature, and pain to the brain.
- Dorsal columns—located posteriorly/medially. These ascending pathways communicate deep touch, proprioception, and vibration to the brain.

The spinal cord branches into 31 pairs of spinal nerves, named for the anatomic location of their origin. This includes 8 cervical nerves (C1–C8) that exit the spinal column above their associated vertebra except for the C8 spinal nerve, which exits between the seventh cervical and first thoracic vertebra. The thoracic, lumbar, and sacral spinal nerves all exit below their associated vertebra.

Although SCI can occur in isolation, it frequently is associated with injuries of the vertebral column. Any underlying spinal disease can significantly increase the risk of injury to the bony spine and consequently the spinal cord. Many examples are associated with aging (like cervical spondylosis and osteoporosis). Spinal arthropathies like ankylosing spondylitis or rheumatoid arthritis may affect younger patients as well.[45,46] Additionally, congenital conditions like the atlantoaxial instability seen in Down syndrome and medication side effects like corticosteroid-induced osteoporosis may place patients at increased risk.[47]

The mechanism of any traumatic neurologic injury may be classified broadly as blunt versus penetrating. Blunt mechanisms are the leading cause of trauma in general and can cause SCI through excessive flexion/extension, rotational movements, shearing, or compressive forces. Penetrating injuries may be due to bullets, knives, or other missiles (like shrapnel) related to the traumatic event. This mechanism classically produces a transection injury of the spinal cord or vertebral fractures with associated SCIs. In rare cases, indirect damage to the spinal cord may occur. High-velocity missiles may cause contusion of the spinal cord as their kinetic energy dissipates despite never physically violating the spinal axis.[48] Case reports describe this phenomenon also occurring with low-velocity bullets.[49]

Classification of Spinal Cord Injuries

The source of SCIs may be primary or secondary. Primary injury encompasses all the initial mechanical insults (eg, compression, shearing, and laceration) affecting nerves at the time of injury. Secondary injury occurs over the following minutes to hours and causes further damage to the spinal cord through edema and additional cellular death. Secondary injury is a complex and poorly understood collection of processes like hypoxia, inflammation, and ischemia but represents an important therapeutic target for emergency physicians and spinal cord specialists.

The degree of injury is classified broadly as complete or incomplete. A complete injury causes total loss of sensation and motor function below the level of injury. Incomplete injuries are highly variable with symptoms that may range from relatively minor to near-complete paralysis. The most widely accepted scale for classifying SCI severity is the American Spinal Injury Association (ASIA) Scale. Grade A is assigned to patients with a complete cord injury, whereas grades B, C, and D identify progressively less severe degrees of incomplete injury. ED providers should be familiar with the ASIA International Standards for Neurological Classification of Spinal Cord Injury (ISNCSCI) worksheet (**Fig. 5**). Its use allows for a rapid and accurate assessment of a patient's deficits, clear communication with specialists, and longitudinal assessment of the patient.

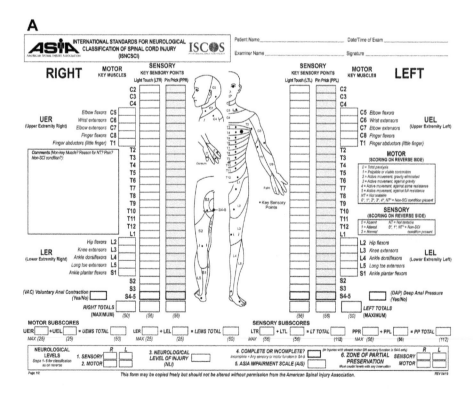

Fig. 5. (*A*) Page 1 of the ISNCSCI worksheet, including dermatomal map and key motor assessments. (*B*) Page 2 of the ISNCSCI worksheet, including motor and sensory grading scales and overall ASIA impairment scale. (*From* ©2020 American Spinal Injury Association; reprinted with permission.)

B

Muscle Function Grading

0 = Total paralysis

1 = Palpable or visible contraction

2 = Active movement, full range of motion (ROM) with gravity eliminated

3 = Active movement, full ROM against gravity

4 = Active movement, full ROM against gravity and moderate resistance in a muscle specific position

5 = (Normal) active movement, full ROM against gravity and full resistance in a functional muscle position expected from an otherwise unimpaired person

NT = Not testable (i.e. due to immobilization, severe pain such that the patient cannot be graded, amputation of limb, or contracture of > 50% of the normal ROM)

0*, 1*, 2*, 3*, 4*, NT* = Non-SCI condition present *

Sensory Grading

0 = Absent   1 = Altered, either decreased/impaired sensation or hypersensitivity

2 = Normal   NT = Not testable

0*, 1*, NT* = Non-SCI condition present *

* Note: Abnormal motor and sensory scores should be tagged with a '*' to indicate an impairment due to a non-SCI condition. The non-SCI condition should be explained in the comments box together with information about how the score is rated for classification purposes (at least normal / not normal for classification).

When to Test Non-Key Muscles:

In a patient with an apparent AIS B classification, non-key muscle functions more than 3 levels below the motor level on each side should be tested to most accurately classify the injury (differentiate between AIS B and C).

Movement	Root level
Shoulder: Flexion, extension, adduction, adduction, internal and external rotation Elbow: Supination	C5
Elbow: Pronation Wrist: Flexion	C6
Finger: Flexion at proximal joint, extension Thumb: Flexion, extension and abduction in plane of thumb	C7
Finger: Flexion at MCP joint Thumb: Opposition, adduction and abduction perpendicular to palm	C8
Finger: Abduction of the index finger	T1
Hip: Adduction	L2
Hip: External rotation	L3
Hip: Extension, abduction, internal rotation Knee: Flexion Ankle: Inversion and eversion Toe: MP and IP extension	L4
Hallux and Toe: DIP and PIP flexion and abduction	L5
Hallux: Adduction	S1

ASIA Impairment Scale (AIS)

A = Complete. No sensory or motor function is preserved in the sacral segments S4-5.

B = Sensory incomplete. Sensory but not motor function is preserved below the neurological level and includes the sacral segments S4-5 (light touch or pin prick at S4-5 or deep anal pressure) AND no motor function is preserved more than three levels below the motor level on either side of the body.

C = Motor incomplete. Motor function is preserved at the most caudal sacral segments for voluntary anal contraction (VAC) OR the patient meets the criteria for sensory incomplete status (sensory function preserved at the most caudal sacral segments S4-5 by LT, PP or DAP), and has some sparing of motor function more than three levels below the ipsilateral motor level on either side of the body. (This includes key or non-key muscle functions to determine motor incomplete status.) For AIS C – less than half of key muscle functions below the single NLI have a muscle grade ≥ 3.

D = Motor Incomplete. Motor incomplete status as defined above, with at least half (half or more) of key muscle functions below the single NLI having a muscle grade ≥ 3.

E = Normal. If sensation and motor function as tested with the ISNCSCI are graded as normal in all segments, and the patient had prior deficits, then the AIS grade is E. Someone without an initial SCI does not receive an AIS grade.

Using ND: To document the sensory, motor and NLI levels, the ASIA Impairment Scale grade, and/or the zone of partial preservation (ZPP) when they are unable to be determined based on the examination results.

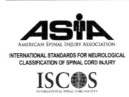

AMERICAN SPINAL INJURY ASSOCIATION

INTERNATIONAL STANDARDS FOR NEUROLOGICAL
CLASSIFICATION OF SPINAL CORD INJURY

ISCOS
INTERNATIONAL SPINAL CORD SOCIETY

Page 2/2

Steps in Classification

The following order is recommended for determining the classification of individuals with SCI.

1. Determine sensory levels for right and left sides.
The sensory level is the most caudal, intact dermatome for both pin prick and light touch sensation.

2. Determine motor levels for right and left sides.
Defined by the lowest key muscle function that has a grade of at least 3 (on supine testing), providing the key muscle functions represented by segments above that level are judged to be intact (graded as a 5).
Note: in regions where there is no myotome to test, the motor level is presumed to be the same as the sensory level, if testable motor function above that level is also normal.

3. Determine the neurological level of injury (NLI).
This refers to the most caudal segment of the cord with intact sensation and antigravity (3 or more) muscle function strength, provided that there is normal (intact) sensory and motor function rostrally respectively.
The NLI is the most cephalad of the sensory and motor levels determined in steps 1 and 2.

4. Determine whether the injury is Complete or Incomplete.
(i.e. absence or presence of sacral sparing)
If voluntary anal contraction = No AND all S4-5 sensory scores = 0 AND deep anal pressure = No, then injury is **Complete**.
Otherwise, injury is Incomplete.

5. Determine ASIA Impairment Scale (AIS) Grade.

Is injury **Complete**?   If YES, AIS=A

NO ↓

Is injury **Motor Complete**? If YES, AIS=B

NO ↓   (No-voluntary anal contraction OR motor function more than three levels below the motor level on a given side, if the patient has sensory incomplete classification)

Are **at least half (half or more)** of the key muscles below the neurological level of injury graded 3 or better?

NO ↓   YES ↓

AIS=C   AIS=D

If sensation and motor function is normal in all segments, AIS=E
Note: AIS E is used in follow-up testing when an individual with a documented SCI has recovered normal function. If at initial testing no deficits are found, the individual is neurologically intact and the ASIA Impairment Scale does not apply.

6. Determine the zone of partial preservation (ZPP).
The ZPP is used only in injuries with absent motor (no VAC) OR sensory function (no DAP, no LT and no PP sensation) in the lowest sacral segments S4-5, and refers to those dermatomes and myotomes caudal to the sensory and motor levels that remain partially innervated. With sacral sparing of sensory function, the sensory ZPP is not applicable and therefore "NA" is recorded in the block of the worksheet. Accordingly, if VAC is present, the motor ZPP is not applicable and is noted as "NA".

Fig. 5. (continued)

Presentation and Examination of Spinal Cord Injuries

Initial evaluation can be challenging, and providers must have a low suspicion for suspecting SCI in trauma patients. Mechanism and associated injuries can be important clues (**Table 5**). High-energy blunt trauma should raise concern, because most SCIs in

Table 5
Classic mechanisms of traumatic spinal cord injuries and commonly associated spinal and systemic injuries

Mechanism	Common Spinal Injuries	Common Associated Injuries
Car accident	Variable	Variable
Motorcycle accident	Thoracic injuries	Head injury (especially if unhelmeted)
Pedestrian struck	Variable	Lower limb fractures
Fall from a height	Thoracolumbar injuries if feet first	Pelvic and lower limb fractures
Diving	C1 burst fracture, C5–C6 fractures	Head injury
Winter sports	Thoracolumbar injuries	Variable
Football/rugby	Cervical injuries	
Gunshot wounds	Variable	Variable

Data from Aito S, D'Andrea M. Clinical Assessment in Spinal Cord Injury. In: Chhabra HS, ed. *ISCoS Textbook on Comprehensive Management of Spinal Cord Injuries.* Wolters Kluwer; 2015.

the United States occur during blunt trauma and as many as 80% of SCI patients have associated polytrauma.[4,50] The emergency provider must remember that SCIs also can result from a low-energy mechanism, especially within vulnerable populations like the elderly.

Associated injuries and contributing factors may limit the ability to get an accurate history. SCIs may occur in the context of substance use and up to 35% of cases may be associated with moderate or severe traumatic brain injury.[51] Thus, providers should assume any confused or unconscious trauma patient to have a possible SCI until proved otherwise.

Patients who can provide a history may describe symptoms concerning for SCIs. Any report of spinal pain, sensory loss, weakness, or other potentially neurologic symptom (eg, urinary retention) should raise concern.

Initial physical examination of a patient with suspected SCI should not differ from that of any other trauma patient. It should follow a protocolized trauma algorithm, such as the primary and secondary surveys of advance trauma life support (ATLS), with additional emphasis on spinal precautions.

The primary survey in the ED may reveal several key complications in severe SCI patients (**Table 6**).

The secondary survey better characterizes the injury or even recognize subtle SCI not identified during the primary survey. Providers should assess major myotomes and dermatomes bilaterally (**Table 7**). Approximately 20% of patients present with a recognizable spinal cord syndrome (**Table 8**).[52]

A rectal examination is required in all cases of potential SCI because decreased tone may be the only presenting abnormality. This examination also is essential for distinguishing incomplete versus complete injuries, which greatly affects prognosis and potentially the timing of interventions. The anal mucocutaneous junction is the lowest dermatome (S4/S5) and should be assessed by light touch and/or deep anal palpation (DAP). DAP is performed by inserting the provider's index finger and applying gentle pressure against the anorectal wall or by squeezing the anus between the examiner's inserted index finger and external thumb. Although DAP is not required for the sensory evaluation, a digital rectal examination is required to assess voluntary contraction of

Table 6	
Key complications of acute spinal cord injury to identify during primary survey	
Primary Survey Component	**Key Assessments**
Airway	• Exclude associated face/neck injuries that may directly compromise the airway (eg, swelling, bleeding, deformity). • Identify if paralysis prevents patient from protecting the airway (eg, insufficient cough to clear secretions).
Breathing	• Use continuous pulse oximetry and capnography. • Insufficient oxygenation and/or ventilation may be due to SCI (eg, paradoxic abdominal breathing) or an alternative injury (eg, pneumothorax, hemothorax, or flail chest).
Circulation	• Assess for systemic hypotension. • Hypotension, with or without associated bradycardia, may be seen in neurogenic shock. • Exclude other potential sources of shock first (eg, hemorrhage).
Disability	• Estimate level and severity of injury as quickly as possible.

Table 7		
Major myotomes and dermatomes		
Spinal Nerve	**Associated Myotome**	**Associated Dermatome**
C5	Elbow flexion (biceps)	
C6	Wrist extension	
C7	Elbow extension (triceps)	
C8	Finger flexion	
T1	Finger abduction	
T4		Nipple
T10		Umbilicus
L2	Hip flexion	
L3	Knee extension	
L4	Ankle dorsiflexion	
L5	Great toe extension	
S1	Plantar flexion	
S2–S4	Voluntary anal contraction	
S4/S5		Anal mucocutaneous junction

the external anal sphincter. The presence of priapism in male patients suggests, but is not required for, diagnosis of complete cord injury.

Diagnostic Evaluation of Spinal Cord Injuries

Laboratory evaluation
There are no laboratory tests specific to the diagnosis of SCI within the ED. Patients with significant blunt or penetrating injuries should empirically receive typical trauma laboratory studies, including any required prior to operative intervention or reversal of coagulopathy. Some laboratory abnormalities may identify potential contributors to secondary injury. Providers should identify and potentially treat

- Anemia
- Significant electrolyte abnormalities
- Hypoxia or hyperoxia

Ongoing research outside the ED uses the presence of inflammatory cytokines within a patient's cerebrospinal fluid to predict the degree of injury and likelihood of neurologic recovery but does not currently have a role in ED diagnosis.[55]

Imaging
Initial imaging should be used to identify unstable bony injuries, especially within the cervical spine. Historically, it was felt plain radiographs were sufficient to detect most bony injuries.[56] These images involve multiple views and can require manipulation of the patient. A significant portion of patients, despite this optimization, does not have sufficient visualization of the entire cervical spine on plain radiography and subsequently require CT.[57] Head-to-head comparisons of plain radiographs and CT are limited, but CT has been promoted consistently in obtunded patients and has a higher sensitivity.[58] National guidelines, such as those from the Eastern Association for the Surgery of Trauma (EAST), and more recent studies support the regular use of cervical CT in appropriate patients.[59–61] Patients with SCI demonstrate neurologic deficits and,

Table 8
Presentation of classic of spinal cord injuries

	Name	Mechanism/Pathology	Presentation	Pearls
Complete	Complete cord injury	Variable mechanisms All tracts damaged	Areflexic flaccid paralysis distal to level of injury Complete less of sensation distal to level of injury	The immediately adjacent dermatome and myotome may have partial function. Males may have transiently high-flow priapism at the time of injury, which rarely requires intervention.[54]
Incomplete	Anterior cord syndrome	Flexion, retropulsion of fracture fragments, or occlusion of the anterior spinal artery Damages anterior 2/3 of the spinal cord (corticospinal and spinothalamic tracts)	Motor function and sensations of pain/temperature are lost (below level of injury). Deep touch, pressure, vibration, and proprioception are preserved.	Poor likelihood of recovery[52]
	Brown-Sequard syndrome	Classically from a penetrating injury Lateral hemisection of spinal cord	True hemisection causes loss of ipsilateral motor function, ipsilateral light touch and proprioception, and contralateral pain and temperature sensation.	Incomplete hemisections are common and cause symptoms related to which tracts are involved.[52] Best prognosis for ambulation[52]
	CCS	Classically from a hyperextension injury Buckling of the ligamentum flavum causes localized injury to the center of the spinal cord	Bilateral weakness, greatest in the upper extremities, and greatest in the distal muscle groups Variable sensory loss	One of the most common SCIs in adults (approximately 10% of cases) Has a favorable prognosis compared with other SCI syndromes[53]
	Conus medullaris syndrome	Traumatic injuries at T12 or L1 causing damage to the sacral cord	Urinary retention and stool incontinence with possible (usually mild) lower extremity involvement (mix of upper and lower motor neuron findings) Saddle anesthesia	Will have both upper and lower motor neuron signs
	Posterior cord syndrome	Mechanisms include hyperextension and occlusion of the posterior spinal artery.	Bilateral loss of vibration and proprioception	Traumatic causes are extremely rare.

Temporary	Spinal shock	Temporary physiologic injury to the spinal cord (nerve pathways remain anatomically intact)	Flaccid paralysis, hypotonia, areflexia Loss of sensory function Loss of autonomic function	Usually lasts hours to days, but weeks also are possible Hypotension is not a defining feature, but it may cause low blood pressure via neurogenic shock.
Non-SCI	Cauda equina syndrome	Injury to lumbosacral nerve roots and therefore not a true SCI	Bladder/bowel dysfunction and possible lower extremity involvement (lower motor signs only) Saddle anesthesia	Often has asymmetric lower extremity weakness[52] Better prognosis for recovery given regenerative properties of nerve roots[52]

therefore, likely already require a head CT in the setting of trauma. It is time efficient and appropriate to pair this head imaging with a cervical CT.

Not all trauma patients require cervical imaging and several well-known clinical decision rules may be used to limit imaging in low-risk patients. The National Emergency X-Radiography Utilization Study (NEXUS) criteria were developed in the late 1990s and validated shortly afterward and demonstrate high sensitivity but relatively poor specificity.[62] The Canadian C-Spine Rule (CCR) was developed shortly afterward and appears to have better sensitivity, better specificity, and an overall lower rate of imaging utilization than the NEXUS criteria.[63] The CCR notably excludes patients 65 years of age or older, which is reasonable given the possibility of significant injury despite a relatively minor mechanism in this demographic.[64] Both of these clinical decision rules exclude patients with neurologic findings, such those expected in SCIs.

Unfortunately, no validated clinical decision rules exist for imaging other areas of the spine and providers should defer to clinical judgment. The American Association for the Surgery of Trauma TL-Spine Multicenter Study Group proposed the following criteria for imaging of the thoracolumbar spine in the setting of trauma[65]:

- Physical examination findings (pain, tenderness, and deformity)
- High-risk mechanism (eg, crush injury, motor vehicle collision with roll-over or ejection, or pedestrian struck)
- Neurologic deficit
- Glasgow coma scale less than 15
- Distracting injury
- Intoxication
- Age greater than 60 years

The American College of Radiology Appropriateness Criteria for suspected spine trauma rate noncontrast CT of the thoracic and lumbar spine as "usually appropriate" in the setting of blunt trauma meeting these criteria.[66] It is important to recognize there is a significant occurrence of noncontiguous vertebral fractures.[67,68] Consequently, the entire spine should be imaged if 1 vertebral column fracture is identified.

CT imaging can suggest SCI but does not routinely allow direct visualization of the spinal cord. MRI is an important adjunct in SCI assessment and captures the spinal cord and associated soft tissue in exquisite detail. SCIs can occur in the absence of vertebral fracture from processes better seen on MRI, such as hemorrhage or edema. Consequently, MRI still should be considered in patients even after a negative CT if concerning features still exist (eg, neurologic deficit).[69] The 2015 EAST guidelines, acknowledging very low-quality evidence, provided a conditional recommendation that cervical collars can be removed from obtunded adult blunt trauma patients after high-quality cervical spine CT.[70]

Decisions about MRI typically should be made in conjunction with a surgical consultant. There are numerous potential indications for MRI in the setting of spinal trauma, such as[71]

- Distinguishing hemorrhagic versus nonhemorrhagic SCIs (important for prognosis)
- Distinguishing acute versus chronic vertebral fractures
- Identifying ligamentous injuries (may be missed on CT)
- Identifying disc herniations (important before some closed reduction attempts)
- Identifying hematomas causing cord compression (important for operative planning and before some closed reduction attempts)

- Identifying vascular injuries that can cause spinal cord infarctions

The term, *SCI without radiographic abnormality (SCIWORA)*, was developed prior to the widespread availability of MRI. It usually is described in pediatric populations. The term, *adult SCIWORA*, is more controversial. Central cord syndrome (CCS), for example, is relatively common and frequently occurs without any vertebral fracture. MRI is essential to the diagnosis and prognosis of such cases.

Management of Spinal Cord Injuries

The initial management of a patient with suspected SCI should not differ from that of any other trauma patient, other than emphasizing stabilization of the spine. Although SCIs can be lethal, such deaths often occur in the prehospital environment secondary to respiratory arrest. The identification and treatment of more common life-threatening injuries (hemorrhage, pneumothorax, splenic laceration, and so forth) take precedent in patients with SCIs who survive to the ED. Providers should follow a standardized trauma algorithm, such as ATLS, to identify and address such injuries.

That said, patients with SCIs are a vulnerable population at risk of unique complications. Providers must promptly take several key steps (**Table 9**) and consider the following therapeutic actions and medical complications:

- Spinal motion restriction
- Respiratory compromise
- Hemodynamic compromise
- Minimizing secondary injury
- Surgical intervention

Table 9 Key management items for patients with acute traumatic spinal cord injury in the emergency department	
Key Step	**Key Details**
Spinal motion restriction	• Apply a cervical collar • Miami J or Philadelphia collar preferred
Medical resuscitation	• Exclude other life-threatening injuries • Obtain definitive airway if indicated • Maintain oxygen saturation >92% • Maintain MAP >85–90 mm Hg
Neurologic examination	• Ideally per the ISNCSCI worksheet • At minimum assess for major motor/sensory deficits, rectal tone/sensation, and an estimated spinal level of deficit
Radiographic evaluation	• CT is appropriate initial imaging • Whole-spine imaging if any vertebral fracture is identified • Obtain MRI if indicated
Early consultation with a surgical specialist	• Assess need for closed reduction • Assess need for early surgical intervention
Avoid steroid administration	• Unless specifically requested after discussion with surgeon or mandated by institutional policy
Transfer (if needed)	• Ideally to a definitive SCI care facility • Consider need for intubation prior to transport

Spinal motion restriction

Most patients with potential SCI arrive with a cervical collar and often on an EMS backboard. Patients should be removed from the backboard as soon as is safely allowed. Cervical collars should remain only for suspected or confirmed cervical fractures and ideally be exchanged from EMS collars to a Miami J collar or equivalent.[72] As emphasized within the 2018 joint policy statement from the American College of Emergency Physicians and the American College of Surgeons Committee on Trauma, the term, *spinal motion restriction*, is preferred to the term, *spinal immobilization*.[73]

Efforts should be made throughout the physical examination and subsequent management to minimize movements of the spine. These includes keeping the patient flat, using log-roll techniques, and maintaining cervical spine support during movement or procedures like intubation. Head of bed elevation still can be accomplished if there is concern of concomitant head injury with reverse Trendelenburg positioning.

Respiratory compromise

A significant proportion of patients with SCI require intubation, especially those with cervical injury.[74] Patients with complete cord injuries above C5 should be intubated prophylactically.[72] Intubation should be performed with manual in-line stabilization in which a second individual maintains the patient's cervical spine in a neutral position after careful removal of the anterior component of the cervical collar.[75] Video-assisted laryngoscopy can be used to maintain a neutral position. This is distinctly different from the sniffing or bed-up–head-elevated positions commonly used during ED intubations. The second provider may approach from either the head or side of the bed. Rapid sequence intubation is appropriate, although fiberoptic intubation also may be considered if time permits.

High cervical spine injuries above C3 typically result in respiratory and subsequently cardiac arrest unless rapidly intubated. Traumatic arrest in the field without signs of alternative causes may provide a clue to a high cervical injury.

Patients with incomplete and/or lower SCIs also may require intubation. Although the phrenic nerve to the diaphragm originates from the C3–C5 spinal nerves, the innervations of additional respiratory and accessory muscles originate lower in the spine. The intercostal muscles, for example, are controlled by the thoracic spinal nerves T1–T11 via intercostal nerves. Loss of the internal intercostals for inhalation can reduce vital capacity and lead to atelectasis and hypoxia. The intercostals are critical to stabilizing the chest wall. Paralysis of these muscles consequently allows the chest wall to contract with activation of the diaphragm, leading to paradoxical abdominal breathing (ie, quad breathing) and a corresponding severe drop in ventilatory ability.

The external intercostals and abdominal wall muscles assist with active exhalation and coughing. Abdominal wall muscles are innervated by a combination of branches from the lower intercostal nerves (T6–T12) and the ilioinguinal/iliohypogastric nerves (L1).[76] Compromise of these muscles can prevent a patient from coughing and clearing secretions adequately. This issue may be exacerbated in acute tetraplegia because these patients may develop increased secretions and bronchial constriction (theorized to be secondary to unopposed vagal activity).[77]

Given the many respiratory complications of acute SCIs, providers should use continuous pulse oximetry and continuous capnography to monitor the oxygenation and ventilatory effort. There are numerous potential indications for intubation in SCIs, and emergency providers should have a low threshold to preemptively establish a definitive airway under controlled conditions (**Table 10**).

Table 10	
Potential indications for intubation in spinal cord injury	
Indication	Details
Severe injury	• Complete SCI of C4 or above
Airway compromise	• Physical compromise • Inability to clear secretions
Work of breathing	• Persistent or increasing tachypnea • Persistent or progressive hypoxemia • Elevated or progressive end-tidal carbon dioxide • Consider in cases of subjective shortness of breath and/or development of paradoxic abdominal breathing
Travel	• Consider preemptively for transfers to other facilities (especially cervical) • Consider ahead of prolonged studies (such as MRI)

Hemodynamic compromise

Cord injuries above T6 can cause hemodynamic compromise. Loss of sympathetic outflow to the peripheral vasculature and heart causes a distributive shock picture with decreased vascular resistance and, sometimes, bradycardia. This process is known as neurogenic shock. The exact incidence is unknown, but 1 review estimated it to occur in 20% of cervical injuries and 7% of thoracic injuries.[78] Bradycardia is not required for diagnosis but tends to occur with more rostral injuries. There are no standardized cutoffs, but several studies have used systolic blood pressure of less than 100 mm Hg and heart rate less than 50 beats per minute to identify neurogenic shock. Hypothermia also may be seen.

Neurogenic shock should be a diagnosis of exclusion. Emergency providers should thoroughly evaluate for other causes of hypotension or bradycardia (eg, hemorrhagic shock, cardiac tamponade, tension pneumothorax, medications, and age). Hypovolemic/hemorrhagic shock (compared to neurogenic) classically demonstrates tachycardia instead of bradycardia, cool skin instead of warm, and reduced urine output instead of normal.

If a diagnosis of neurogenic shock still is suspected, then patients should initially receive intravenous fluids (or transfusion, if indicated) to mitigate the underlying vasodilatory effects.[79] Intractable hypotension should be treated further with vasopressors. Historically, patients with neurogenic shock received phenylephrine or dopamine. More recent guidelines recommend norepinephrine as the first-line agent because of its more favorable side-effect profile.[72] Providers should target a mean arterial pressure (MAP) of 85 to 90 mm Hg. Atropine may be used for bradycardia.

Minimizing secondary injury

Damage to the spinal cord continues after the initial injury. Emergency providers should take steps to minimize this ongoing harm. Key principles include avoiding any physiologic extremes, such as hypoxia/hyperoxia or hyperthermia. Hypotension should be corrected. The role of therapeutic hypothermia in SCIs is unclear and without evidence to recommend routine use at this time, but it remains an active area of research.[80,81] Regardless of this research, fever should be avoided.

Current guidelines recommend a MAP goal greater than 85 mm Hg for all patients with acute traumatic SCIs.[82] Several early uncontrolled case series arbitrarily used this value for 7 days.[83,84] Subsequent study has continued to suggest neurologic improvement in patients who avoid MAPs less than 85 but still consists of uncontrolled case series and retrospective cohorts with an overall low quality of evidence.[85,86] Given current recommendations, ED patients with SCIs who are below this target should receive intravenous fluids and, if necessary, vasopressors to maintain this blood pressure goal. As discussed previously, norepinephrine is the preferred agent if vasopressor support is required. There are at least 2 ongoing randomized controlled trials comparing the traditional MAP goals of 85 mm Hg to 90 mm Hg to lower targets of 65 mm Hg to 70 mm Hg.[81]

Corticosteroids historically were assumed to have a regular role in minimizing secondary injury after SCIs with near ubiquitous use despite never being studied outside of animal models. Subsequent studies on this topic, typically using methylprednisolone, have generated controversial results. The National Acute Spinal Cord Injury Study (NASCIS) I was one of the first randomized controlled trials to look at minimizing secondary injury but only included alternative doses of methylprednisolone without a placebo because of the untested but prevailing assumption of benefit.[87] NASCIS II included a placebo arm but did not show benefit in the primary analysis.[88] Subsequent subgroup analysis suggested some motor benefit to those receiving methylprednisolone within the first 8 hours of injury. This finding prompted NASCIS III, which again excluded a true placebo group and instead further assessed timing (within 3 hours vs within 8 hours of injury, respectively) and duration (24 hours vs 48 hours, respectively).[89]

Subsequent meta-analyses has questioned the net benefit of such protocols given the relatively mild reported motor benefit and competing concerns of side effects.[90,91] The previous trials have shown or suggested higher rates of wound infections, severe pneumonia, sepsis, and gastrointestinal complications.[55] In recent years, the use of corticosteroids in SCIs has decreased significantly and most related surgical or trauma societies either have recommended against use or that insufficient evidence exists to recommend this therapy.[82,92,93] The AO Spine 2017 guidelines remain the lone major exception and still propose methylprednisolone be considered if initiated within 8 hours of a cervical injury.[94]

Surgical interventions

Emergency providers should discuss cases early with a surgical specialist once an injury has been identified. Approximately 80% of patients in the National Spinal Cord Injury Statistical Center's registry required at least 1 major surgical intervention (internal fixation, laminectomy, neural canal restoration, or open reduction) during their index hospitalization.[40] Unfortunately, the exact indications and timing for surgery and/or closed reduction are not well defined and remain an active area of research. The need for timely decompression and/or stabilization of an SCI in the setting of polytrauma should be balanced against any additional potentially life-threatening injuries.

The goal is to minimize additional secondary injury through decompression and prevent subsequent acute injuries through stabilization. In some cases, this may be achieved by closed reduction. This technique is appropriate in awake individuals with a reliable neurologic examination and cervical injuries amenable to traction reduction, including certain fractures, subluxations, and/or dislocations. It can be performed with a halo ring (for lighter traction weights) or Gardner-Wells skull tongs (capable of handling higher weights).[95] This technique is not appropriate for those with calvarial injury or abnormality (eg, fracture, prior bony cranial intervention, or congenital abnormality) or those with degenerative diseases of the spine or injuries that may worsen with longitudinal traction (eg, hangman fracture). Closed reduction still may be attempted in some obtunded patients after a prereduction MRI.[96]

The need for immediate surgical intervention should be determined through consultation with an emergency provider's local neurosurgical or spine specialist. Practice patterns can vary, but common indications include ongoing compression of the spinal cord, progressive neurologic deficits, and/or unstable spinal injuries. Historically there was concern that early intervention was associated with increased complications and poorer outcomes. More recent research has suggested that early intervention, which unfortunately has variable definitions between 8 hours and 72 hours, may benefit outcomes without any significant increase in complications.[81] Some surgeons still may prefer a delayed approach in complete SCI and CCS, although this practice also has been challenged recently with AO Spine weakly recommending in 2017 that early surgery be considered for CCS.[97,98]

SUMMARY

Traumatic injuries to the nervous system remain a worldwide challenge. It is imperative emergency providers maintain a low index of suspicion for both PNIs and SCIs, especially in the context of polytrauma, because these diagnoses carry significant implications for morbidity and mortality in these patients. Although some patients may be managed conservatively, it is crucial emergency providers identify cases requiring emergent intervention and be familiar with the most significant consequences.

CLINICS CARE POINTS

- The ulnar and peroneal nerves are the most commonly injured peripheral nerves in the upper and lower extremities, respectively.
- Peripheral nerve injury should prompt consideration of associated fractures and arterial injuries.
- Sharp nerve transections should be repaired within 3 days, open/ragged injuries within 3 weeks, and closed injuries within 3 months.
- Use tools like continuous capnography to monitor for respiratory insufficiency after acute spinal cord injury. Maintain a low threshold for intubation.
- Fluid resuscitation and, if needed, norepinephrine should be used to treat neurogenic shock and/or achieve higher mean arterial pressure goals.
- Acute traumatic spinal cord injuries should be discussed promptly with a specialist as early intervention may be beneficial.

DISCLOSURE

The authors have nothing to disclose.

REFERENCES

1. Foster CH, Karsy M, Jensen MR, et al. Trends and cost-analysis of lower extremity nerve injury using the national inpatient sample. Neurosurgery 2019;85(2):250–6.
2. Lad SP, Nathan JK, Schubert RD, et al. Trends in median, ulnar, radial, and brachioplexus nerve injuries in the United States. Neurosurgery 2010;66(5):953–60.
3. Tapp M, Wenzinger E, Tarabishy S, et al. The epidemiology of upper extremity nerve injuries and associated cost in the US Emergency Departments. Ann Plast Surg 2019;83(6):676–80.
4. National spinal cord injury Statistical center, Facts and Figures at a glance. Birmingham (AL): University of Alabama at Birmingham; 2020.
5. Lekovic GP, Harrington TR. Litigation of missed cervical spine injuries in patients presenting with blunt traumatic injury. Neurosurgery 2007;60(3):513–6.

6. Ferrante MA. The assessment and management of peripheral nerve trauma. Curr Treat Options Neurol 2018;20(7):25.

7. Noble J, Munro CA, Prasad VS, et al. Analysis of upper and lower extremity peripheral nerve injuries in a population of patients with multiple injuries. J Trauma 1998;45(1):116–22.

8. Huckhagel T, Nüchtern J, Regelsberger J, et al. Nerve trauma of the lower extremity: evaluation of 60,422 leg injured patients from the TraumaRegister DGU® between 2002 and 2015. Scand J Trauma Resusc Emerg Med 2018; 26(1):1–8.

9. Huckhagel T, Nüchtern J, Regelsberger J, et al. Nerve injury in severe trauma with upper extremity involvement: evaluation of 49,382 patients from the TraumaRegister DGU® between 2002 and 2015. Scand J Trauma Resusc Emerg Med 2018;26(1):76.

10. Stone L, Keenan MA. Peripheral nerve injuries in the adult with traumatic brain injury. Clin Orthop Relat Res 1988;233:136–44.

11. Olivo R, Tsao B. Peripheral Nerve Injuries in Sport. Neurol Clin 2017;35(3): 559–72.

12. Fix JD. Neuroanatomy. 4th edition. Philadelphia, PA: Wolters Kluwer/Lippincott Williams & Wilkins; 2008. p. 80–8.

13. Mahan MA. Nerve stretching: a history of tension. J Neurosurg 2020;132(1): 252–9.

14. Seddon HJ. A classification of nerve injuries. Br Med J 1942;2(4260):237–9.

15. Sunderland S. The anatomy and physiology of nerve injury. Muscle Nerve 1990; 13(9):771–84.

16. Bijon C, José J, Diaz H, et al. Nerve injuries to the volar aspect of the hand : a comparison of the reliability of the Weber static test versus the gauze test. Injury 2017;48(11):2582–5.

17. Thai JN, Pacheco JA, Margolis DS, et al. Evidence-based comprehensive approach to forearm arterial laceration. West J Emerg Med 2015;16(7):1127–34.

18. Stanec S, Tonković I, Stanec Z, et al. Treatment of upper limb nerve war injuries associated with vascular trauma. Injury 1997;28(7):463–8.

19. Campbell WW. Evaluation and management of peripheral nerve injury. Clin Neurophysiol 2008;119(9):1951–65.

20. Grant GA, Goodkin R, Kliot M. Evaluation and surgical management of peripheral nerve problems. Neurosurgery 1999;44(4):825–39, discussion 839–40.

21. Bassilios Habre S, Bond G, Jing XL, et al. The surgical management of nerve gaps: present and future. Ann Plast Surg 2018;80(3):252–61.

22. Wang E, Inaba K, Byerly S, et al. Optimal timing for repair of peripheral nerve injuries. J Trauma Acute Care Surg 2017;83:875–81.

23. Smith BW, Sakamuri S, Spain DA, et al. An update on the management of adult traumatic nerve injuries-replacing old paradigms: a review. J Trauma Acute Care Surg 2019;86(2):299–306.

24. Kenney RJ, Hammert WC. Physical examination of the hand. J Hand Surg Am 2014;39(11):2324–34.

25. Ohana M, Moser T, Moussaouï A, et al. Current and future imaging of the peripheral nervous system. Diagn Interv Imaging 2014;95(1):17–26.

26. Chambers JA, Hiles CL, Keene BP. Brachial plexus injury management in military casualties: who, what, when, why, and how. Mil Med 2014;179(6):640–4.

27. Purger DA, Sakamuri S, Hug NF, et al. Imaging of damaged nerves. Clin Plast Surg 2020;47(2):245–59.

28. Holzgrefe RE, Wagner ER, Singer AD, et al. Imaging of the peripheral nerve: concepts and future direction of magnetic resonance neurography and ultrasound. J Hand Surg Am 2019;44(12):1066–79.
29. Marquez Neto OR, Leite MS, Freitas T, et al. The role of magnetic resonance imaging in the evaluation of peripheral nerves following traumatic lesion: where do we stand? Acta Neurochir (Wien) 2017;159(2):281–90.
30. Visalli C, Cavallaro M, Concerto A, et al. Ultrasonography of traumatic injuries to limb peripheral nerves: technical aspects and spectrum of features. Jpn J Radiol 2018;36(10):592–602.
31. Ali ZS, Pisapia JM, Ma TS, et al. Ultrasonographic evaluation of peripheral nerves. World Neurosurg 2016;85:333–9.
32. Mallon S, Starcevic V, Rheinboldt M, et al. Sonographic evaluation of peripheral nerve pathology in the emergency setting. Emerg Radiol 2018;25(5):521–31.
33. Brown JM, Yablon CM, Morag Y, et al. US of the peripheral nerves of the upper extremity: a landmark approach. Radiographics 2016;36(2):452–63.
34. Yablon CM, Hammer MR, Morag Y, et al. US of the peripheral nerves of the lower extremity: a landmark approach. Radiographics 2016;36(2):464–78.
35. Zaidman CM, Seelig MJ, Baker JC, et al. Detection of peripheral nerve pathology comparison of ultrasound and MRI. Neurology 2013;80(18):1634–40.
36. Padua L, Di Pasquale A, Liotta G, et al. Ultrasound as a useful tool in the diagnosis and management of traumatic nerve lesions. Clin Neurophysiol 2013;124(6):1237–43.
37. Toia F, Gagliardo A, D'Arpa S, et al. Preoperative evaluation of peripheral nerve injuries: what is the place for ultrasound? J Neurosurg 2016;125(3):603–14.
38. Robinson LR. Predicting recovery from peripheral nerve trauma. Phys Med Rehabil Clin N Am 2018;29(4):721–33.
39. Robinson LR. How electrodiagnosis predicts clinical outcome of focal peripheral nerve lesions. Muscle Nerve 2015;(September):321–33.
40. National Spinal Cord Injury Statistical Center. Annual statistical report for the spinal cord injury model systems. Birmingham (AL): University of Alabama at Birmingham; 2019. Available at: https://www.nscisc.uab.edu. Last access: December 2019.
41. Kumar R, Lim J, Mekary RA, et al. Traumatic spinal injury: global epidemiology and worldwide volume. World Neurosurg 2018;113:e345–63.
42. Lee BB, Cripps R, New P, et al. Demographic profile of spinal cord injury. In: Chhabra HS, editor. ISCoS Textbook on comprehensive management of spinal cord injuries. New Delhi, India: Wolters Kluwer; 2015. p. 36–51.
43. Frostell A, Hakim R, Thelin EP, et al. A review of the segmental diameter of the healthy human spinal cord. Front Neurol 2016;7(DEC):1–13.
44. Ulbrich EJ, Schraner C, Boesch C, et al. Normative MR cervical spinal canal dimensions. Radiology 2014;271(1):172–82.
45. Chaudhary SB, Hullinger H, Vives MJ. Management of acute spinal fractures in ankylosing spondylitis. ISRN Rheumatol 2011;2011:150484.
46. Ghazi M, Kolta S, Briot K, et al. Prevalence of vertebral fractures in patients with rheumatoid arthritis: revisiting the role of glucocorticoids. Osteoporos Int 2012;23(2):581–7.
47. Wong SPY, Mok CC. Management of glucocorticoid-related osteoporotic vertebral fracture. Osteoporos Sarcopenia 2020;6(1):1–7.
48. Mirovsky Y, Shalmon E, Blankstein A, et al. Complete paraplegia following gunshot injury without direct trauma to the cord. Spine (Phila Pa 1976) 2005;30(21):2436–8.

49. Klack F, Tassin C, Cotton F, et al. Gunshot injury without direct injury to the cord may lead to complete paraplegia. Eur J Trauma Emerg Surg 2011;37:49–51.
50. Burney RE, Maio RF, Maynard F, et al. Incidence, characteristics, and outcome of spinal cord injury at trauma centers in North America. Arch Surg 1993;128(5): 596–9.
51. Iida H, Tachibana S, Kitahara T, et al. Association of head trauma with cervical spine injury, spinal cord injury, or both. J Trauma 1999;46(3):450–2.
52. McKinley W, Santos K, Meade M, et al. Incidence and outcomes of spinal cord injury clinical syndromes. J Spinal Cord Med 2007;30(3):215–24.
53. Brooks NP. Central cord syndrome. Neurosurg Clin N Am 2017;28(1):41–7.
54. Todd NV. Priapism in acute spinal cord injury. Spinal Cord 2011;49(10):1033–5.
55. Badhiwala JH, Wilson JR, Kwon BK, et al. A review of clinical trials in spinal cord injury including biomarkers. J Neurotrauma 2018;35(16):1906–17.
56. Davis JW, Phreaner DL, Hoyt DB, et al. The etiology of missed cervical spine injuries. J Trauma 1993;34(3):342–6.
57. Gale SC, Gracias VH, Reilly PM, et al. The inefficiency of plain radiography to evaluate the cervical spine after blunt trauma. J Trauma 2005;59(5):1121–5.
58. Holmes JF, Akkinepalli R. Computed tomography versus plain radiography to screen for cervical spine injury: a meta-analysis. J Trauma 2005;58(5):902–5.
59. Como JJ, Diaz JJ, Dunham CM, et al. Practice management guidelines for identification of cervical spine injuries following trauma: update from the eastern association for the surgery of trauma practice management guidelines committee. J Trauma 2009;67(3):651–9.
60. Mathen R, Inaba K, Munera F, et al. Prospective evaluation of multislice computed tomography versus plain radiographic cervical spine clearance in trauma patients. J Trauma 2007;62(6):1427–31.
61. Bailitz J, Starr F, Beecroft M, et al. CT should replace three-view radiographs as the initial screening test in patients at high, moderate, and low risk for blunt cervical spine injury: a prospective comparison. J Trauma 2009;66(6):1605–9.
62. Hoffman JR, Mower WR, Wolfson AB, et al. Validity of a set of clinical criteria to rule out injury to the cervical spine in patients with blunt trauma. National Emergency X-Radiography Utilization Study Group. N Engl J Med 2000;343(2):94–9.
63. Stiell IG, Clement CM, McKnight RD, et al. The Canadian C-spine rule versus the NEXUS low-risk criteria in patients with trauma. N Engl J Med 2003;349(26): 2510–8.
64. Paykin G, O'Reilly G, Ackland HM, et al. The NEXUS criteria are insufficient to exclude cervical spine fractures in older blunt trauma patients. Injury 2017; 48(5):1020–4.
65. Inaba K, Nosanov L, Menaker J, et al. Prospective derivation of a clinical decision rule for thoracolumbar spine evaluation after blunt trauma: an American Association for the Surgery of Trauma Multi-Institutional Trials Group Study. J Trauma Acute Care Surg 2015;78(3):459–67.
66. Beckmann NM, West OC, Nunez Jr D, et al. ACR Appropriateness Criteria® Suspected Spine Trauma. Available at: https://Acsearch.Acr.Org/Docs/69359/Narrative/. American College of Radiology. Accessed January 7, 2020.
67. Keenen TL, Antony J, Benson DR. Non-contiguous spinal fractures. J Trauma 1990;30(4):489–91.
68. Mugesh Kanna R, Chandrasekar ●, Gaike V, et al. Multilevel non-contiguous spinal injuries: incidence and patterns based on whole spine MRI. Eur Spine J 2016; 25(4):1163–9.

69. Inaba K, Byerly S, Bush LD, et al. Cervical spinal clearance: a prospective Western Trauma Association Multi-institutional Trial. J Trauma Acute Care Surg 2016; 81(6):1122–30.
70. Patel MB, Humble SS, Cullinane DC, et al. Cervical spine collar clearance in the obtunded adult blunt trauma patient: a systematic review and practice management guideline from the Eastern Association for the Surgery of Trauma. J Trauma Acute Care Surg 2015;78(2):430–41.
71. Kumar Y, Hayashi D. Role of magnetic resonance imaging in acute spinal trauma: a pictorial review. BMC Musculoskelet Disord 2016;17:310.
72. Stein DM, Knight WA 4th. Emergency neurological life support: traumatic spine injury. Neurocrit Care 2017;27(Suppl 1):170–80.
73. Fischer PE, Perina DG, Delbridge TR, et al. Spinal motion restriction in the trauma patient - a joint position statement. Prehosp Emerg Care 2018;22(6):659–61.
74. Gardner BP, Watt JW, Krishnan KR. The artificial ventilation of acute spinal cord damaged patients: a retrospective study of forty-four patients. Paraplegia 1986;24(4):208–20.
75. Austin N, Krishnamoorthy V, Dagal A. Airway management in cervical spine injury. Int J Crit Illn Inj Sci 2014;4(1):50–6.
76. Beaussier M. Innervation of the abdominal wall and viscera. In: Atchabahian A, Gupta R, editors. The anesthesia guide. The McGraw-Hill Companies, Inc; 2013. p. 646–9.
77. Galeiras Vázquez R, Rascado Sedes P, Mourelo Fariña M, et al. Respiratory management in the patient with spinal cord injury. Biomed Res Int 2013;2013:168757.
78. Guly HR, Bouamra O, Lecky FE. The incidence of neurogenic shock in patients with isolated spinal cord injury in the emergency department. Resuscitation 2008;76(1):57–62.
79. Dave S, Cho JJ. Neurogenic shock. Treasure Island (FL): StatPearls Publishing; 2020.
80. Martirosyan NL, Patel AA, Carotenuto A, et al. The role of therapeutic hypothermia in the management of acute spinal cord injury. Clin Neurol Neurosurg 2017;154: 79–88.
81. Donovan J, Kirshblum S. Clinical trials in traumatic spinal cord injury. Neurotherapeutics 2018;15(3):654–68.
82. Walters BC, Hadley MN, Hurlbert RJ, et al. Guidelines for the management of acute cervical spine and spinal cord injuries: 2013 update. Neurosurgery 2013; 60(CN_suppl_1):82–91.
83. Wolf A, Levi L, Mirvis S, et al. Operative management of bilateral facet dislocation. J Neurosurg 1991;75(6):883–90.
84. Vale FL, Burns J, Jackson AB, et al. Combined medical and surgical treatment after acute spinal cord injury: results of a prospective pilot study to assess the merits of aggressive medical resuscitation and blood pressure management. J Neurosurg 1997;87(2):239–46.
85. Catapano JS, John Hawryluk GW, Whetstone W, et al. Higher mean arterial pressure values correlate with neurologic improvement in patients with initially complete spinal cord injuries. World Neurosurg 2016;96:72–9.
86. Evaniew N, Mazlouman SJ, Belley-Côté EP, et al. Interventions to optimize spinal cord perfusion in patients with acute traumatic spinal cord injuries: a systematic review. J Neurotrauma 2020;37(9):1127–39.
87. Bracken MB, Collins WF, Freeman DF, et al. Efficacy of methylprednisolone in acute spinal cord injury. JAMA 1984;251(1):45–52.

88. Bracken MB, Shepard MJ, Collins WF, et al. A randomized, controlled trial of methylprednisolone or naloxone in the treatment of acute spinal-cord injury. Results of the Second National Acute Spinal Cord Injury Study. N Engl J Med 1990;322(20):1405–11.

89. Bracken MB, Shepard MJ, Holford TR, et al. Methylprednisolone or tirilazad mesylate administration after acute spinal cord injury: 1-year follow up. results of the third National Acute Spinal Cord Injury randomized controlled trial. J Neurosurg 1998;89(5):699–706.

90. Evaniew N, Noonan VK, Fallah N, et al. Methylprednisolone for the treatment of patients with acute spinal cord injuries: a propensity score-matched cohort study from a Canadian Multi-Center Spinal Cord Injury Registry. J Neurotrauma 2015; 32:1674–83.

91. Liu Z, Yang Y, He L, et al. High-dose methylprednisolone for acute traumatic spinal cord injury: a meta-analysis. Neurology 2019;93(9):e841–50.

92. Schroeder GD, Kwon BK, Eck JC, et al. Survey of Cervical Spine Research Society members on the use of high-dose steroids for acute spinal cord injuries. Spine (Phila Pa 1976) 2014;39(12):971–7.

93. Hurlbert RJ, Hadley MN, Walters BC, et al. Pharmacological therapy for acute spinal cord injury. Neurosurgery 2013;72(Suppl 2):93–105.

94. Fehlings MG, Wilson JR, Tetreault LA, et al. A clinical practice guideline for the management of patients with acute spinal cord injury: recommendations on the use of methylprednisolone sodium succinate. Glob Spine J 2017;7(3 Suppl): 203S–11S.

95. Daffner S. Halo application and closed skeleton reduction of cervical dislocations. In: Fehlings MG, editor. Essentials of spinal cord injury. New York, NY: Thieme Publishing; 2013. p. 117–9.

96. Gelb DE, Hadley MN, Aarabi B, et al. Initial closed reduction of cervical spinal fracture-dislocation injuries. Neurosurgery 2013;72(SUPPL.2):73–83.

97. Piazza M, Schuster J. Timing of surgery after spinal cord injury. Neurosurg Clin N Am 2017;28(1):31–9.

98. Fehlings MG, Tetreault LA, Wilson JR, et al. A clinical practice guideline for the management of patients with acute spinal cord injury and central cord syndrome: recommendations on the timing (≤24 hours versus >24 hours) of decompressive surgery. Glob Spine J 2017;7(3_supplement):195S–202S.

Modern Neuroimaging Techniques in Diagnosing Transient Ischemic Attack and Acute Ischemic Stroke

Karen Greenberg, DO[a], Julie Bykowski, MD[b],*

KEYWORDS

- Stroke • TIA • Ischemia • Infarct • Large vessel occlusion • MRA • CT perfusion
- MR perfusion

KEY POINTS

- Noncontrast CT is the first-line imaging of acute stroke symptoms to assess for intracranial hemorrhage and evidence of edema related to ischemia.
- Head and neck CTA is useful in evaluation of acute stroke symptoms to detect LVO, dissection, or significant intracranial arterial stenoses.
- Diffusion-weighted brain MRI is the most sensitive method to confirm acute ischemia; however, patients may be unable to have MRI.
- CT and MR perfusion parameters have been established through clinical trials to stratify risk for revascularization in acute ICA and proximal MCA occlusion.
- Multiple vendors provide AI software to help expedite stroke imaging review. All are an aid to the physician rather than stand-alone diagnostic tool.

Neuroimaging should be obtained for all patients suspected of having acute ischemic stroke or transient ischemic attack. Noncontrast head computed tomography (CT) scans are used to exclude hemorrhage, evaluate for early brain injury, and exclude stroke mimics. CT angiography assists in identifying proximal vessel occlusions, dissection, or high-grade arterial stenoses. Additional imaging techniques have emerged to improve selection of patients likely to benefit from therapies. Artificial intelligence applications assist in acute stroke imaging assessment, identifying acute hemorrhage, and predicting risk of endovascular intervention in acute large vessel occlusion. Each should be considered an aid rather than stand-alone diagnostic tool.

---

[a] Neurologic Emergency Department, Global Neurosciences Institute, Crozer Chester Medical Center, 3100 Princeton Pike, Building 3, Suite D, Lawrenceville, NJ 08648, USA; [b] Department of Radiology, UC San Diego Health, 200 West Arbor Drive, San Diego, CA 92013, USA
* Corresponding author.
E-mail address: jbykowski@health.ucsd.edu

Emerg Med Clin N Am 39 (2021) 29–46
https://doi.org/10.1016/j.emc.2020.09.002
0733-8627/21/© 2020 Elsevier Inc. All rights reserved.

emed.theclinics.com

INTRODUCTION

Neuroimaging should be obtained for all patients suspected of having acute ischemic stroke (AIS) or transient ischemic attack (TIA). Noncontrast head computed tomography (CT) scans are used to exclude hemorrhage, to evaluate for early brain injury, and to exclude stroke mimics, such as tumor. CT angiography (CTA) can assist in identifying proximal vessel occlusions, dissection, or high-grade arterial stenoses, which may be responsible for the ischemic deficit. Additional CT and magnetic resonance imaging (MRI) techniques have emerged to improve selection of patients likely to benefit from therapies, such as intravenous thrombolysis or mechanical thrombectomy.

American Heart Association (AHA) guidelines[1] and the American College of Radiology (ACR) Appropriateness Criteria[2] emphasize access to emergent brain imaging before initiating stroke therapy. It is crucial to remember that brain and neurovascular imaging studies represent a single moment in time within a dynamic process and must be interpreted in conjunction with clinical changes.

There are an increasing number of artificial intelligence (AI) applications that may assist in the acute stroke imaging assessment, to identify acute hemorrhage, and to predict risk of endovascular intervention in acute large vessel occlusion (LVO). These applications are marketed as a resource when there is a lack of timely, available expertise for CT scan interpretation. Each should be considered an aid, however, rather than stand-alone diagnostic tool. Medicolegal concerns regarding liability for AI misdiagnosis, a physician not acting on an AI finding, remain to be resolved.[3,4]

DISCUSSION
Noncontrast Head Computed Tomography

Rapid and accurate detection of stroke by emergency clinicians at the time of first contact is crucial for timely initiation of appropriate treatment of AIS patients. Noncontrast head CT is the preferred imaging study for evaluation of acute stroke symptoms because of widespread availability, rapid scan times, and ease of detecting intracranial hemorrhage.[5] There is level 1 evidence that all patients with suspected acute stroke should receive emergent brain imaging on arrival, before initiating acute stroke therapy.[1] Effective protocols and communication have confirmed that a median door-to-imaging time of 20 minutes or less can be accomplished across different hospital settings.[6–8]

Imaging findings
An advantage of noncontrast head CT is the conspicuity of acute hemorrhage as bright signal relative to the gray of the brain parenchyma (**Fig. 1**). Acute hemorrhage represents only 8% to 15% acute strokes, associated most commonly with hypertension; however, it also may be due to underlying arterial abnormalities, venous occlusion, cavernoma, and cerebral amyloid.

CT has poor sensitivity (20%–75%) and better specificity (56%–100%) in determining early ischemic changes within 6 hours to 8 hours; therefore, the diagnosis of acute stroke remains a clinical decision.[9] Early infarct signs on noncontrast head CT are subtle and include loss of gray–white matter, cortical sulcal effacement, focal parenchymal hypoattenuation, and the insular ribbon or obscuration of the sylvian fissure (**Fig. 2**). Both underestimation and overestimation of early infarct signs are common even in a controlled setting.[10,11]

Evaluation for the subtle changes in gray–white matter definition in acute ischemia is difficult on CT, and preset options for stroke windows (40 WW:40 WL) displays (**Fig. 3**) or alternate settings have been used for many years to enhance visual perception.

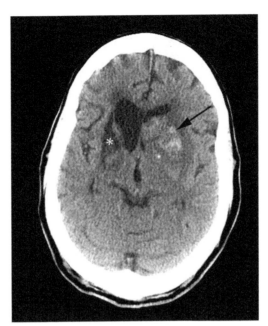

Fig. 1. Acute intracranial hemorrhage. Noncontrast head CT shows hyperintense acute hypertensive hemorrhagic in the left basal ganglia (*arrow*) with local mass effect on the lateral ventricle. The frontal horn of the right lateral ventricle is expanded in compensation given encephalomalacia from prior hypertensive hemorrhagic infarct (*asterisk*).

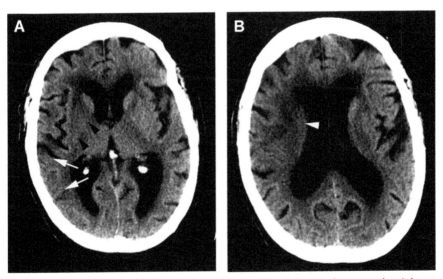

Fig. 2. AIS. Noncontrast head CT show loss of gray–white definition between the right putamen and internal capsule (*A* [*arrowheads*]), along the right temporal lobe cortex (*A* [*arrows*]) and the right caudate body (*B* [*arrowhead*]) in this patient with acute right MCA infarct.

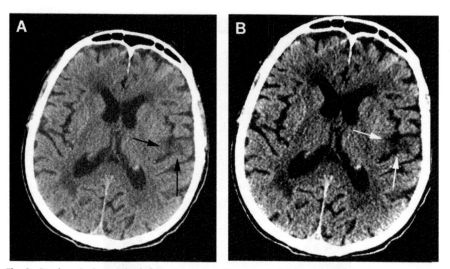

Fig. 3. Stroke windows. The left posterior insular acute infarct is a subtle finding on noncontrast head CT (*A* [*arrows*]). The same image viewed with stroke window settings (*B* [*arrows*]) improves the visual perception of the hypoattenuation of the infarct from the normal adjacent brain.

Small studies suggest review may be adequate using a smartphone or laptop to identify features that influence intervention[12]; however, these do not have wider validation. The ACR maintains technical standards for image quality and review, which do not include mobile devices.[13] AHA guidelines include that sites without in-house imaging interpretation expertise should have an approved teleradiology system for timely review of brain imaging.[1] Several vendors have received Food and Drug Administration (FDA) clearance for AI applications to aid in detection of intracranial hemorrhage and work list/provider alert systems to help reduce time to decision making.[14–18]

In the setting of acute stroke symptoms, identification of a focally dense (bright) artery on noncontrast CT should prompt emergent vascular imaging correlation (**Fig. 4**). Vascular hyperdensity can indicate the presence of red-cell thrombus; however, it has been shown to be only 52% sensitive detecting LVO in a meta-analysis, including Third International Stroke trial patients.[19] Smaller single-site series have reported increased sensitivity to 75% for basilar thromboses and 76% for M1 thrombosis.[20] False-positive dense vessels include patients with underlying vessel atherosclerosis or more diffuse dense vessels due to hemoconcentration.

Implications for treatment

Early infarct signs on noncontrast head CT are not a contraindication to treatment with intravenous thrombolysis nor is the presence of a hyperdense artery sign.[1] Analysis from the National Institute of Neurological Disorders and Stroke (NINDS) rt-PA Acute Stroke Trial[21] found that early CT signs of infarction were not independently associated with increased risk of adverse outcome after intravenous alteplase treatment within 3 hours of onset of symptoms, and patients treated with alteplase did better whether or not they had early CT signs. Vascular evaluation is not required for the decision to treat with alteplase.

The Alberta Stroke Program Early CT Score (ASPECTS) 10-point scale was developed to assess noncontrast head CT for early ischemic changes in patients suspected to have middle cerebral artery (MCA) LVO.[22] It has been used as an eligibility criterion

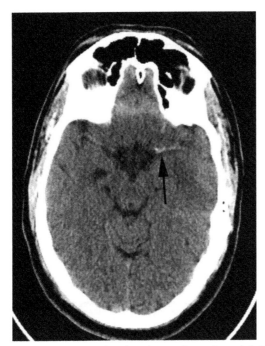

Fig. 4. Dense arterial sign. Noncontrast head CT shows a hyperdense left MCA (*arrow*) in this patient with presentation NIHSS = 20. Patient was treated with alteplase and M1 thrombectomy and discharged to home 2 days later with NIHSS = 2.

for mechanical thrombectomy clinical trials for anterior circulation stroke and adapted into the clinical setting as a predictor of functional outcome and risk of symptomatic hemorrhagic conversion. Points are deducted for visible gray–white matter loss in each of the following areas: 3 supraganglionic (frontal operculum, anterior temporal lobe, and posterior temporal lobe), 3 subganglionic (anterior, lateral, and posterior MCA), the caudate, lentiform nucleus, insula, and internal capsule. Patients with scores of 7 or less were more likely to have adverse outcomes (death and dependence). Although inter-rater variability exists, it rarely has an impact on the dichotomization above/below a score of 7.[23]

Computed Tomography Angiogram

To date, no clinical score has become widely accepted as an eligible prehospital marker for LVO and the need for mechanical thrombectomy in ischemic stroke. The best combination of sensitivity and specificity is achieved by a National Institutes of Health Stroke Scale (NIHSS) score cutoff between 7 and 10 for LVO or between 11 and 14 for mechanical thrombectomy.[24]

Because CTA is well suited to assess for clot that may be accessible for endovascular therapy, this has become more integrated into the acute stroke evaluation,[25] with some centers even endorsing "CTA for All" protocols.[26] There remains continued debate, however, regarding use and overuse of CTA, particularly for patients with low NIHSS or at centers without access to emergent endovascular therapy, given the cost, contrast, and radiation exposure.[27]

Anticipating CTA as part of the acute stroke evaluation, emergency department clinicians should have a brief discussion with the patient and/or family regarding the benefit of contrast to determine if the patient is a candidate for neurointervention to minimize lasting brain injury versus the risk of exacerbating existing severe renal insufficiency and rare (0.04%) but unpredictable severe adverse reactions. Patients with a prior allergic-like reaction to contrast have approximately 5-times the risk if re-exposed.[28] Hospitals should have protocols in place regarding contrast use in stroke codes, because obtaining glomerular filtration rate results delays intervention.

Imaging findings

Axial images are readily available at the time of the scan, allowing for detection of changes in caliber or contrast density within the extracranial and intracranial arteries as well as assessment of luminal plaque. LVO results in an abrupt cutoff of the contrast enhancement within the artery (**Fig. 5**). Proximal M2 occlusions may be difficult to perceive on the axial images, given anatomic variations in MCA bifurcation within the MCA and sylvian fissures; therefore, 3-dimensional (3-D) maximum intensity projection (MIP) reconstructions of the arteries can help expedite review.

Multiphase CTA has been proposed as a method to assess collateral circulation in stroke patients with LVO, as an alternative to CT perfusion. The traditional head and neck CTA represents the first of 3 phases of the multiphase CTA examination. The 2

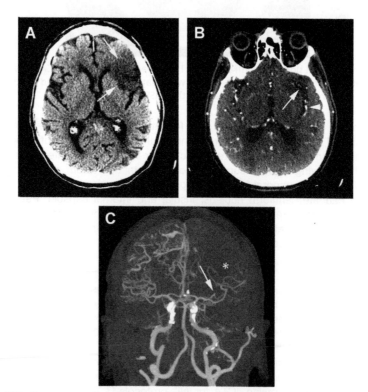

Fig. 5. LVO. Noncontrast head CT shows hypoattenuation and loss of gray–white matter definition in the left frontal operculum and insula (*A* [*arrows*]). Source images from CTA confirm lack of contrast within the left proximal M2 branch (*B* [*arrow*]) and contrast within left sylvian branches (*B* [*arrowhead*]). MIP reconstructions better display the left superior division proximal M2 occlusion (*C* [*arrow*]) and paucity of distal left MCA branches (*asterisk*) compared with contralateral normal side.

additional scans are of the head only, in the equilibrium phase (8 seconds after first CTA) and the late venous phase (16 seconds after first CTA). This results in additional radiation exposure to the brain and eyes.[29] There is no additional contrast given; however, due to rapid sequence of timing, high suspicion for LVO is required at the time of scan initiation; otherwise, this is exposing patients to radiation unnecessarily. For multiphase CTA, the 3 phases must be evaluated concurrently to compare the extent of pial arterial enhancement across the time points in the area of the vessel occlusion compared with the asymptomatic contralateral hemisphere. Clot burden and collateral scores have been proposed as independent predictors for endovascular triage; however, have been limited to small studies or retrospective data sets.[30–33]

AI applications have entered the international marketplace, designed to alert clinicians to possibility of LVO and to generate clot burden scores.[17,18] Although small studies and conference proceedings have shown these applications may function with comparable accuracy to a neuroradiologist, they are not approved to replacing a physician's review of the scan.

Infarcts along the border zone of the major intracranial vascular territories should prompt close evaluation for atherosclerotic stenoses of the proximal vessels (**Fig. 6**). Soft atherosclerotic plaque is dark on CTA. Calcified plaque is bright on CT

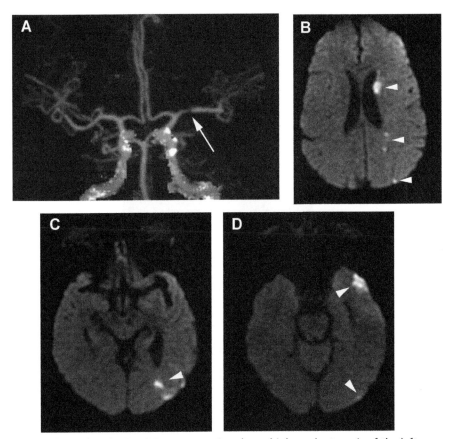

Fig. 6. Atherosclerosis. CTA 3-D reconstruction shows high-grade stenosis of the left proximal M1 segment (A [arrow]), which remains patent. Subsequent diffusion-weighted MRI (B-D) confirms the distribution of hyperintense acute infarcts along the border zone of the left ACA/MCA and MCA/PCA vascular territories (B–D [arrowheads]).

and is conspicuous even relative to the arterial enhancement. Through-plane recon-structions can be created with scanner-based and third-party software options, to verify the extent of any luminal stenosis.

Internal carotid dissection commonly presents as a flame-shaped tapering of the contrast, due to nonenhancing thrombus obstructing the vessel lumen (**Fig. 7**). Non-obstructive carotid and vertebral artery dissection is more subtle, detected by flat-tening of the normal round cross-section of the vessel due to eccentric thrombus beneath the intimal flap.

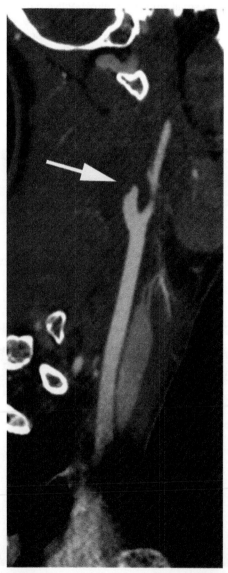

Fig. 7. Internal carotid artery (ICA) dissection. CTA reconstructions centered on the vessel lumen show the flame-shaped cutoff of the acute right ICA dissection (*arrow*), with thrombus related to intimal injury resulting in arterial occlusion.

It is important to remember venous thrombosis as a potential source for ischemic and hemorrhagic stroke. Although CTA is optimized for arterial assessment, there often is sufficient enhancement to exclude venous sinus thrombosis. If this is suspected as the etiology, however, it is prudent to notify the radiologist and technologist so they may adapt the bolus-to-scan timing. The empty delta sign is specific to clot within the superior sagittal sinus (**Fig. 8**); however, the same principle applies to the other sinuses, with the filling defect as a dark area within otherwise enhancing venous sinuses. Normal variants of arachnoid granulations and anatomic asymmetry of cortical and deep venous drainage can mimic thrombus.

Implications for treatment
In 2015, studies, including MR CLEAN[34], EXTEND-IA[35], REVASCAT[36], ESCAPE[37], and SWIFT PRIME[38], demonstrated the superiority of endovascular thrombectomy versus standard care alone among patients with acute stroke when performed within 6 hours to 12 hours of symptom onset. The benefits of the intervention declined as the time

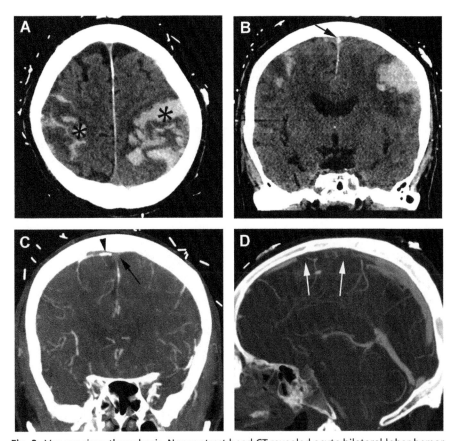

Fig. 8. Venous sinus thrombosis. Noncontrast head CT revealed acute bilateral lobar hemorrhage (A [asterisks]). On coronal view, hyperdense thrombus also was visible in the superior sagittal sinus (B [arrow]), corresponding to the empty delta sign of nonfilling of the sinus on postcontrast imaging (C [arrow]) compared with the enhancing adjacent cortical vein (C [arrowhead]). The CTA performed during the stroke code had sufficient venous filling to confirm thrombosis of the midthird of the superior sagittal sinus (D [arrows]).

from onset increased.[34-38] A subset of acute stroke patients, however, exhibits brain tissue that is ischemic but not yet infarcted. These patients have a disproportionately severe clinical deficit compared with the amount of infarcted tissue on imaging. ESCAPE also used collateral circulation filling of 50% or more of the MCA territory, preferentially defined on multiphase CTA, as an eligibility factor for thrombectomy.

Expedited Magnetic Resonance Imaging and Magnetic Resonance Angiography

Direct-to-MRI or expedited MRI access during stroke codes has been successfully implemented at many facilities. All patients must be screened for implants and intra-cranial or intraorbital metal prior to entering the MRI scanner. Some devices may be safely imaged in 1.5T or 3T magnetic resonance (MR) scanners using specific proto-cols[39]; however, they may require vendor support. It, therefore, is essential to have a pathway for clinical decision management that does not include MRI.

Diffusion-weighted MR imaging (DWI) is the most accurate imaging technique to identify an AIS,[40-42] detecting cytotoxic edema due to ischemia. DWI may not confirm an acute infarct in approximately 7% of patients, such as in posterior circulation ischemia, with small strokes in the brainstem, or when MRI is done within 6 hours of symptom onset.[43]

Imaging findings

DWI must be interpreted with the apparent diffusion coefficient (ADC) map, where acute ischemia is hyperintense (bright) on DWI and hypointense (dark) on ADC (**Fig. 9**). Over the subsequent 2 weeks, the acute DWI and ADC changes

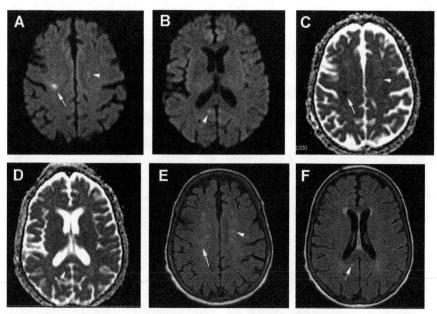

Fig. 9. Infarcts of varying ages on MRI. DWI identified 3 separate hyperintense foci (A [ar-row and arrowhead]; B [arrow]). ADC images confirmed diffusion restriction only for the acute infarct in the posterior right frontal lobe (C [arrow]). The right occipital lesion was iso-intense on ADC (D [arrow]) corresponding to subacute infarct. The left frontal lesion was ADC hyperintense (C [arrowhead]) reflecting chronic infarct T2 shine through. FLAIR images did not have corresponding signal changes for the acute infarct (E [arrow]); however, the lesions were visible for the subacute (F [arrow]) and chronic (E [arrowhead]) infarcts.

pseudonormalize,[44] which can help distinguish recent infarcts of varying ages. DWI signal can be distorted by intracranial hemorrhage; therefore, correlation with additional sequences is essential.

Fluid-attenuated inversion recovery (FLAIR) is a fluid-sensitive sequence that suppresses cerebrospinal fluid signal to increase conspicuity of areas of parenchymal vasogenic edema, prior infarcts, and gliosis.[45] Evidence of acute ischemia on FLAIR generally lags DWI by several hours.

Susceptibility-weighted imaging exploits the magnetic properties of deoxygenated hemoglobin to identify intravascular thrombus[46,47] and may help clarify calcified thromboemboli[48] and prior intracranial hemorrhage[49] as well as asymmetry to the veins that are compensating within the area at risk for infarct expansion.[50]

Intracranial MRA is performed most often with noncontrast time-of-flight and inflow-related techniques to minimize venous signal. Antegrade flowing arterial blood is bright and the remainder of structures are dark, which also facilitate creation of 3-D reconstructions. Contrast-enhanced techniques may confer some benefit in determining thrombus length.[51]

Neck MRA can be performed with noncontrast techniques; however, because both turbulence at the carotid bifurcation and slow flow proximal to an obstruction can result in signal loss, contrast-enhanced angiography also may be performed for extracranial arterial assessment. When dissection is suspected, axial black-blood T1-weighted sequences can be added.[52,53] On black-blood imaging, early subacute thrombus (intracellular methemoglobin) is hyperintense (bright), therefore, conspicuous, due to the saturation of the remaining structures. Hyperacute blood clot is isointense to normal brain signal and not as perceptible using this technique.

Implications for treatment

Although imaging confirmation of ischemia is not required for acute stroke intervention, DWI is the most accurate imaging method to clarify acute ischemia from other potential sources for symptoms.[42] Reversal of DWI signal, or normalization of signal in a previously diffusion-restricting lesion, may occur in small infarct volume with recanalization[54,55]; however, DWI remains the best predictor of the ultimate infarct.[56]

Approximately 20% to 25% of ischemic strokes are preceded by transient ischemic symptoms.[57] A suspected TIA should be evaluated urgently where appropriate specialist expertise and imaging are available, and DWI is the preferred test. A patient with transient symptoms who has even a very small ischemic brain lesion on DWI would be diagnosed with a minor ischemic stroke. If MRI is not available, CTA head and neck could be considered as part of TIA work-up, recognizing the limitation that CTA gives information about the vessels but not if tissue is ischemic.

In patients with noncardioembolic ischemic stroke, aspirin is the most effective treatment to reduce the risk of recurrent stroke during the first 3 months, and it is the only antiplatelet therapy that has been shown to reduce the risk of recurrent disabling ischemic stroke. Clopidogrel should be added to aspirin for 3 weeks, per AHA guidelines.[57] If atrial fibrillation or a cardiac source of embolism is detected, oral anticoagulation should be initiated without delay. If carotid stenosis of 50% or more is found to be the cause, the patient should be referred for possible carotid endarterectomy.

Computed Tomography and Magnetic Resonance Perfusion

Perfusion imaging is based on a series of repeated scans through the anterior circulation over approximately 1 minute after a bolus of contrast. These techniques have emerged to define the area at risk for progressive infarct if reperfusion is not achieved. A pitfall of contrast bolus perfusion is decreased cardiac output, which requires the technologist to adjust the scan timing to avoid missing the bolus. Generally, this is recognized at the time of preceding CTA. Although CT is more accessible than MRI, CT has additional radiation exposure, in total bringing the total dose of noncontrast head CT, contrast CTA and contrast CT perfusion to approximately 6 times that of the noncontrast head CT alone.[29]

A variety of perfusion parameters can be extracted from a series of scans tracking a bolus of contrast through the MCA vascular territory from arteries through parenchyma to the veins. The Clinical Mismatch in the Triage of Wake Up and Late Presenting Strokes Undergoing Neurointervention With Trevo (DAWN)[58] and the Endovascular Therapy Following Imaging Evaluation for Ischemic Stroke (DEFUSE 3) trials[59] were based on the ischemic core, measured as tissue with cerebral blood flow less than 30% relative to that of the contralateral (normal) side, and the at-risk territory measured based on maximum time to peak greater than 6 seconds. These are only surrogate measures, may be more reliable for larger infarcts,[60] and can have both false-positive and false-negative results.[35]

Image review

To interpret, images must be postprocessed by software, which can generate color overlay maps and provide calculations based on preset parameters and thresholds (**Fig. 10**). Several vendors have released automated postprocessing systems to

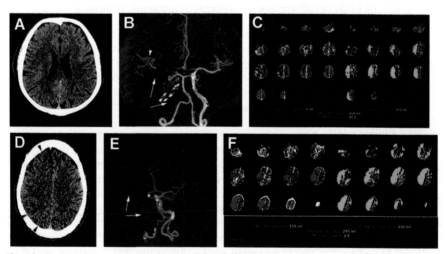

Fig. 10. Companion cases regarding the use of CT perfusion postprocessing for eligibility for thrombectomy in the expanded treatment window. A 62-year old man awoke with left-sided weakness. Initial head CT did not show early ischemic signs (*A*); however, CTA showed absence of contrast corresponding to right ICA and MCA occlusion (*B* [*arrows*]), with some collateral sylvian branch flow (*B* [*arrowhead*]). CT perfusion postprocessing indicated small ischemic core (*C* [*pink*]) and perfusion mismatch (*C* [*green*]) with volume/ratio meeting criteria for endovascular intervention. Thrombectomy was successful. A 56-year old man awoke with left-sided weakness. Initial noncontrast CT showed loss of gray–white differentiation in the right ACA and MCA territories (*D* [*arrowheads*]) and CTA showed absence of contrast corresponding to right ICA and MCA occlusion (*E* [*arrows*]). CT perfusion postprocessing showed an ischemic core greater than 70 mL (*F* [*pink*]), therefore not meeting criteria for endovascular intervention.

reduce time from image acquisition to treatment decision.[17,18] Although different calculation methods have similar end results,[61] there have not been head-to-head comparisons of the different vendors' products.[62] Visual inspection by a radiologist of the color maps is essential for recognizing pitfalls of automated calculations, such as underestimation of infarcts due to parameter settings as well as review of the time-attenuation curves to identify any technical complications during the scan.[63]

Implications for treatment

Intravenous alteplase The FDA only approves the administration of alteplase up to 3 hours after the onset of AIS symptoms. The AHA/American Stroke Association (ASA), however, approves the administration of alteplase up to 4.5 hours after the onset of AIS symptoms and has been standard evidence-based practice since 2009.[64] In 2018 and 2019, 2 trials: WAKEUP and EXTEND, have suggested that the treatment window may be extended in patients who are shown to have ischemic but not yet infarcted brain tissue on imaging. The WAKEUP trial used MRI imaging[65] and the EXTEND trial used both MR and CT perfusion.[66]

The EXTEND trial[66] involved patients presenting 4.5 hours to 9 hours after symptom onset or awakening with stroke symptoms who had mismatch on CT or MR perfusion between hypoperfused (Tmax >6 s) to infarct core (<30% relative cerebral blood volume compared with contralateral), volume ratio of greater than 1:2, an absolute difference greater than 10 mL, and an infarct core lesion volume of less than or equal to 70 mL. Among the patients in the EXTEND trial who had ischemic stroke and salvageable brain tissue, the use of intravenous alteplase resulted in a higher percentage of patients with no or minor neurologic deficits than the use of placebo. There were more cases of symptomatic cerebral hemorrhage (6%) in the alteplase group than in the placebo group; 6% is the same symptomatic cerebral hemorrhage rate from the original NINDS trial.[21]

Endovascular thrombectomy In 2018 and 2019, 2 extended time window trials, DAWN and the DEFUSE 3 trial, were published.[58,59] These trials used CT or MR perfusion imaging to prove that patients with documented emergency LVO and limited infarcted brain tissue identified on advanced imaging who underwent endovascular therapy in treatment windows later than 6 hours had better functional outcomes than patients treated with standard medical therapy alone. The powerful treatment effect was maintained for appropriately selected populations less than or equal to 16 hours (in DEFUSE 3) and 24 hours (in DAWN) from last known well time.

In response to these new data, the AHA/ASA acute stroke guidelines for 2018 recommend thrombectomy less than or equal to 24 hours under trial inclusion criteria—a position embraced by neurointerventional societies.[1] The DAWN trial used a selection paradigm that assigned a pretreatment core infarct threshold by perfusion imaging (maximum of 50 mL) based on patient age and presenting NIHSS. DEFUSE 3 was more inclusive, taking patients broadly with pretreatment core infarct volumes less than or equal to 70 mL who had substantial penumbral volumes on perfusion imaging. Both trials provide evidence for offering endovascular thrombectomy up to 24 hours after onset and are part of the AHA/ASA guidelines.[1]

SUMMARY

For patients with suspected ischemic stroke, the goals of acute neuroimaging are to exclude hemorrhage, exclude stroke mimics, detect signs of early infarction, identify LVO, and determine core infarct and extent of penumbra in those cases. Noncontrast head CT is the preferred initial imaging study for evaluation of acute stroke symptoms.

CTA provides a rapid assessment to detect LVO. MRI with DWI is superior to CT for the detection of acute ischemia and the exclusion of stroke mimics, although it is not widely available for acute evaluation. CT and MR perfusion have emerged as means to extend the therapeutic window for thrombectomy in some patients with anterior circulation LVO. AI products are available to expedite stroke imaging review; however, they are intended to be used as an adjunct to physicians and not as stand-alone diagnostic tools.

CLINICS CARE POINTS

- Noncontrast CT is useful in evaluation of acute stroke symptoms to assess for intracranial hemorrhage and evidence of edema related to ischemia.
- Head and neck CTA is useful in evaluation of acute stroke symptoms to detect LVO, dissection, or significant intracranial arterial stenoses.
- Diffusion-weighted brain MRI is the most sensitive method to confirm acute ischemia; however, patients may be unable to have MRI due to metal implants/devices or claustrophobia or if they are disoriented and unable to follow instructions how to stay safe in the MRI scanner.
- Multiphase CTA can help assess extent of collateral perfusion in patients with suspicion for LVO; however, it incurs additional radiation exposure.
- CT perfusion and MR perfusion parameters have been established through clinical trials to stratify risk for revascularization in patients with acute ICA and proximal MCA occlusion.
- Multiple vendors provide AI software to help expedite stroke imaging review. All remain considered an aid to the physician rather than stand-alone diagnostic tool.

DISCLOSURE

Dr K. Greenberg: Speakers Bureau, Genentech. Dr J. Bykowski: Medical Advisory Board, Spiral Therapeutics.

REFERENCES

1. Powers WJ, Rabinstein AA, Ackerson T, et al. Guidelines for the Early Management of Patients With Acute Ischemic Stroke: 2019 Update to the 2018 Guidelines for the Early Management of Acute Ischemic Stroke: A Guideline for Healthcare Professionals From the American Heart Association/American Stroke Association. Stroke 2019;50(12):e344-418 [published correction appears in Stroke. 2019 Dec;50(12):e440-e441].
2. Expert Panel on Neurologic Imaging, Salmela MB, Mortazavi S, et al. ACR Appropriateness Criteria® Cerebrovascular Disease. J Am Coll Radiol 2017;14(5S): S34-S61.
3. National Institute for Health and Care Excellence (NICE). Medtech innovation briefing (MIB207). Artificial intelligence for analysing CT brain scans 2020. Available at: https://www.nice.org.uk/advice/mib207/resources/artificial-intelligence-for-analysing-ct-brain-scans-pdf-2285965396121029. Accessed June 4, 2020.
4. Jaremko JL, Azar M, Bromwich R, et al. Canadian association of radiologists white paper on ethical and legal issues related to artificial intelligence in radiology. Can Assoc Radiol J 2019;70(2):107-18.
5. Zerna C, Thomalla G, Campbell BCV, et al. Current practice and future directions in the diagnosis and acute treatment of ischemic stroke. Lancet 2018;392:1247.

6. Aghaebrahim A, Streib C, Rangaraju S, et al. Streamlining door to recanalization processes in endovascular stroke therapy. J Neurointerv Surg 2017;9(4):340–5.
7. Messé SR, Khatri P, Reeves MJ, et al. Why are acute ischemic stroke patients not receiving IV tPA? Results from a national registry. Neurology 2016;87(15):1565–74.
8. Zaidi SF, Shawver J, Espinosa Morales A, et al. Stroke care: initial data from a county-based bypass protocol for patients with acute stroke. J Neurointerv Surg 2017;9(7):631–5.
9. Lansberg MG, Albers GW, Beaulieu C, et al. Comparison of diffusion-weighted MRI and CT in acute stroke. Neurology 2000;54(8):1557–61.
10. Hacke W, Kaste M, Fieschi C, et al. Intravenous thrombolysis with recombinant tissue plasminogen activator for acute hemispheric stroke. The European Cooperative Acute Stroke Study (ECASS). JAMA 1995;274(13):1017–25.
11. Wardlaw JM, Mielke O. Early signs of brain infarction at CT: observer reliability and outcome after thrombolytic treatment–systematic review. Radiology 2005;235(2):444–53.
12. Salazar AJ, Useche N, Bermúdez S, et al. Evaluation of the accuracy equivalence of head CT interpretations in acute stroke patients using a smartphone, a laptop, or a medical workstation. J Am Coll Radiol 2019;16(11):1561–71.
13. American College of Radiology. ACR-AAPM-SIIM Technical Standard for Electronic Practice of Medical Imaging. 2017. Available at: https://www.acr.org/-/media/ACR/Files/Practice-Parameters/elec-practice-medimag.pdf. Accessed June 4, 2020.
14. AIDoc. Available at: https://www.aidoc.com/. Accessed June 11, 2020.
15. AI1 Solutions. Available at: https://www.zebra-med.com/. Accessed June 11, 2020.
16. ACCIPIO Ix. Available at: https://www.maxq.ai/. Accessed June 11, 2020.
17. RAPID AI. Available at: https://www.rapidai.com/. Accessed June 11, 2020.
18. VIZ.AI. Available at: https://www.viz.ai/solutions/. Accessed June 11, 2020.
19. Mair G, Boyd EV, Chappell FM, et al. Sensitivity and specificity of the hyperdense artery sign for arterial obstruction in acute ischemic stroke. Stroke 2015;46(1):102–7.
20. Lim J, Magarik JA, Froehler MT. The CT-Defined Hyperdense Arterial Sign as a Marker for Acute Intracerebral Large Vessel Occlusion. J Neuroimaging 2018;28(2):212–6.
21. National Institute of Neurological Disorders and Stroke rt-PA Stroke Study Group. Tissue plasminogen activator for acute ischemic stroke. N Engl J Med 1995;333(24):1581–7.
22. Barber PA, Demchuk AM, Zhang J, et al. Validity and reliability of a quantitative computed tomography score in predicting outcome of hyperacute stroke before thrombolytic therapy. ASPECTS Study Group. Alberta Stroke Programme Early CT Score. Lancet 2000;355(9216):1670–4 [published correction appears in Lancet 2000 Jun 17;355(9221):2170].
23. Pexman JH, Barber PA, Hill MD, et al. Use of the Alberta Stroke Program Early CT Score (ASPECTS) for assessing CT scans in patients with acute stroke. AJNR Am J Neuroradiol 2001;22(8):1534–42.
24. Beume LA, Hieber M, Kaller CP, et al. Large vessel occlusion in acute stroke. Stroke 2018;49(10):2323–9.
25. Pérez de la Ossa N, Carrera D, Gorchs M, et al. Design and validation of a prehospital stroke scale to predict large arterial occlusion: the rapid arterial occlusion evaluation scale. Stroke 2014;45(1):87–91.

26. Mayer SA, Viarasilpa T, Panyavachiraporn N, et al. CTA-for-all: impact of emergency computed tomographic angiography for all patients with stroke presenting within 24 hours of onset. Stroke 2020;51(1):331–4.
27. Douglas V, Shamy M, Bhattacharya P. Should CT angiography be a routine component of acute stroke imaging? Neurohospitalist 2015;5(3):97–8.
28. ACR Committee on Drugs and Contrast Media. ACR manual on contrast media. Reston, Virginia, USA: American College of Radiology; 2020. Available at: https://www.acr.org/-/media/ACR/Files/Clinical-Resources/Contrast_Media.pdf%20ACR%20contrast%20manual%202020. Accessed June 4, 2020.
29. Mnyusiwalla A, Aviv RI, Symons SP. Radiation dose from multidetector row CT imaging for acute stroke. Neuroradiology 2009;51(10):635–40.
30. Tan JC, Dillon WP, Liu S, et al. Systematic comparison of perfusion-CT and CT-angiography in acute stroke patients. Ann Neurol 2007;61(6):533–43.
31. Tan IY, Demchuk AM, Hopyan J, et al. CT angiography clot burden score and collateral score: correlation with clinical and radiologic outcomes in acute middle cerebral artery infarct. AJNR Am J Neuroradiol 2009;30(3):525–31.
32. Menon BK, d'Esterre CD, Qazi EM, et al. Multiphase CT angiography: a new tool for the imaging triage of patients with acute ischemic stroke. Radiology 2015;275(2):510–20.
33. Boers AMM, Sales Barros R, Jansen IGH, et al. Value of quantitative collateral scoring on CT angiography in patients with acute ischemic stroke. AJNR Am J Neuroradiol 2018;39(6):1074–82.
34. Berkhemer OA, Fransen PS, Beumer D, et al. A randomized trial of intraarterial treatment for acute ischemic stroke. N Engl J Med 2015;372(1):11–20 [published correction appears in N Engl J Med. 2015 Jan 22;372(4):394].
35. Campbell BC, Mitchell PJ, Kleinig TJ, et al. Endovascular therapy for ischemic stroke with perfusion-imaging selection. N Engl J Med 2015;372(11):1009–18.
36. Jovin TG, Chamorro A, Cobo E, et al. Thrombectomy within 8 hours after symptom onset in ischemic stroke. N Engl J Med 2015;372(24):2296–306.
37. Goyal M, Demchuk AM, Menon BK, et al. Randomized assessment of rapid endovascular treatment of ischemic stroke. N Engl J Med 2015;372(11):1019–30.
38. Saver JL, Goyal M, Bonafe A, et al. Stent-retriever thrombectomy after intravenous t-PA vs. t-PA alone in stroke. N Engl J Med 2015;372(24):2285–95.
39. Shellock FG. Reference manual for magnetic resonance safety, implants, and devices: 2020 edition. Playa Del Ray, CA, USA: Biomedical Research Publishing Group; 2020. Available at: http://www.mrisafety.com/. Accessed June 4, 2020.
40. Beauchamp NJ Jr, Barker PB, Wang PY, et al. Imaging of acute cerebral ischemia. Radiology 1999;212(2):307–24.
41. Fiebach JB, Schellinger PD, Jansen O, et al. CT and diffusion-weighted MR imaging in randomized order: diffusion-weighted imaging results in higher accuracy and lower interrater variability in the diagnosis of hyperacute ischemic stroke. Stroke 2002;33(9):2206–10.
42. Schellinger PD, Bryan RN, Caplan LR, et al. Evidence-based guideline: The role of diffusion and perfusion MRI for the diagnosis of acute ischemic stroke: report of the Therapeutics and Technology Assessment Subcommittee of the American Academy of Neurology. Neurology 2010;75(2):177–85 [published correction appears in Neurology. 2010 Sep 7;75(10):938].
43. Edlow BL, Hurwitz S, Edlow JA. Diagnosis of DWI-negative acute ischemic stroke: A meta-analysis. Neurology 2017;89(3):256–62.
44. Schlaug G, Siewert B, Benfield A, et al. Time course of the apparent diffusion coefficient (ADC) abnormality in human stroke. Neurology 1997;49(1):113–9.

45. Okuda T, Korogi Y, Shigematsu Y, et al. Brain lesions: when should fluid-attenuated inversion-recovery sequences be used in MR evaluation? Radiology 1999;212(3):793–8.
46. Cho KH, Kim JS, Kwon SU, et al. Significance of susceptibility vessel sign on T2*-weighted gradient echo imaging for identification of stroke subtypes. Stroke 2005;36(11):2379–83.
47. Gonzalez RG, Schaefer P. In: Gonzalez RG, Hirsch JA, Koroshetz WJ, et al, editors. Conventional MRI and MR angiography of stroke. Berlin: Springer; 2006. p. 115–37.
48. Wu Z, Mittal S, Kish K, et al. Identification of calcification with MRI using susceptibility-weighted imaging: a case study. J Magn Reson Imaging 2009; 29(1):177–82.
49. Fiehler J, Albers GW, Boulanger JM, et al. Bleeding risk analysis in stroke imaging before thromboLysis (BRASIL): pooled analysis of T2*-weighted magnetic resonance imaging data from 570 patients. Stroke 2007;38(10):2738–44.
50. Darwish EAF, Abdelhameed-El-Nouby M, Geneidy E. Mapping the ischemic penumbra and predicting stroke progression in acute ischemic stroke: the overlooked role of susceptibility weighted imaging. Insights Imaging 2020;11(1):6.
51. Dhundass S, Savatovsky J, Duron L, et al. Improved detection and characterization of arterial occlusion in acute ischemic stroke using contrast enhanced MRA. J Neuroradiol 2020;47(4):278–83.
52. Hunter MA, Santosh C, Teasdale E, et al. High-resolution double inversion recovery black-blood imaging of cervical artery dissection using 3T MR imaging. AJNR Am J Neuroradiol 2012;33(11):E133–7.
53. Al-Smadi AS, Abdalla RN, Elmokadem AH, et al. Diagnostic accuracy of high-resolution black-blood MRI in the evaluation of intracranial large-vessel arterial occlusions. AJNR Am J Neuroradiol 2019;40(6):954–9.
54. Fiehler J, Knudsen K, Kucinski T, et al. Predictors of apparent diffusion coefficient normalization in stroke patients. Stroke 2004;35(2):514–9.
55. Asdaghi N, Campbell BC, Butcher KS, et al. DWI reversal is associated with small infarct volume in patients with TIA and minor stroke. AJNR Am J Neuroradiol 2014;35(4):660–6.
56. Lövblad KO, Baird AE, Schlaug G, et al. Ischemic lesion volumes in acute stroke by diffusion-weighted magnetic resonance imaging correlate with clinical outcome. Ann Neurol 1997;42(2):164–70.
57. Amarenco P. Transient ischemic attack. N Engl J Med 2020;382(20):1933–41.
58. Nogueira RG, Jadhav AP, Haussen DC, et al. Thrombectomy 6 to 24 hours after stroke with a mismatch between deficit and infarct. N Engl J Med 2018;378(1): 11–21.
59. Albers GW, Marks MP, Kemp S, et al. Thrombectomy for stroke at 6 to 16 hours with selection by perfusion imaging. N Engl J Med 2018;378(8):708–18.
60. Amukotuwa S, Straka M, Aksoy D, et al. Cerebral blood flow predicts the infarct core: new insights from contemporaneous diffusion and perfusion imaging. Stroke 2019;50(10):2783–9.
61. Abels B, Villablanca JP, Tomandl BF, et al. Acute stroke: a comparison of different CT perfusion algorithms and validation of ischaemic lesions by follow-up imaging. Eur Radiol 2012;22(12):2559–67.
62. Mokli Y, Pfaff J, dos Santos DP, et al. Computer-aided imaging analysis in acute ischemic stroke – background and clinical applications. Neurol Res Pract 2019; 1:23.

63. Laughlin B, Chan A, Tai WA, et al. RAPID automated CT perfusion in clinical practice. Pract Neurol 2019;38–50.
64. Del Zoppo GJ, Saver JL, Jauch EC, et al. American Heart Association Stroke Council. Expansion of the time window for treatment of acute ischemic stroke with intravenous tissue plasminogen activator: a science advisory from the American Heart Association/American Stroke Association. Stroke 2009;40(8):2945–8 [published correction appears in Stroke. 2010 Sep;41(9):e562].
65. Thomalla G, Simonsen CZ, Boutitie F, et al. MRI-guided thrombolysis for stroke with unknown time of onset. N Engl J Med 2018;379(7):611–22.
66. Ma H, Campbell BCV, Parsons MW, et al. Thrombolysis guided by perfusion imaging up to 9 hours after onset of stroke. N Engl J Med 2019;380(19):1795–803.

Neurologic Emergencies at the Extremes of Age

Danya Khoujah, MBBS, MEHP[a,b,]*, Megan J. Cobb, MD, DPT[a,c]

KEYWORDS

- Pediatric • Altered mental status • Geriatric • Trauma • Encephalitis • Stroke

KEY POINTS

- In a child with fever and altered mental status, consider anti–*N*-methyl-ᴅ-aspartate receptor encephalitis and acute disseminated encephalomyelitis in the differential diagnosis.
- Nonconvulsive status epilepticus is associated with higher mortality, longer pediatric intensive care unit stays, and increased long term disability.
- Age alone is not a contraindication for intravenous tissue-type plasminogen activator administration within 3 hours.
- Acute worsening in Parkinson's disease is usually due to a medication change, infection, or missed subdural hemorrhage.
- Meningitis in older adults presents atypically and has worse outcomes than the general population.

INTRODUCTION

Neurologic conditions, both common and emergent, present to the emergency department (ED) daily. The diagnosis and management of such conditions can be more complex at the extremes of age than in the average adult. In the pediatric population, neurologic emergencies are somewhat rare and some may require emergent consultation, as summarized in **Box 1**.

On the opposite end of the age spectrum, older adults disproportionately require emergency care, and the combination of geriatric physiologic changes with increased comorbidities leads to atypical presentations and worsened outcomes.[1,2] The unique considerations regarding emergency department (ED) presentation and management of stroke and altered mental status (AMS) in both age groups, in addition to seizures

[a] Department of Emergency Medicine, University of Maryland School of Medicine, 110 S Paca St, 6th Floor, Suite 200, Baltimore, MD 21201, USA; [b] Department of Emergency Medicine, MedStar Franklin Square Medical Center, 9000 Franklin Square Dr, Baltimore, MD 21237, USA; [c] Maryland Emergency Medicine Network, Upper Chesapeake Emergency Medicine, 500 Upper Chesapeake Drive, Bel Air, MD 21014, USA
* Corresponding author. Department of Emergency Medicine, University of Maryland School of Medicine, 110 S Paca St, 6th Floor, Suite 200, Baltimore, MD 21201, USA
E-mail address: dkhoujah@gmail.com
Twitter: @DanyaKhoujah (D.K.)

Emerg Med Clin N Am 39 (2021) 47–65
https://doi.org/10.1016/j.emc.2020.09.003
0733-8627/21/© 2020 Elsevier Inc. All rights reserved.
emed.theclinics.com

Box 1
Pediatric conditions requiring emergent neurology consultation

- High suspicion for stroke, regardless of intent to use tissue-type plasminogen activator
- Autoimmune encephalitis
- Acute demyelinating encephalomyelitis
- Acute peripheral neurologic deficit, that is, acute flaccid myelitis, Guillain–Barré syndrome, acute brachial neuritis
- Transverse myelitis
- Any suspected seizure at <1 year of age
- Reported or observed seizure activity with reports of loss of milestones or other systemic symptoms
- Newly documented neurologic deficits/symptoms or first time seizure with concerns regarding timely follow-up
- Refractory status epilepticus, convulsive or nonconvulsive

---

and intracranial hemorrhage in pediatrics, and Parkinson's disease and meningitis in the geriatric population are discussed.

NEUROLOGIC EMERGENCIES IN THE PEDIATRIC PATIENT
Pediatric Neurologic Examination

Although not "little adults," our pediatric patients are not aliens either. Their neurologic systems are, however, still in development and in need of a different approach for examination. The normal range for each component varies by age, environmental exposure, and any underlying congenital malformations or diseases. The physical examination begins from the moment you see the patient. Observe how alert or withdrawn they are, or how they respond to their caregiver's voice. Note the muscle tone and posture of the infant or child, and their response to touch. Understand the child's baseline behavior from the accompanying caregiver and compare it with your assessment to uncover any abnormalities. An effective mnemonic for a gross neurologic evaluation of the child is *TICLS*: Tone, Interaction, Consolability (irritability), Look (gaze), Speech (including jargon or cry), as one arm of the Pediatric Assessment Triangle[3] (**Table 1**).

Table 1
Pediatric neurologic examination: the TICLS mnemonic

	Element	Exam Questions
T	Tone	Do they appear floppy or limp? Head lag? Response when touched?
I	Interaction	Resistance to exam? Smile or grin? Acknowledgment of providers?
C	Consolability	Are they irritable or fussy? Consoled by caregiver presence or affection? Pitch of the cry?
L	Look	Pupillary size? Eye contact? Fixed or roaming gaze? Conjugate or disconjugate? Tracking?
S	Speech	Age appropriate babble or jargon? Age appropriate sentences? Oriented or confused? Speech slurring?

Data from Horeczko T, Enriquez B, McGrath NE, Gausche-Hill M, Lewis RJ. The Pediatric Assessment Triangle: Accuracy of Its Application by Nurses in the Triage of Children. *J Emerg Nurs.* 2013;39(2):182-189.

Pediatric Acute Ischemic Stroke

Clinical presentation

In the pediatric population, stroke is rare and can be more difficult to recognize than in the adult population. Children younger than 5 years of age are the most likely to experience acute ischemic stroke (AIS) among pediatric patients. AIS in young children is more likely to present with global neurologic impairment, such as seizure or AMS, than in adults.[4] Up to 50% of infants and young children with AIS may present with AMS, fever, and/or seizure. Older children and teens are more likely to present with focal neurologic deficits similar to those in adults. Considering AIS in the list of differential diagnoses of seizure or AMS, especially in infants and younger children, can improve time to diagnosis. Delay in diagnosis up to 24 hours from the time of presentation is common, even though patients often present within 6 hours from time of onset.[4]

Examination should begin promptly with observation of the patient and quantification of neurologic deficits as soon as they are identified or reported by the caregiver. A noncontrast computed tomography (CT) scan of the brain and point-of-care glucose are just as important in children as in adults. Rapid use of the Pediatric National Institute of Health Stroke Scale should be included in patients ages 6 years and younger to quantify neurologic deficits and guide the decision to use thrombolytics, particularly if the score is greater than or equal to 6.[4,5] The Pediatric National Institute of Health Stroke Scale is partially completed by the physician's observation of the child's behavior and responses in the ED given that it is difficult for many younger children to follow the instructions of the examination. Other age-specific modifications are summarized in **Box 2**.

Thrombolytics

After ruling out intracranial hemorrhage using a CT scan, tissue-type plasminogen activator (tPA) can be given in consultation with the pediatric neurologist and/or

---

Box 2
National Institutes of Health Stroke Scale Modifications in Pediatric Patients

- Orientation – Ask age and point to family member
- Commands – Blink eyes and touch nose
- Gaze – Assessed with horizontal gaze only
- Visual fields – Finger counting if >6 years old, or visual threat if <6 years old
- Facial palsy – Scored same as adults
- Motor strength – If unable to follow commands, score by spontaneous or elicited movement, that is, assisted weight bearing may demonstrate 1 leg weaker than the other
- Ataxia – Ask to reach or kick toy in examiner's hand
- Sensation – Pinprick testing, or observe for spontaneous response to pinprick
- Language – Assess with stated words, naming pictures[a]
- Dysarthria – Repeating words or sentences, ask about baseline speech impediment
- Extinction/inattention – Scored similarly to adults

[a] Must understand baseline verbal skills.

Data from Ichord RN, Bastian R, Abraham L, et al. Interrater reliability of the Pediatric National Institutes of Health Stroke Scale (PedNIHSS) in a multicenter study. *Stroke.* 2011;42(3):613-617.

pediatric intensivist, if available, who will be accepting the patient. MRI of the brain is the preferred imaging for detailed examination of brain parenchyma; however, it is not required before tPA administration. Thrombolytics should not be delayed for an MRI if the physician's suspicion for AIS is reasonably high, but certain institutional algorithms may require demonstration of acute vascular occlusion before giving tPA.[4] Goal administration time is of less than 4.5 hours from the time of onset, and early administration is more likely to result in improved outcomes. The pediatric tPA dosing is the same as that in adults: 0.9 mg/kg with 10% administered as a bolus followed by 90% as an infusion over 60 minutes.[4] In vitro data show that the thrombus composition of children's plasma contains less fibrin as compared with adults, resulting in higher recanalization rates with tPA.[4] A small study to review efficacy and safety of tPA in children was published in 2019; there was no clinically significant intracranial hemorrhage after tPA administration in 26 children. One patient experienced severe epistaxis requiring intubation, but details regarding epistaxis evaluation and management are of limited description. There were 2 patients with cerebral petechiae found on follow-up MRI within the area of infarction, but this did not seem to limit their recovery. Overall, the estimated risk profile of tPA in pediatric stroke is 2.1% when given within 4.5 hours from time of onset.[5]

Thrombectomy
There is limited evidence supporting thrombectomy in patients under 18 years of age; however, it may be performed on patients under certain circumstances. Expert opinion, based on extrapolated adult data, encourages its consideration within 6 hours of symptoms onset in select patients. Technical limitations include the smaller size of peripheral and intracranial vessels, as well as increased concerns for radiation risk and contrast load.[4]

Stroke in sickle cell disease
Sickle cell disease accounts for a large portion of disease burden in pediatric stroke, particularly in African American children. The time of greatest risk for stroke in a patient with sickle cell disease is between 2 and 5 years of age.[4] Given that many of these strokes are silent in nature, the only clinical signs may be early hand dominance, speech delays, or learning disabilities. When AIS in sickle cell disease is symptomatic, it is theorized that, owing to the development of higher pain tolerance, headache is a less frequently reported symptom of AIS in sickle cell disease as compared with AIS patients without sickle cell disease.[6] In patients presenting with an acute neurologic deficit, immediate treatment is needed (**Box 3**). In patients with a baseline hemoglobin (Hgb) of less than 10 g/dL, urgent transfusion of 10 mL/kg of packed red blood cells for a goal Hgb of 10 g/dL or sickle cell percentage of less than 15% is indicated, to be given within 6 hours of symptom onset.[4] If the baseline Hgb is greater than 10 mg/dL, exchange transfusion must be performed. Repeat transfusion may be needed but Hgb should not go above 11 g/dL, and post-transfusion Hgb measured at approximately 2 hours after to assess risk hyperviscosity syndrome, which may occur with rapid overcorrection of the Hgb.[4] Hyperviscosity syndrome may lead to cerebral venous sinus thrombosis or multifocal infarcts. Pain and hydration status should be addressed as they would in other vasoocclusive crises. The emergency physician should also look for additional underlying precipitating factors contributing to the acute presentation, such as infection, dehydration, trauma, hypoxia, or acidosis. Ultimately, the patient will require emergent transfer to higher level care and consultation with pediatric hematology if available.

Box 3
Stroke management in pediatric patient with sickle cell disease

Special considerations in sickle cell disease

- When AIS suspected, prompt transfusion is needed
- Goal time to transfusion: <6 hours from onset of symptoms
- Start with 10 mL/kg of packed red blood cells, goal Hgb 10 g/dL or <15% sickled Hgb
- May need exchange transfusion if baseline Hgb is close to 10 g/dL
- Avoid hypervolemia and hyperviscosity syndrome from overtransfusing
- For Hgb >12 g/dL, consider phlebotomy to decrease total blood volume (consult with hematology for recommended volume removal)
- Consider aggravating factors that may contribute to acute sickling or clinical presentation

Abbreviation: Hgb, hemoglobin.

Data from Ferriero DM, Fullerton HJ, Bernard TJ, et al. Management of stroke in neonates and children: A scientific statement from the American Heart Association/American stroke association. *Stroke.* 2019;50(3):E51-E96; Guilliams KP, Kirkham FJ, Holzhauer S, et al. Arteriopathy Influences Pediatric Ischemic Stroke Presentation, but Sickle Cell Disease Influences Stroke Management. *Stroke.* 2019;50(5):1089-1094.

Intracranial Hemorrhage

Many principles of adult care should be readily applied in the management of traumatic and nontraumatic intracranial hemorrhage in pediatric patients. Prioritization of the airway, breathing, and circulation, monitoring of vitals, and assessing blood glucose are necessary.[7] Airway management in the setting of profound mental status change is of paramount importance. Patients with suspected intracranial hemorrhage should then undergo a CT scan of the head to assess severity of intracranial bleeding. There should be an ongoing focus to optimize oxygenation, ventilation, and blood pressure.[4] Ideal parameters for arterial oxygen and carbon dioxide levels, as well as glucose, are similar to those for adults; however, target blood pressure is less clear. In cases of cerebral edema or impending herniation, administration of either mannitol or hypertonic saline is equally acceptable, and the physician should consider their variable effects on blood pressure[7] (**Table 2**). Seizure activity should be treated aggressively. Antiepileptics are commonly used prophylactically owing to concerns of transient intracranial pressure spikes during convulsions, but there is little evidence to support the safety and efficacy of this practice.[4] After patient stabilization, identification of intracranial hemorrhage, and initiation of supportive measures, communication with nearest pediatric neurosurgery and intensive care should ensue to arrange for transfer.

Fever and Altered Mental Status

Bacterial meningitis should not be the only diagnosis considered when a pediatric patient presents with fever and AMS. Other important diagnoses are summarized in **Box 4**.

Acute disseminated encephalomyelitis and anti–N-methyl-D-aspartate receptor encephalitis
Acute disseminated encephalomyelitis (ADEM) is an acute multifocal demyelinating disease presenting with fever, acute AMS, and neuromotor dysfunction, such as

Table 2
Pediatric management of elevated intracranial pressure

Osmotic Agent	Dose	Frequency	Adverse Effects
Mannitol	0.25–1.00 g/kg IV over 20 min	Up to every 4–6 h	Hypovolemia Acute renal failure Diuresis Decreased BP
Hypertonic saline (3%)	2–5 mL/kg IV given over 10–20 min	Can start continuous infusion of 0.1–1.0 mL/kg/h	Rebound cerebral edema Osmotic demyelination syndrome[a] Increased BP

Abbreviation: BP, blood pressure.
[a] Formerly known as central pontine myelinosis.
Data from Kliegman RM, Stanton BF, St Geme JWI, Schor NF, Behrman RE. *Nelson Textbook of Pediatrics.* 20th ed.; 2016; Kochanek PM, Tasker RC, Carney N, et al. Guidelines for the Management of Pediatric Severe Traumatic Brain Injury, Third Edition: Update of the Brain Trauma Foundation Guidelines, Executive Summary. *Neurosurgery.* 2019;84(6):1169-1178; Stopa BM, Dolmans RG, Broekman ML, et al. Hyperosmolar Therapy in Pediatric Severe Traumatic Brain Injury—A Systematic Review. Critical Care Medicine 2019; 47(12): e1022-e1031.

seizures. Patients are commonly young males, ages 5 to 8 years old, with recent viral illness or immunization. The illness can be idiopathic.[8,9] Patients often seem to be quite ill, and symptoms can progress in hours to days, lasting up to several weeks. The clinical picture is extremely similar to acute bacterial meningitis and a distinguishing feature is contrast-enhanced MRI revealing bilateral, multifocal, asymmetric enhancing lesions on T2-weighted or fluid-attenuated inversion recovery images.[10] Lumbar puncture findings are not diagnostic in ADEM and may reveal elevated proteins and lymphocytic pleocytosis. More important, a lumbar puncture should be done to rule out infectious meningoencephalitis and xanthochromia from intracranial hemorrhage.[8,9]

Box 4
Clinical considerations for pediatric AMS and fever

- Infectious meningitis
- Infectious encephalitis
- ADEM
- Hemophagocytic lymphohistiocytosis
- Anti-NDMAR encephalitis
- Other autoimmune encephalitis
- Stroke (infants and toddlers)
- Toxic ingestions
  - Sympathomimetic
  - Anticholinergic
- Thyrotoxicosis
- Paraneoplastic syndromes

* Not all inclusive.

Anti–*N*-methyl-ᴅ-aspartate receptor (NMDAR) encephalitis is insidious in onset; symptoms progress over weeks. It is more common in prepubertal males or postpubertal females. Classified as an autoimmune encephalitis, second most common only to ADEM, it is typically preceded by a febrile viral-like syndrome. It progresses over the following days to week, and develops into light switch acutely fluctuating mental status changes, dyskinesia, seizures, fever, and autonomic instability.[9] Caregivers may report that the patient does not remember events of the day, has a delay or decrease in expressive language, seems to be restless with tremors or repetitive movements, and may hallucinate. Young children may present with increased frequency of unprovoked tantrums.[11] Given the overlap in symptoms between anti-NMDAR encephalitis and initial presentation of schizophrenia or other psychoses, a thorough history is critical. Early behavioral and mental status changes are often mistaken for a new behavioral or psychiatric disorder, which highlights the importance of a thorough assessment to exclude an underlying organic etiology for the presentation of such patients before psychiatry consultation. When suspected, a full assessment should include a brain MRI, to rule out other entities such as ADEM, and lumbar puncture, to test specifically for anti-NMDAR antibodies.

Both ADEM and anti-NMDAR encephalitis require a high index of suspicion, aggressive seizure control, and early initiation of steroids. Empiric treatment for bacterial and viral meningitis should be given as well. Second- and third-line therapies such as intravenous immunoglobulin, plasmapheresis, and biologic agents such as cyclophosphamide and rituximab are effective, however not indicated in acute ED management. Postpubertal girls (or girls >14 years old) suspected of having anti-NMDAR encephalitis should undergo abdomen and pelvis MRI for the evaluation of possible ovarian mass, because an ovarian teratoma is discovered in up to 40% of these patients.[9]

Extracranial causes of altered mental status

Given the sensitivity of children's nervous systems, the astute physician must also consider that fever and AMS may be a consequence of disease outside of the central nervous system. One of the most common to remember is hypoglycemia, which is not a direct cause of fever, but may be a consequence of febrile illness and concomitant hypermetabolic state. Point-of-care glucose testing should be considered the sixth vital sign for any ill-appearing, altered, or vomiting child. Inborn errors of metabolism such as fatty acid oxidation disorders, carnitine transport disorder, or mitochondrial disease may also present with AMS owing to the metabolic derangements of even a minor febrile illness. Endocrinopathy-like thyrotoxicosis and pheochromocytoma should also be considered, particularly in the setting of tachycardia and hypertension for age. Finally, any anticholinergic or sympathomimetic toxidrome can also present with elevated temperatures and AMS.

Seizures

Seizures are a common clinical entity that emergency physicians must be competent in identifying and managing. Febrile, post-traumatic, and rebound seizures after medication noncompliance are all quite common; however, there are some additional considerations for seizure in pediatrics of which physicians must be aware.

Neonatal seizures

Neonatal seizures occur in 1.0 to 3.5 per 1000 live births, and can have significant consequences if misdiagnosed or mismanaged.[12] The neonatal seizure is defined as seizure activity in a patient less than 28 days old, and can be difficult to recognize owing to the immaturity of the central nervous system. Generalized seizure activity may present only with mouthing, horizontal eye deviation, blinking, decreased responsiveness, or single limb extension, not with the classic tonic–clonic activity of a more mature brain.[9] Common causes include hypoxic–ischemic encephalopathy, ischemic and hemorrhagic perinatal stroke, electrolyte disturbance, structural brain abnormality, abusive head trauma, or infections. The first-line treatment for neonatal seizures is phenobarbital 20 mg/kg, but if there is a delay in administration, a benzodiazepine can be given.[12] Second-line therapy includes fosphenytoin, levetiracetam, midazolam, and lidocaine (**Table 3**). In refractory neonatal seizures, pyridoxine may be also be effective in some metabolic errors.[9]

Nonconvulsive status epilepticus
Nonconvulsive status epilepticus is another clinical entity of which to be vigilant. Delayed recognition often leads to prolonged hospitalization, prolonged intensive care stays, and long-term morbidity. Nonconvulsive status epilepticus should be in the differential diagnosis when the presenting problem is abrupt onset of lethargy, decreased responsiveness, or AMS, or may be the consequence of inadequate seizure control. Nonconvulsive status epilepticus can also occur after a patient has been intubated for airway protection, has received paralytics, but continues to have epileptiform brain activity. When suspected, a spot electroencephalography is indicated, if available. A trial of a short-acting antiepileptic medication such as midazolam and close observation for change in mental status may also reveal the clinical condition.[12]

NEUROLOGIC EMERGENCIES IN THE GERIATRIC PATIENT
Acute Ischemic Stroke

Prevalence
Stroke is the leading cause of disability in the United States and mostly affects the geriatric population; three-quarters of strokes occur in patients 65 or older,[13] and one-third are in patients greater than 80 years.[14] AIS in older adults is more likely to be secondary to a cardioembolic source (such as atrial fibrillation) than in their younger counterparts.[14,15]

Presentation
Older adults are more likely to have underlying disability at baseline, present atypically, present later to care, and receive less evidence-based care than their younger counterparts.[2,16–18] Some atypical presentations are summarized in **Box 5**. Physicians should maintain a low threshold for suspecting strokes in older adults and obtaining emergent brain imaging for stroke-like and atypical presentations alike.

Table 3
Medications for neonatal seizures

Drug	Dose	Common Adverse Effects
Phenobarbital	20 mg/kg loading dose (max 40 mg/kg)	Respiratory depression, hypotension
Phenytoin	20 mg/kg loading dose	Arrhythmia, central nervous system depression, hypotension
Midazolam	Depends on additional medications being used. Maximum dosing 0.15 mg/kg	Respiratory depression, hypotension May increase length of stay and risk of mortality
Levetiracetam	20 mg/kg	Somnolence

Data from El-Dib M, Soul JS. The use of phenobarbital and other anti-seizure drugs in newborns. *Semin Fetal Neonatal Med.* 2017;22(5):321-327.

Box 5
Atypical AIS presentations in older adults

- AMS
- Dizziness
- Falls
- Headache
- Nausea and vomiting
- Reduced mobility or difficulty walking
- Seizure
- Syncope
- Urinary incontinence

Data from Arch AE, Weisman DC, Coca S, Nystrom K V., Wira CR, Schindler JL. Missed Ischemic Stroke Diagnosis in the Emergency Department by Emergency Medicine and Neurology Services. *Stroke.* 2016;47(3):668-673; Muangpaisan W, Hinkle JL, Westwood M, Kennedy J, Buchan AM. Stroke in the very old: clinical presentations and outcomes. *Age Ageing.* 2008;37(4):473-475; Pare JR, Kahn JH. Basic neuroanatomy and stroke syndromes. *Emerg Med Clin North Am.* 2012;30(3):601-615; Goyal M, Menon BK, van Zwam WH, et al. Endovascular thrombectomy after large-vessel ischaemic stroke: a meta-analysis of individual patient data from five randomised trials. *Lancet.* 2016;387(10029):1723-1731.

Treatment

Treating older adults with systemic tPA or endovascular therapy is a complex decision; they are more likely to have stroke-related death and disability than their younger counterparts, whether they receive treatment or not.[19] The improvement in outcome owing to revascularization treatment seems to be preserved in appropriately selected older adults,[18,20,21] although they may be more likely to have hemorrhagic complications after treatment.[22] Age alone is not a reason to withhold revascularization treatment in older adults.

Systemic thrombolytics

Intravenous tPA has been extensively studied and is standard of care for AIS up to 4.5 hours of last known well with certain exclusions.[23] The data for safety and efficacy of tPA within the 3-hour window are relatively robust, even in patients 80 years or older.[21] However, the evidence is not as clear for the extended time window from 3.0 to 4.5 hours in patients greater than 80 years of age. Although recommended by the American Heart Association as a Level IIa recommendation,[23] based mostly on the Third International Stroke Trial data, experts caution against the use of tPA for octogenarians within the extended window.[24–26] As noted elsewhere in this article, older adults are more likely to have worse outcomes after a stroke and it may be reasonable to quote a higher rate of complications when discussing tPA with the patient and/or family, because the rate of symptomatic intracranial hemorrhage seems to be closer to 10% to 13%, in contrast with 5% to 8% in the younger patients.[22]

Endovascular thrombectomy

AIS secondary to a large vessel occlusion is unlikely to respond to IV tPA.[27] Endovascular thrombectomy (EVT) is the standard of care in patients presenting with anterior circulation large vessel occlusions within 6 hours, and up to 24 hours in those having a mismatch between the infarct and ischemia on imaging.[23] The American Heart Association guidelines do not cite an upper age limit for EVT,[23] because studies have shown no heterogeneity of treatment effects by age.[18] The patients included in these studies were carefully selected; they all had a good premorbid function with little or no disability. Additionally, some studies excluded older patients (>80 years of age) with larger infarcts because they are more likely to have a poor outcome.[28] Patients with moderate to severe disability at baseline are currently not candidates for EVT, given the scarcity of data in this population.[19] This criterion effectively excludes one-third of octogenarians presenting with AIS.[29] The strict selection criteria of the EVT studies informing the guidelines limits the translation of the positive effects of EVT into clinical care.[30] It is worth noting that the procedure itself may be more technically difficult in older adults given the tortuosity of vasculature and impairment of collaterals. However, it is unclear if this difficulty increases the risk of complications such as dissection.

Altered Mental Status

AMS, a disturbance in brain function manifested by altered consciousness and/or cognition, is common in older ED patients. One-quarter of older adults in the ED have some form of AMS, whether acute or chronic,[31] a percentage that doubles in patients 85 years or older.[32]

Dementia

Dementia is a gradual and progressive significant impairment of one or more cognitive domains, severe enough to interfere with independence in everyday activities.[33] When this impairment is modest and does not limit independence, it is termed "mild cognitive impairment."[33] There are many causes for dementia (**Table 4**) that may coexist at times.[33]

Although dementia is usually diagnosed in the outpatient setting, a patient's first presentation may be in the ED. It is estimated that the number of older adults living with Alzheimer disease, the most common cause of primary dementia, will triple between 2010 and 2050.[14] Furthermore, one-half of the cases of dementia are missed in the outpatient setting.[34] Formal cognitive testing is necessary to exclude dementia, especially in high-functioning individuals, because AMS may not be readily apparent. The Mini-Mental Status Exam is the most widely known cognitive test and may not be feasible in the ED setting owing to its length and complexity.[35] Alternative cognitive tests that have been validated in the ED are summarized in **Box 6** and have varying

Table 4 Causes of dementia	
Primary (Neurodegenerative)	**Secondary**
Alzheimer disease	Vascular (multi-infarct) dementia
Dementia with Lewy Bodies	Trauma
Frontotemporal lobar degeneration	Infectious
Parkinson's disease	HIV
Huntington disease	Syphilis
	Prion disease
	Drugs and toxins
	Vasculitis
	Intracranial mass/hemorrhage

Abbreviation: HIV, human immunodeficiency virus.
Data from American Psychiatric Association. *Diagnostic and Statistical Manual of Mental Disorders.* Fifth Edit. Arlington, VA: American Psychiatric Association; 2013.

Box 6
Cognitive tests that may be used in the ED

- Mini-Mental Status
- Mini-Mental Status-2: Brief Version
- Quick Confusion Scale
- Brief Alzheimer's Screen
- Short Blessed Test
- Ottawa 3DY
- Caregiver Completed AD8

Data from Carpenter CR, Bassett ER, Fischer GM, Shirshekan J, Galvin JE, Morris JC. Four sensitive screening tools to detect cognitive dysfunction in geriatric emergency department patients: brief Alzheimer's Screen, Short Blessed Test, Ottawa 3DY, and the caregiver-completed AD8. *Acad Emerg Med.* 2011;18(4):374-384; Folstein MF, Folstein SE, McHugh PR. "Mini-mental state". A practical method for grading the cognitive state of patients for the clinician. *J Psychiatr Res.* 1975;12(3):189-198. Folstein MF, Folstein SE, White T, Messer MA. Mini-Mental State Examination, 2nd edition. 2010. Psychological Assessment Resources, Florida; Stair TO, Morrissey J, Jaradeh I, Zhou TX, Goldstein JN. Validation of the Quick Confusion Scale for mental status screening in the emergency department. *Intern Emerg Med.* 2007;2(2):130-132.

---

sensitivity, specificity, and usefulness in the ED. Dementia-like illness may occur secondary to depression, hypothyroidism, vitamin B_{12} deficiency, or normal pressure hydrocephalus.[36] If a safe disposition can be ensured and no other acute medical conditions are uncovered (including superimposed delirium, see below), the workup for chronic AMS can be continued as an outpatient.

Delirium
Delirium is another form of cognitive impairment commonly encountered in the ED and is easily missed.[37,38] Delirium is an acute medical emergency and should be treated as such, because it is associated with worsening morbidity (including long-term cognitive effects) and mortality, especially if undiagnosed.[37,39] Delirium may be hypoactive, hyperactive, or mixed, with the hypoactive subtype most frequently missed and therefore associated with the worst outcomes.[40] The hallmark of delirium is inattention, and diagnostic criteria are listed in **Fig. 1**.[33]

Delirium occurs in vulnerable patients with predisposing factors, who are then exposed to 1 or more precipitating insults (**Table 5**). Obtaining a collateral history and a comprehensive medication list are essential. At-risk older adults should be screened for delirium during their ED visit using a validated delirium screening tool such as the Delirium Triage Screen[41,42] (**Fig. 2**). Those who screen positive should then have the diagnosis confirmed using the brief Confusion Assessment Method, which is a stepwise approach through the diagnostic criteria of delirium, or other highly specific tool.[41,42] Flowsheets and videos for both tools are available on the ED Delirium Website (http://eddelirium.org/).

Patients with delirium should have the underlying cause uncovered using a thorough assessment and focused investigations. In addition to treating the underlying cause, there are many nonpharmacologic methods to manage delirium and prevent it, such as providing frequent reorientation, increasing familiar interactions with loved ones, avoiding unnecessary tethering to monitors, and ensuring that patients have their glasses and hearing aids.[42] In the case of hyperactive delirium imminently affecting

All of the following criteria:

Disturbance in Attention

Reduced ability to direct, focus, sustain, and shift attention

Disturbance in Cognition

One or more of the following:
- Memory deficit
- Disorientation
- Language disturbance
- Disturbance in visuospatial ability
- Disturbance in perception

Disturbance in Awareness

Reduced orientation to the environment

- Acute (hours to days), is a change from baseline attention and awareness, and fluctuates in severity during the course of a day.

- Not better explained by a pre-existing established neurocognitive disorder.

- Does not occur in the context of a coma or severely reduced level of arousal.

- Is a direct physiological consequence of another medical condition, substance intoxication or withdrawal, exposure to a toxin, or is due to multiple etiologies.

Fig. 1. Diagnostic criteria for delirium. (*Data from* the Diagnostic and Statistical Manual of Mental Disorders, Fifth Edition, (Copyright 2013). *American Psychiatric Association.*)

the safety of the patient and/or health care staff, low-dose atypical antipsychotics, such as risperidone or quetiapine, are recommended over other medications.[43] Most patients with delirium will require admission to the hospital for further management and patient safety. Differentiating between delirium and dementia can be

Table 5 Causes of delirium	
Precipitating Insults	**Predisposing Factors**
Infections	Age
Medications/toxins	Dementia
Iatrogenic	Underlying neurologic or psychiatric disorder
Intracranial diseases	(eg, stroke, seizure, schizophrenia)
(eg, stroke, infection, seizure)	Hearing or visual impairment
Cardiovascular diseases	Alcohol or drug use disorder
(eg, acute coronary syndrome)	
Metabolic disorder (eg, uremia)	
Endocrine disorder (eg, thyroid disorder)	
Dehydration	

Data from Wilber ST, Ondrejka JE. Altered Mental Status and Delirium. *Emerg Med Clin North Am.* 2016;34(3):649-665.

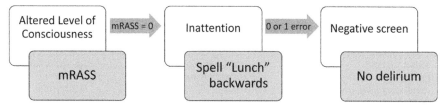

Fig. 2. Delirium triage screen. mRASS, modified Richmond Agitation and Sedation Scale. (*Data from* Geriatric emergency department guidelines. *Ann Emerg Med.* 2014;63(5):e7-25; Han JH, Wilson A, Vasilevskis EE, et al. Diagnosing delirium in older emergency department patients: validity and reliability of the delirium triage screen and the brief confusion assessment method. *Ann Emerg Med.* 2013;62(5):457-465.)

complex, especially because dementia is the most common condition predisposing to delirium.[44] A simple comparison is presented in **Table 6**.

Parkinson's Disease

Parkinson's disease is a neurodegenerative disorder affecting 1% of the population above the age of 60 years.[45] Parkinson's disease is due to a dopaminergic deficiency in the striatum owing to Lewy bodies, which manifests as a variety of motor, autonomic, and psychiatric symptoms,[46,47] and are summarized in **Table 7**.

Patients with Parkinson's disease may be seen in the ED for falls and trauma, medication side effects, acute worsening of symptoms, and psychiatric issues.[48] Falls are common in patients with Parkinson's disease; two-thirds of patients with Parkinson's disease have fallen at least once and 40% have fallen recurrently.[49] Falls occur secondary to a combination of postural instability, postural dizziness, and unstable gait. After excluding significant injuries from the fall, gait stability should be assessed before discharge to ensure a safe disposition,[42] which may require an assessment by a physical therapist.

Medications frequently used for Parkinson's disease treatment and their side effects are summarized in **Table 8**. Levodopa, the mainstay of Parkinson's disease treatment, has a short half-life and fluctuations in its level can cause noticeable symptom worsening. A patient's scheduled home dose should be administered while in the ED for any reason, unless otherwise contraindicated. This factor is also relevant in patients receiving levodopa as a continuous intestinal infusion through a percutaneous endoscopic gastrostomy with a jejunal extension tube who present with malfunction of the tube. Taking a careful medication history is necessary in older adults with Parkinson's

Table 6		
Comparison between dementia and delirium		
	Dementia	**Delirium**
Time course	Chronic (months to years)	Acute (hours to days)
Course	Progressive	Fluctuating
Consciousness	Intact (except in late stages)	Altered
Autonomic disturbance	Absent	May be present
Reversibility	Usually irreversible	Usually reversible

Data from American Psychiatric Association. *Diagnostic and Statistical Manual of Mental Disorders, Fifth Edition.* Washington, DC: American Psychiatric Association; 2013.

Table 7
Symptoms and signs of Parkinson's disease

Motor	Autonomic	Psychiatric
Resting tremor[a]	Postural dizziness (hypotension	Hallucinations
Rigidity[a] (smooth [lead pipe] or	and tachycardia)	Dementia
oscillatory [cog-wheel])	Sweating	Depression
Bradykinesia/akinesia[a]	Constipation	Sleep disorders
Postural instability[a]	Urinary incontinence or retention	Impulse control
Dystonia	Sialorrhea	disorder
Dysphagia		
Stuttering		
Gait disorder		
Masked facies		

[a] Hallmark symptoms, commonly summarized as TRAP (tremor, rigidity, akinesia, postural instability).
Data from Armstrong MJ, Okun MS. Diagnosis and Treatment of Parkinson Disease: A Review. *JAMA.* 2020;323(6):548-560; Zesiewicz TA. Parkinson Disease. *Continuum.* 2019;25(4):896-918.

Table 8
Medications commonly used to treat Parkinson's disease

Class	Examples	Side Effects
Dopamine replacement[a]	Levodopa[b]	Dyskinesia
		Motor fluctuation
		(on–off phenomenon)
		Wearing off
Dopamine agonists[a]	Ropinirole	Hallucinations
	Pramipexole	Somnolence or sleep attacks
	Apomorphine (parenteral)	Edema
		Orthostatic hypotension
		Dizziness
Monoaminoxidase B inhibitors	Selegiline	Nausea
	Rasalgiline	Sleep disturbance
	Safinamide	
	Zonisamide	
Anticholinergics	Trihexyphenidyl	Delirium
	Benztropine	Urinary retention
		Constipation
		Dry mouth
Catechol-o-methyl-transferase Inhibitors	Tolcapone	Liver toxicity
	Entacapone	Diarrhea
	Opicapone	
NMDAR agonist	Amantadine	Hallucinations
		Edema
		Orthostatic hypotension

[a] Similar side effects with differing frequency.
[b] Frequently combined with a peripheral decarboxylase inhibitors (eg, carbidopa) to decrease nausea and prolong half-life.
Data from Armstrong MJ, Okun MS. Diagnosis and Treatment of Parkinson Disease: A Review. *JAMA.* 2020;323(6):548-560; Miyasaki JM, Martin W, Suchowersky O, Weiner WJ, Lang AE. Practice parameter: Initiation of treatment for Parkinson's disease: An evidence-based review: Report of the quality standards subcommittee of the American Academy of Neurology. *Neurology.* 2002;58(1):11-17.

disease, given the propensity of polypharmacy in older adults and the relatively high likelihood of adverse drug events from anti-Parkinsonian medications.[42,50,51] Dopamine receptor blockers, such as antipsychotics and some antiemetics, are best avoided in a patient with Parkinson's disease because they worsen the movement disorder.[52]

Sudden deterioration in a patient with Parkinson's disease occurs secondary to changes in the medication regimen or the addition of new medications, metabolic derangements, concurrent infection (such as urinary tract infection or pneumonia), malfunction of a deep brain stimulator (if present), or a chronic subdural hematoma from a missed fall.[48] Patients present with worsening of rigidity, bradykinesia, and postural instability, and may be completely akinetic. This finding may be associated with dysphagia and dysautonomia as well.[48]

A unique side effect of acutely discontinuing dopaminergic medications is Parkinsonism hyperpyrexia syndrome, which presents similarly to neuroleptic malignant syndrome and should be considered in patients with Parkinson's disease presenting with AMS and a fever. It is clinically indistinguishable from neuroleptic malignant syndrome, with the only difference being the absence of exposure to neuroleptics. Treatment is supportive and includes the reintroduction of antiparkinsonian medications.[48]

Meningitis

Immunosenescence, the decreased ability to fight infections owing to age, renders geriatric patients more prone to infections, different organisms, atypical presentations, and worse outcomes.[53] Therefore, meningitis is more likely to occur in older adults than in their younger counterparts[54,55] and is more likely to be bacterial.[56] Older adults present with less typical symptoms of meningitis when compared with the general population; they are less likely to have a fever,[55,57] neck stiffness,[55,58] rash,[55] or leukocytosis[59] and are more likely to have AMS.[55,60] Older adults are more likely to have a delay in receiving antibiotics[55] and a worsened outcome.[54,55,59,60] Common organisms are listed in **Box 7**.[54,55,60,61] Antibiotics should be started as soon as the diagnosis is suspected, even before completing a lumbar puncture. Empiric antibiotics should include vancomycin and a third-generation cephalosporin (such as ceftriaxone)

Box 7
Common causative organisms for bacterial meningitis in older adults

Streptococcus pneumoniae[a]

Neisseria meningitidis[b]

Listeria monocytogenes[a]

Haemophilus influenzae

Group B streptococcus

Gram-negative rods (eg, *Escherichia coli, Klebsiella*)[a]

[a] More likely to occur in older adults than their younger counterparts. [b] Less likely to occur in older adults than their younger counterparts.

Data from Domingo P, Pomar V, de Benito N, Coll P. The spectrum of acute bacterial meningitis in elderly patients. *BMC Infect Dis.* 2013;13:108; Thigpen MC, Whitney CG, Messonnier NE, et al. Bacterial Meningitis in the United States, 1998–2007. *N Engl J Med.* 2011;364(21):2016-2025; Tunkel AR, Hartman BJ, Kaplan SL, et al. Practice Guidelines for the Management of Bacterial Meningitis. *Clin Infect Dis.* 2004;39(9):1267-1284; Weisfelt M, Van De Beek D, Spanjaard L, Reitsma JB, De Gans J. Community-Acquired Bacterial Meningitis in Older People. *J Am Geriatr Soc.* 2006;54(10):1500-1507.

as in younger patients, in addition to ampicillin, to cover for possible *Listeria*,[61] and acyclovir, to cover for herpes simplex virus.[62] Older adults will require a head CT scan before obtaining a lumbar puncture to exclude an abscess, mass, or other etiologies of their presentation.[61,63] Cerebrospinal fluid findings will be nonspecific in herpes encephalitis and the etiology will only be revealed with targeted polymerase chain reaction testing.[62]

CLINICAL CARE POINTS

- The management of pediatric stroke is in the 3 Ts: tPA, transfusion, and transfer.
- Use standard weight-based dosing of tPA in pediatric stroke, with limited research thus far demonstrating both safety and efficacy.
- In fever and AMS, consider alternative diagnoses such as anti-NMDA encephalitis or ADEM in children.
- Nonconvulsive status epilepticus is associated with higher mortality, longer pediatric intensive care unit stays, and increased long-term disability.
- Advanced age alone is not a contraindication for IV tPA within 3 hours or EVT
- Delirium is frequently missed and should be screened for using the Delirium Triage Screen.
- Acute worsening in Parkinson's disease is usually due to a medication change, infection, or missed subdural hemorrhage.
- Meningitis in older adults presents atypically and has worse outcomes than the general population.

DISCLOSURE

The authors have nothing to disclose.

REFERENCES

1. Hofman MR, Hanenberg F, Sierevelt I, et al. Elderly patients with an atypical presentation of illness in the emergency department. Neth J Med 2017;75:241–6.
2. Muangpaisan W, Hinkle JL, Westwood M, et al. Stroke in the very old: clinical presentations and outcomes. Age Ageing 2008;37(4):473–5.
3. Horeczko T, Enriquez B, McGrath NE, et al. The Pediatric Assessment Triangle: accuracy of its application by nurses in the triage of children. J Emerg Nurs 2013;39(2):182–9.
4. Ferriero DM, Fullerton HJ, Bernard TJ, et al. Management of stroke in neonates and children: a scientific statement from the American Heart Association/American stroke association. Stroke 2019;50(3):E51–96.
5. Amlie-Lefond C, Shaw DWW, Cooper A, et al. Risk of Intracranial Hemorrhage Following Intravenous tPA (Tissue-Type Plasminogen Activator) for Acute Stroke Is Low in Children. Stroke 2020;51(2):542–8.
6. Guilliams KP, Kirkham FJ, Holzhauer S, et al. Arteriopathy Influences Pediatric Ischemic Stroke Presentation, but Sickle Cell Disease Influences Stroke Management. Stroke 2019;50(5):1089–94.
7. Meyer PG, Ducrocq S, Carli P. Pediatric neurologic emergencies. Curr Opin Crit Care 2001;7(2):81–7.
8. Nishiyama M, Nagase H, Tomioka K, et al. Clinical time course of pediatric acute disseminated encephalomyelitis. Brain Dev 2019;41(6):531–7.
9. Kliegman RM, Stanton BF, St Geme JWI, et al. Nelson textbook of pediatrics. 20th edition. Phialdelphia, PA: Elsevier; 2016.

10. Saigal G, Ezuddin NS, Vega G de la. Neurologic Emergencies in Pediatric Patients Including Accidental and Nonaccidental Trauma. Neuroimaging Clin N Am 2018;28(3):453–70.
11. Suthar R, Saini AG, Sankhyan N, et al. Childhood Anti-NMDA Receptor Encephalitis. Indian J Pediatr 2016;83(7):628–33.
12. El-Dib M, Soul JS. The use of phenobarbital and other anti-seizure drugs in newborns. Semin Fetal Neonatal Med 2017;22(5):321–7.
13. Hall MJ, Levant S, DeFrances CJ. Hospitalization for stroke in U.S. hospitals, 1989-2009. NCHS Data Brief 2012;(95):1–8.
14. Virani SS, Alonso A, Benjamin EJ, et al. Heart disease and stroke statistics—2020 update: a report from the American Heart Association 2020. Circulation 2020; 141(9):e139–596.
15. Ay H, Arsava EM, Andsberg G, et al. Pathogenic Ischemic Stroke Phenotypes in the NINDS-Stroke Genetics Network. Stroke 2014;45(12):3589–96.
16. Arch AE, Weisman DC, Coca S, et al. Missed Ischemic Stroke Diagnosis in the Emergency Department by Emergency Medicine and Neurology Services. Stroke 2016;47(3):668–73.
17. Pare JR, Kahn JH. Basic neuroanatomy and stroke syndromes. Emerg Med Clin North Am 2012;30(3):601–15.
18. Goyal M, Menon BK, van Zwam WH, et al. Endovascular thrombectomy after large-vessel ischaemic stroke: a meta-analysis of individual patient data from five randomised trials. Lancet 2016;387(10029):1723–31.
19. Jayaraman MV, McTaggart RA. Endovascular Treatment of Anterior Circulation Large Vessel Occlusion in the Elderly. Front Neurol 2017;8:713.
20. Emberson J, Lees KR, Lyden P, et al. Effect of treatment delay, age, and stroke severity on the effects of intravenous thrombolysis with alteplase for acute ischaemic stroke: a meta-analysis of individual patient data from randomised trials. Lancet 2014;384(9958):1929–35.
21. Wardlaw JM, Murray V, Berge E, et al. Thrombolysis for acute ischaemic stroke. Cochrane Database Syst Rev 2014;(7):CD000213.
22. Hemphill JC 3rd, Lyden P. Stroke thrombolysis in the elderly: risk or benefit? Neurology 2005;65(11):1690–1.
23. Powers WJ, Rabinstein AA, Ackerson T, et al. Guidelines for the early management of patients with acute ischemic stroke: 2019 update to the 2018 guidelines for the early management of acute ischemic stroke a guideline for healthcare professionals from the American Heart Association/American Stroke Association. Stroke 2019;50(12):E344–418.
24. Sandercock P, Wardlaw JM, Lindley RI, et al. The benefits and harms of intravenous thrombolysis with recombinant tissue plasminogen activator within 6 h of acute ischaemic stroke (the third international stroke trial [IST-3]): a randomised controlled trial. Lancet 2012;379(9834):2352–63.
25. Hacke W, Kaste M, Bluhmki E, et al. Thrombolysis with alteplase 3 to 4.5 hours after acute ischemic stroke. N Engl J Med 2008;359(13):1317–29.
26. Demaerschalk BM, Kleindorfer DO, Adeoye OM, et al. Scientific Rationale for the Inclusion and Exclusion Criteria for Intravenous Alteplase in Acute Ischemic Stroke A Statement for Healthcare Professionals from the American Heart Association/American Stroke Association. Stroke 2016;47(2):581–641.
27. Riedel CH, Zimmermann P, Jensen-Kondering U, et al. The importance of size: successful recanalization by intravenous thrombolysis in acute anterior stroke depends on thrombus length. Stroke 2011;42(6):1775–7.

28. Nogueira RG, Jadhav AP, Haussen DC, et al. Thrombectomy 6 to 24 hours after stroke with a mismatch between deficit and infarct. N Engl J Med 2017;378(1): 11–21.

29. Chandra RV, Leslie-Mazwi TM, Oh DC, et al. Elderly patients are at higher risk for poor outcomes after intra-arterial therapy. Stroke 2012;43(9):2356–61.

30. Alawieh A, Chatterjee A, Feng W, et al. Thrombectomy for acute ischemic stroke in the elderly: a "real world" experience. J Neurointerv Surg 2018;10(12): 1209–17.

31. Hustey FM, Meldon SW. The prevalence and documentation of impaired mental status in elderly emergency department patients. Ann Emerg Med 2002;39(3): 248–53.

32. Boustani M, Peterson B, Hanson L, et al. Screening for dementia in primary care: a summary of the evidence for the U.S. Preventive Services Task Force. Ann Intern Med 2003;138(11):927–37.

33. American Psychiatric Association. Diagnostic and statistical manual of mental disorders. 5th edition. Arlington (VA): American Psychiatric Association; 2013.

34. Valcour VG, Masaki KH, Curb JD, et al. The detection of dementia in the primary care setting. Arch Intern Med 2000;160(19):2964–8.

35. Folstein MF, Folstein SE, McHugh PR. "Mini-mental state". A practical method for grading the cognitive state of patients for the clinician. J Psychiatr Res 1975; 12(3):189–98.

36. Craft S, Cholerton B, Reger M. Chapter 62. Cognitive changes associated with normal and pathological aging. In: Halter JB, Ouslander JG, Tinetti ME, et al, editors. Hazzard's Geriatric medicine and gerontology, 6e. New York: The McGraw-Hill Companies; 2009. Available at: http://accessmedicine.mhmedical.com/content.aspx?aid=5121585.

37. Han JH, Shintani A, Eden S, et al. Delirium in the emergency department: an independent predictor of death within 6 months. Ann Emerg Med 2010;56(3): 244–52.e1.

38. Boucher V, Lamontagne M-E, Nadeau A, et al. Unrecognized incident delirium in older emergency department patients. J Emerg Med 2019;57(4):535–42.

39. Kennedy M, Enander RA, Tadiri SP, et al. Delirium risk prediction, healthcare use and mortality of elderly adults in the emergency department. J Am Geriatr Soc 2014;62(3):462–9.

40. Jackson TA, Wilson D, Richardson S, et al. Predicting outcome in older hospital patients with delirium: a systematic literature review. Int J Geriatr Psychiatry 2016;31(4):392–9.

41. Han JH, Wilson A, Vasilevskis EE, et al. Diagnosing delirium in older emergency department patients: validity and reliability of the delirium triage screen and the brief confusion assessment method. Ann Emerg Med 2013;62(5):457–65.

42. American College of Emergency Physicians, American Geriatrics Society, Emergency Nurses Association, et al. Geriatric emergency department guidelines. Ann Emerg Med 2014;63(5):e7–25.

43. Shenvi C, Kennedy M, Austin CA, et al. Managing delirium and agitation in the older emergency department patient: the ADEPT Tool. Ann Emerg Med 2019; 75(2):136–45.

44. Han JH, Zimmerman EE, Cutler N, et al. Delirium in older emergency department patients: recognition, risk factors, and psychomotor subtypes. Acad Emerg Med 2009;16(3):193–200.

45. de Lau LML, Breteler MMB. Epidemiology of Parkinson's disease. Lancet Neurol 2006;5(6):525–35.

46. Zesiewicz TA. Parkinson Disease. Continuum (Minneap Minn) 2019;25(4): 896–918.
47. Armstrong MJ, Okun MS. Diagnosis and treatment of Parkinson disease: a review. JAMA 2020;323(6):548–60.
48. Prasad S, Pal PK. When time is of the essence: managing care in emergency situations in Parkinson's disease. Parkinsonism Relat Disord 2019;59:49–56.
49. Allen NE, Schwarzel AK, Canning CG. Recurrent falls in Parkinson's Disease: a systematic review. Parkinsons Dis 2013;2013:906274. Brauer S, editor.
50. Hohl CM, Dankoff J, Colacone A, et al. Polypharmacy, adverse drug-related events, and potential adverse drug interactions in elderly patients presenting to an emergency department. Ann Emerg Med 2001;38(6):666–71.
51. Miyasaki JM, Martin W, Suchowersky O, et al. Practice parameter: initiation of treatment for Parkinson's disease: an evidence-based review: report of the Quality Standards Subcommittee of the American Academy of Neurology. Neurology 2002;58(1):11–7.
52. American Geriatrics Society 2019 Updated AGS Beers Criteria® for Potentially Inappropriate Medication Use in Older Adults. J Am Geriatr Soc 2019;67(4): 674–94.
53. Liang SY. Sepsis and Other Infectious Disease Emergencies in the Elderly. Emerg Med Clin North Am 2016;34(3):501–22.
54. Thigpen MC, Whitney CG, Messonnier NE, et al. Bacterial Meningitis in the United States, 1998–2007. N Engl J Med 2011;364(21):2016–25.
55. Domingo P, Pomar V, de Benito N, et al. The spectrum of acute bacterial meningitis in elderly patients. BMC Infect Dis 2013;13:108.
56. Delerme S, Castro S, Viallon A, et al. Meningitis in elderly patients. Eur J Emerg Med 2009;16(5):273–6.
57. Shah K, Richard K, Edlow JA. Utility of lumbar puncture in the afebrile vs. febrile elderly patient with altered mental status: a pilot study. J Emerg Med 2007; 32(1):15–8.
58. Choi C. Bacterial meningitis in aging adults. Clin Infect Dis 2001;33(8):1380–5.
59. Lai W-A, Chen S-F, Tsai N-W, et al. Clinical characteristics and prognosis of acute bacterial meningitis in elderly patients over 65: a hospital-based study. BMC Geriatr 2011;11(1):91.
60. Weisfelt M, Van De Beek D, Spanjaard L, et al. Community-acquired bacterial meningitis in older people. J Am Geriatr Soc 2006;54(10):1500–7.
61. Tunkel AR, Hartman BJ, Kaplan SL, et al. Practice guidelines for the management of bacterial meningitis. Clin Infect Dis 2004;39(9):1267–84.
62. Anderson RS, Liang SY. Infectious diseases in the elderly. In: Kahn JH, Magauran BG Jr, Olshaker JS, editors. Geriatric emergency medicine: principles and practice. Cambridge University Press; 2014. p. 254–62.
63. Hasbun R, Abrahams J, Jekel J, et al. Computed tomography of the head before lumbar puncture in adults with suspected meningitis. N Engl J Med 2001;345(24): 1727–33.

Headache in the Emergency Department

Avoiding Misdiagnosis of Dangerous Secondary Causes, An Update

Ryan Raam, MD*, Ramin R. Tabatabai, MD, MACM

KEYWORDS

- Secondary headaches • Emergency medicine • Misdiagnosis

KEY POINTS

- There are several dangerous secondary causes of headaches that emergency physicians must consider in patients presenting with acute headache.
- Careful history and physical examination targeted at these important secondary causes of headache will help to avoid misdiagnosis in these patients.
- Secondary headaches are rare, "can't miss" diagnoses with often variable and atypical presentations.

NATURE OF THE PROBLEM/DEFINITION

Headache is the seventh most common chief complaint in the emergency department (ED), comprising approximately 2.5% of all ED visits in the United States.[1] Depending on its underlying cause, headache can be broadly categorized as either primary or secondary. The International Classification of Headache Disorders (ICHD) identifies primary headaches as migraine, tension-type, cluster, or one of the other trigeminal autonomic cephalgias.[2] Primary headaches comprise the vast majority of all headaches.[3] Secondary headaches are defined as those due to a distinctive underlying disorder, such as trauma, infection, or malignancy.[2] Evaluation of the patient with headache in the ED is focused on the alleviation of pain and the consideration of dangerous secondary causes.

A sophisticated clinical approach must be used to determine which patients require expedited neuroimaging or further diagnostic evaluation for potential secondary

This article is an update of an article published in *Emergency Medicine Clinics of North America*, Volume 34, Issue 4, November 2016, pages 695-716.
Keck School of Medicine of USC, LAC+USC Emergency Medicine Residency, 1200 North State Street #1011, Los Angeles, CA 90033, USA
* Corresponding author.
E-mail address: ryan.raam@med.usc.edu

headache. An in-depth understanding of several specific pathologic entities, many of them rare, is necessary to identify serious disease without the overuse of diagnostic resources in patients with primary and benign presentations.[4] Moreover, in some cases, misdiagnosis of a particular type of secondary headache may lead to treatment that is deleterious to the patient.

GENERAL APPROACH TO THE PATIENT WITH HEADACHE

The first goal of the emergency physician (EP), if the patient is stable, will be targeted toward relieving the patient's pain. Individual studies and consensus recommendations advise treating primary headaches preferentially with nonopioid medications (American College of Emergency Physician [ACEP] Level A Recommendation).[5] It is important to note that primary and secondary headaches cannot reliably be differentiated based on response to analgesic therapy.[6] A multitude of life-threatening causes of secondary headache, including subarachnoid hemorrhage (SAH) and cervical artery dissection (CeAD), has been reported to respond to simple analgesic and antimigraine medications.[7–14] As the patient's pain is being addressed, the EP considers secondary causes that warrant further workup and intervention. **Table 1** illustrates the most critical secondary diagnoses to consider in the patient with undifferentiated headache, along with key clinical features, and diagnostic and treatment considerations.

The 2008 ACEP clinical policy on acute headache evaluation describes 4 specific groups that deserve special attention and may warrant neuroimaging in the ED setting (**Table 2**).[6] Although the authors advocate adherence to these guidelines, they aim to highlight additional high-risk presentations and diagnoses, each of which should be evaluated within its own unique clinical context. In 2019, ACEP revisited the topic of headache in the ED to address related questions from the 2009 guidelines (**Table 3**). These recommendations are also addressed in this article, as is pertinent.[5]

DANGEROUS CAUSES OF SECONDARY HEADACHE
Subarachnoid Hemorrhage

SAH is among the most important considerations in patients presenting with headache. Onset can occur during physical exertion, such as exercise or during coitus, but such a trigger is noted in only approximately 20% of cases.[15] The classic clinical picture is one of sudden and severe headache that is maximal at onset.[16] Approximately 8% of patients presenting to the ED with a thunderclap headache are diagnosed with SAH.[17,18] The timeframe for what is considered thunderclap varies in the literature, up to even 1 hour in some studies.[19–21] However, the ICHD defines it as peaking within seconds to a minute.[2] Agreement between providers on the presence of a "thunderclap headache" for a particular patient is poor.[18] Other important clinical features include vomiting, neck stiffness, seizure, neurologic deficits, syncope, and alteration in mental status or coma.[19]

Although a thunderclap headache is a hallmark symptom for SAH, other causes of secondary headache should also be considered based on the patient's presentation, including cerebral venous thrombosis, CeAD, hemorrhagic stroke, posterior reversible encephalopathy syndrome, acute angle closure glaucoma (AACG), pituitary apoplexy, third ventricle colloid cysts, and reversible cerebral vasoconstriction syndrome.

In recent years, the Ottawa Subarachnoid Hemorrhage Rule has been derived and validated with a sensitivity of 100%, to aid the clinician in evaluating patients for SAH.[19,20,22,23] In addition, other studies have shown that it is possible to rule out SAH without lumbar puncture (LP) if a third-generation (or higher) computed tomographic (CT) scan is performed within 6 hours of symptom onset of a thunderclap

Table 1
Dangerous causes of secondary headache

Diagnosis	Clinical Features	Diagnostic Testing	Interventions	Additional Comments
Subarachnoid hemorrhage (SAH)	Severe, sudden onset headache Different than other headaches	CT Head Lumbar puncture	Neurosurgical consultation Blood pressure control Nimodipine Ventriculostomy	CT has highest sensitivity in first 6 h, then decreases after that Important to consider other causes of thunderclap headache
Cervical artery dissection (CeAD) Internal carotid artery dissection (ICAD) OR Vertebral artery dissection (VAD)	New onset head, neck, or facial pain ICAD: Anterior circulation ischemia, Horner syndrome, cranial nerve abnormalities, or monocular vision loss VAD: Posterior circulation ischemia	CT Head/Neck angiography	Anticoagulation vs antiplatelet Consider thrombolytics in early ischemic stroke and extracranial dissection	Neurologic symptoms can be delayed after headache onset Rule out concomitant SAH before initiating anticoagulation Traumatic mechanism in 40%
Giant cell arteritis (GCA)	Headache in age >50 Polymyalgia rheumatica association Temporal artery abnormalities on examination Jaw claudication Visual loss (mainly monocular) Fevers	ESR (cannot rule out if normal) Temporal artery biopsy	Systemic glucocorticoid therapy	When suspicion high, start steroid therapy while awaiting ESR/biopsy results Consider GCA and perform thorough head, neck, and ophthalmologic evaluation in elderly patients with fever of unknown source
Cerebral venous thrombosis (CVT)	Headache + signs of increased ICP or focal neurologic deficits	CT or MR venogram	Anticoagulation Endovascular thrombectomy if progressive symptoms despite anticoagulation	Highest risk if history of oral contraceptive, pregnancy/postpartum, thrombophilia

(continued on next page)

Table 1
(continued)

Diagnosis	Clinical Features	Diagnostic Testing	Interventions	Additional Comments
Idiopathic intracranial hypertension (IIH)	Most common in young, obese women in third or fourth decade of life Headache, vision loss, papilledema, transient visual obscurations, pulsatile tinnitus	Neuroimaging to rule out other space-occupying lesions Lumbar puncture with opening pressure >20 mm Hg	Weight loss Acetazolamide or Furosemide Optic nerve fenestration or CNS shunt if progressive vision loss	Cranial VI (abducens) palsy in at-risk patient population is suggestive Treat to prevent visual loss in 25% of patients
Acute angle closure glaucoma (AACG)	Acute onset monocular pain, headache, redness, decreased vision ± nausea vomiting Mid-fixed dilated pupil, "steamy cornea"	Ocular pressure >21 mm Hg (most often >30 mm Hg)	Ophthalmologic consultation Pressure-lowering eye drops Systemic osmotic therapy	Perform an eye examination on alert patients with dilated pupil and sudden onset severe headache (can mimic SAH with posterior communicating artery aneurysm)
Bacterial meningitis	Fever, headache, altered mental status, nuchal rigidity	Lumbar puncture (± CT Head, see 2008 ACEP Clinical Policy on Acute Headache)	IV antibiotics Consider IV dexamethasone	Jolt accentuation, Brudzinski sign, Kernig sign, nuchal rigidity all are poorly sensitive physical examination findings
Preeclampsia	Headache in pregnancy >20 +/– visual symptoms, abdominal pain, chest pain, shortness of breath, vomiting	Systolic blood pressure >140 mm Hg or diastolic blood pressure >110 on 2 occasions + Any of the following: Proteinuria, thrombocytopenia, renal insufficiency, impaired liver function, pulmonary	Obstetric consultation Urgent delivery if severe symptoms Blood pressure management IV Magnesium	Must consider diagnosis up to 6 wk postpartum, highest risk in first week postdelivery

			edema, cerebral or visual disturbances	
Pituitary apoplexy	Severe headache Visual complaints, vomiting +/− hypopituitarism	CT Head noncontrast for hemorrhage MRI for pituitary mass	Neurosurgical consultation Systemic glucocorticoids for any adrenal insufficiency	Ocular paresis can occur, affecting CN III, IV, or VI (most commonly CN III)
Carbon monoxide poisoning	Flulike illness; worse each morning Mild: headache, nausea, myalgia, dizzy Severe: confusion, syncope, neurologic deficits, death	Arterial blood gas cooximetry	Non-rebreather oxygen +/− hyperbaric oxygen chamber therapy	Consider when multiple patients from same household have similar symptoms Hyperbaric oxygen therapy is indicated for neurologic or cardiovascular signs and above certain cutoffs
Space-occupying lesions	Progressively worsening headache History of malignancy Worse in morning or in head-down position	CT Head MRI	Neurosurgical consultation ICP-lowering therapies Lesion-specific therapies	Emergent ICP-lowering therapies may include elevating head of bed, diuretics, and hyperventilation Lesion-specific therapies may include operative intervention, corticosteroids, and antimicrobial agents
Occult trauma	Signs of abuse or neglect Anticoagulation or coagulopathy	CT Head	Neurosurgical consultation	Patients in at-risk populations (eg, abuse) may not volunteer a history of trauma
Reversal cerebral vasoconstriction syndrome (RCVS)	Thunderclap headaches resolving within minutes or hours	CT or MR angiography	Supportive care, monitoring in	Ischemic or hemorrhagic strokes can occur in 20% of patients

(continued on next page)

Table 1
(continued)

Diagnosis	Clinical Features	Diagnostic Testing	Interventions	Additional Comments
	Multiple recurrent sudden, severe exacerbations are highly suggestive		neurosurgical intensive care unit	Postpartum period is a risk factor (occurs in other patient populations as well)
Cerebellar infarction	Headache with dizziness Cerebellar signs Cranial nerve abnormalities	CT Head MRI	Neurologic/neurosurgical consultation	Although CT Head is insensitive for infarction, it is helpful initially to rule out hemorrhage and identify life-threatening edema and mass effect

Table 2
2008 American College of Emergency Physician clinical policy: which patients with headache require neuroimaging in the ED?

Patient Presentation	Recommendation Level
Headache + new abnormal findings in a neurologic examination (eg, focal deficit, altered mental status, altered cognitive function)	Level B Recommendation [a](emergent noncontrast head CT)
New sudden-onset severe headache	Level B Recommendation [a](emergent noncontrast head CT)
HIV-positive patients with a new type of headache	Level B Recommendation [a](emergent noncontrast head CT)
Age >50 with new headache but with normal neurologic examination	Level C Recommendation [b](urgent noncontrast head CT)

Routine studies are indicated when the study is not considered necessary to make a disposition in the ED.
[a] *Emergent studies* are those essential for a timely decision regarding potentially life-threatening or severely disabling entities.
[b] *Urgent studies* are those that are arranged before discharge from the ED (scan appointment is included in the disposition).
Edlow JA, Panagos PD, Godwin SA, Thomas TL, Decker WW; American College of Emergency Physicians. Clinical policy: critical issues in the evaluation and management of adult patients presenting to the emergency department with acute headache. Ann Emerg Med. 2008 Oct;52(4):407-36.

headache, and interpreted by a radiologist experienced with cranial CT.[21,24–26] The most recent 2019 ACEP Clinical Policy on headaches supports the use of the aforementioned approaches to evaluate SAH in patients who present to the ED (Level B Recommendations).[5]

Currently, the gold standard in the diagnosis of SAH is by cerebrospinal fluid (CSF) analysis. However, in the event that a patient requires further testing after a negative noncontrast head CT, both LP and CT angiography (CTA) of the head are reasonable options to rule out SAH (ACEP Level C Recommendation).[5,27,28] Both have pros and cons that limit their diagnostic yield. Traumatic LPs complicate the interpretation of the CSF results, which may lead to even further testing. CTA has very good sensitivity for detecting aneurysms larger than 3 mm, potentially identifying more than 99% of aneurysmal SAH.[29,30] However, this approach has the unintended consequence of identifying asymptomatic aneurysms that do not require neurosurgical intervention.[31–33] A shared decision-making model informing the patient of potential risks and benefits of each diagnostic approach should be used on an individual basis.

Cervical Artery Dissection

CeAD is an important but difficult cause of headache to diagnose in the ED. CeAD includes both internal carotid artery dissection (ICAD) and vertebral artery dissection (VAD). ICAD is estimated as the underlying cause of 2% of all cases of stroke and up to 24% of strokes in children and young adults.[34–36] Both subtypes of CeAD are linked to preceding cervical trauma, such as vigorous physical activity, coughing, sneezing, or chiropractic manipulation in approximately 40% of cases, although recent studies question the association of chiropractic cervical manipulation and CeAD.[37,38] Headache in CeAD is a prominent symptom in approximately 70% of cases, but patients also may present with isolated neck or facial pain on the ipsilateral side of the dissected artery.[39,40] Perhaps the biggest obstacle to prompt diagnosis of CeAD is the delayed onset of neurologic symptoms, with median times ranging from

Table 3
2019 American College of Emergency Physician clinical policy: which patients with headache require neuroimaging in the ED?

Patient Presentation	Recommendation Level
In the adult ED patient presenting with acute headache, are there risk-stratification strategies that reliably identify the need for emergent neuroimaging?	Level B Recommendation Use the Ottawa Subarachnoid Hemorrhage Rule as a decision rule that has high sensitivity to rule out SAH, but low specificity to rule in SAH, for patients presenting to the ED with a normal neurologic examination result and peak headache severity within 1 h of onset of pain symptoms
In the adult ED patient treated for acute primary headache, are nonopioids preferred to opioid medications?	Level A Recommendation Preferentially use nonopioid medications in the treatment of acute primary headaches in ED patients
In the adult ED patient presenting with acute headache, does a normal noncontrast head CT scan performed within 6 h of headache onset preclude the need for further diagnostic workup for SAH?	Level B Recommendation Use a normal noncontrast head CT[a] performed within 6 h of symptom onset in an ED headache patient with a normal neurologic examination, to rule out nontraumatic SAH
In the adult ED patient who is still considered to be at risk for SAH after a negative noncontrast head CT, is CTA of the head as effective as lumbar puncture to safely rule out SAH?	Level C Recommendation Perform lumbar puncture or CTA to safely rule out SAH in the adult ED patient who is still considered to be at risk for SAH after a negative noncontrast head CT result Use shared decision making to select the best modality for each patient after weighing the potential for false positive imaging and the pros and cons associated with lumbar puncture

[a] Minimum third-generation scanner.
American College of Emergency Physicians Clinical Policies Subcommittee (Writing Committee) on Acute Headache:, Godwin SA, Cherkas DS, et al. Clinical Policy: Critical Issues in the Evaluation and Management of Adult Patients Presenting to the Emergency Department With Acute Headache. Ann Emerg Med 2019;74(4):e41-e74.

4 days in patients with ICAD and 14.5 hours in patients with VAD.[39,41] Further complicating the situation, patients older than 60 years may not present with the aforementioned traditional symptoms and risk factors.[42]

In the large, observational CADISP (Cervical Artery Dissection and Ischemic Stroke Patients) study, patients with ICAD presented with cerebral ischemic symptoms 73% of the time and patients with VAD presented with cerebral ischemic symptoms in 90% of cases.[43] Patients with ICAD typically present with anterior circulation ischemic symptoms (painful complete or partial Horner syndrome, painful cranial nerve XII palsy, painful sudden onset pulsatile tinnitus, and permanent or transient monocular vision loss secondary to ischemia), whereas VAD classically presents with posterior circulation ischemic deficits (dizziness/vertigo with or without neurologic deficits, such as ataxia, diplopia, and dysarthria).[2,44] In ICAD, cranial nerve palsies are less common, but the hypoglossal (XII) nerve is most frequently affected in isolation or in combination with other lower cranial nerves IX to XI.[45] CeAD that presents with head-ache, or facial or neck pain alone is especially challenging. In these cases, the only clinical clues may lie in a concerning mechanism and a typical pattern of pain.

Diagnosis is confirmed via MRI/magnetic resonance angiography (MRA) or CTA.[46,47] The sensitivity for ultrasound in the diagnosis of CeAD ranges from 70% to 86%, and therefore, the provider should pursue more advanced CTA or MRA studies if clinical suspicion exists.[48] Ideally, if the diagnosis can be made before the development of neurologic deficits, a window of opportunity exists to prevent a poor clinical outcome.[49]

Giant Cell Arteritis

Giant cell arteritis (GCA), or temporal arteritis, is a vasculitis of medium and large ves-sels and is the most common cause of systemic vasculitis in patients older than 50 in North America and Europe.[50] The most important risk factor in GCA is age, as disease almost never develops in patients younger than 50, with most patients developing GCA after 70 years of age.[51–53]

Headache is the most critical clinical feature, occurring in 83% of patients with GCA. The American College of Rheumatology classification for diagnosis of GCA requires 3 of the following 5 diagnostic criteria: age ≥50 years, new-onset localized headache, temporal artery tenderness or decreased temporal artery pulse, erythrocyte sedimen-tation rate (ESR) ≥ 50 mm/h, and abnormal temporal artery biopsy.[54] ESR levels may suggest the presence of GCA, but 5% of patients with biopsy-confirmed GCA can have normal ESR levels. Therefore, a negative ESR cannot reliably rule out the dis-ease.[52,55] C-reactive protein greater than 2.45 mg/dL and thrombocytosis greater than 400,000 increase the likelihood of a positive biopsy for GCA and may be helpful in the diagnosis, but similar to ESR, a normal result does not definitively rule out the diagnosis.[56]

Other important features include the presence of Polymyalgia rheumatica, temporal artery abnormalities (tender, nodular, swollen, thickened arteries, and/or decreased pulse), jaw claudication, fevers, and visual loss.[57] The presence of unexplained ane-mia or constitutional symptoms of fever, weight loss, or malaise may also provide additional clues. In a review of elderly patients with fever of unknown origin, GCA was the most frequent specific ultimate diagnosis, accounting for 17% of cases.[58]

Imaging studies, such as ultrasound or MRI of the temporal artery, at an institution with experience in these techniques, may play some role in the future for diagnosis of this disease.[59,60] However, the utility of these imaging studies in routine clinical care is not yet clear.

Transient monocular visual impairment or diplopia can be an early manifestation of GCA, although in 10% of patients, binocular visual changes are present.[61] If GCA is strongly suspected, empiric treatment with corticosteroids should be started and ophthalmology consult for temporal artery biopsy should be obtained. Initiation of ste-roid therapy should not be delayed in awaiting temporal biopsy if suspicion for GCA is high, as biopsy results will not be affected for at least 1 week.[62]

Cerebral Vein and Sinus Thrombosis

Cerebral vein and sinus thrombosis (CVT) is a rare form of stroke that can occur at any age with a mean age of approximately 40 years.[63] Oral contraceptive use (especially in obese patients) and thrombophilia are common risk factors for development of CVT.[64] Several additional risk factors have been identified, including pregnancy and postpartum states, malignancy, as well as infections, particularly those involving the ears, sinus, mouth, face, and neck.[63,65]

In the large multicenter cerebral venous thrombosis (VENOST) study, headache was the most common presenting complaint in cases of CVT, occurring in approximately 90% of cases.[66] It is the sole symptom, however, in only 25% of cases.[63,66,67] The headache is most typically slow and progressive in onset but may have a thunderclap presentation in a minority of patients.[68,69] The average time delay from presentation to diagnosis is 7 days, and a careful evaluation for signs of increased intracranial pressure (ICP) or focal brain injury is needed to identify patients with CVT.[63] Signs of increased ICP, such as papilledema or a cranial nerve VI (abducens) palsy, may suggest superior sagittal sinus thrombosis, the most commonly affected location in CVT.[70] A wide range of additional focal neurologic deficits can develop depending on the location of infarction or secondary hemorrhage, including aphasia, unilateral or bilateral weakness, and altered mental status. Rapid neurologic deterioration with stupor and coma has been noted in up to 18% of cases, whereas seizures are found in up to 40% of patients.[63] Finally, one-third of patients with CVT develop intracerebral hemorrhage, placing them at risk for worse outcomes.[66,71]

Several metaanalyses have investigated the utility of D-dimer in screening patients for CVT. Results are variable between the analyzed studies, with sensitivities ranging from 58% to 97%.[72,73] Given the high variability and low sensitivities in some studies, a normal D-dimer should not be relied on for ruling out CVT. Initial neuroimaging will often include CT or MRI of the brain. Unfortunately, neither CT nor MRI effectively rule out CVT, and further workup with CT or MR venography is recommended when clinical suspicion is high.[74]

Idiopathic Intracranial Hypertension

Idiopathic intracranial hypertension (IIH) is characterized by an elevation of ICP (CSF >20 cm H_2O), with normal ventricles and CSF analysis and in the absence of space-occupying lesions.[75] It is most common in young, obese women in the third or fourth decade of life.[76] Headaches in IIH can be severe and disabling, and there is a risk of permanent visual loss in the absence of therapeutic intervention.[77] Headaches occur in most patients with IIH with variable, nonspecific features. Associated symptoms include transient visual obscurations, pulsatile tinnitus, photopsia, and occasional radicular shoulder and arm pains.[76] Transient visual obscurations are described as brief episodes of monocular or binocular visual loss followed by full recovery.[78] Pulsatile tinnitus is seen in approximately one-half of patients and is likely due to turbulent blood flow through a stenotic venous sinus.[76] Physical examination should involve a search for papilledema, peripheral visual field defects, and unilateral or bilateral cranial nerve VI (abducens) palsy. The key to diagnosis in IIH is an elevated opening pressure by LP in the absence of space-occupying lesions on neuroimaging. There is a link between IIH and CVT; a negative CT or MRI in combination with elevated opening pressures may warrant further workup with venography to evaluate for potential CVT.[79]

Acute Angle Closure Glaucoma

AACG develops when the anterior chamber angle is narrowed, obstructing the flow of aqueous humor and leading to increased intraocular pressure (IOP). Patients older than 50 years are at risk for AACG, and its peak incidence occurs in patients older than 70.[80] Pupillary dilation resulting from any cause (eg, a dimly lit room) can precipitate an attack.

Clinically, patients present with abrupt-onset eye pain, blurry vision, and headache. They may additionally complain of nausea and vomiting. The typical physical examination reveals a mid-fixed dilated pupil with decreased visual acuity, injected conjunctiva, and corneal edema.[81] Ocular pressures greater than 21 mm Hg are necessary to make the diagnosis, and IOP is typically 30 mm Hg or higher. Once identified, medical and surgical therapy should be targeted at reducing the IOP to prevent permanent visual loss.[82]

Bacterial Meningitis

Meningitis can result from a bacterial, viral, fungal, parasitic, or noninfectious cause. Of these, bacterial meningitis is of particular concern and is associated with high mortality (approximately 15%).[83]

The classic triad of altered mental status, fever, and neck stiffness is present in only 44% of cases.[84] However, 99% of patients with bacterial meningitis will have at least 1 of these 3 classic symptoms, and 95% present with 2 of the following: headache, fever, neck stiffness, altered mental status.[84] Many patients with bacterial meningitis have preceding ear, sinus, or lung infections.[85]

Physical examination findings for bacterial meningitis have included the Kernig sign, Brudzinski sign, nuchal rigidity, and jolt accentuation.[86] A prospective analysis of these tests for meningitis found that jolt accentuation has a sensitivity of 21% with a specificity of 82%. Nuchal rigidity was found to have a sensitivity of 13% with a specificity of 80%. Kernig and Brudzinski signs both were found to have very low sensitivities of 2% with specificities of 97% and 98%, respectively.[87] Although these findings may help suggest the diagnosis of bacterial meningitis, the absence of these findings cannot rule out the disease, and CSF analysis is necessary for appropriate evaluation. Treatment with antimicrobials should not be delayed for CT, LP, or CSF results.[88]

Traditionally, a CT scan of the brain has been considered standard practice before performing an LP in order to identify central lesions that may theoretically increase the risk of postprocedure brainstem herniation. However, certain patient subsets are at increased risk for elevated ICP, and these patients should likely undergo neuroimaging before LP (ACEP Level C Recommendation; see **Table 2**). Specifically, cranial CT before LP should be considered in any patient with any of the following features: 60 years or older, immune-compromised, history of central nervous system (CNS) disease, recent seizures, altered mental status, focal neurologic deficit, or papilledema, as these patients may have a higher potential risk of brain herniation with LP.[88–90] Adherence to these criteria should be strongly considered to expedite time to diagnosis and treatment without increasing cost and unnecessary exposure of the patient to radiation.[91]

Preeclampsia

Preeclampsia is considered in the newly hypertensive patient after 20 weeks' gestation up to 6 weeks postpartum and affects approximately 5% of all pregnancies.[92] A systolic blood pressure greater than 140 mm Hg or diastolic blood pressure greater than 90 mm Hg on 2 occasions in combination with either proteinuria or end-organ damage is diagnostic.[93] The American College of Obstetricians and Gynecologists (ACOG) updated their criteria in 2013, and proteinuria is no longer an essential component for diagnosis if new onset of any of the following findings is present: thrombocytopenia, renal insufficiency, impaired liver function, pulmonary edema, or cerebral or visual disturbance.[93] Any patient at greater than 20 weeks' gestation meeting the ACOG criteria with new-onset headache should be identified as having preeclampsia, and urgent consultation and treatment should be considered. In addition, a high index of suspicion should be maintained for the diagnoses of preeclampsia and eclampsia, as up to one-third of pregnant patients with new-onset or atypical headaches will carry the diagnosis of preeclampsia.[94,95]

Pituitary Apoplexy

Pituitary apoplexy is an acute ischemic or hemorrhagic infarction of the pituitary gland, occurring in patients with pituitary adenomas.[96] Underlying risk factors for apoplexy are identified in only 25% to 40% of patients, and they include pregnancy, head trauma, pituitary radiation, major surgery, and treatment with dopamine agonists.[96–98]

The clinical presentation of pituitary apoplexy is widely variable, from benign to catastrophic. The typical patient complains of severe headache, vomiting, and visual complaints. The headache can often present as sudden and severe in its onset, mimicking SAH.[99] Patients also may present with infectious-type symptoms of fever, meningeal irritation, and alteration in mental status. The visual symptoms can manifest as decreased visual acuity or visual field defects in 75% of patients, with ocular paresis occurring in approximately 70%.[98] Ocular paresis can develop as a result of compression of the cavernous sinus and associated cranial nerves III, IV, and VI. Of these, cranial nerve III (oculomotor) is most susceptible to compression.[99] Finally, at time of presentation, patients may demonstrate evidence of hypopituitarism, and any evidence of glucocorticoid deficiency in the form of hypoglycemia, hypotension, or hyponatremia will require replacement with intravenous (IV) hydrocortisone.[98] The initial diagnostic test for evaluation of pituitary apoplexy will often be a noncontrast CT of the head to rule out SAH. Although noncontrast CT is sensitive for acute hemorrhage, MRI should be pursued if CT is negative to detect infarction.[100,101]

Carbon Monoxide Poisoning

Carbon monoxide (CO) poisonings account for approximately 50,000 ED visits per year in the United States.[102] CO poisoning is a dangerous underlying cause of headache; most cases are related to smoke inhalation, but faulty furnaces, inadequate ventilation of heating sources, and exposure to engine exhaust are also important causes.[103] Mild exposures may cause headaches, myalgias, dizziness, and neuropsychological impairment.[104,105] More severe exposures can result in alteration of mental status, focal neurologic deficits, loss of consciousness, or death.[103] Delayed neurologic sequelae and neuropsychiatric effects also may result.[106,107]

In the ED, the patient with headache and recent potential exposure must be evaluated for CO poisoning, particularly when multiple household members or pets also are ill. Pulse oximetry (Spo_2) is unable to distinguish between oxyhemoglobin and carboxyhemoglobin and thus cannot reliably screen for CO exposure.[108] Therefore, co-oximetry via serum blood gas analysis is needed to measure elevated carboxyhemoglobin levels. Once identified, oxygen by non-rebreather mask should be initiated and consideration given to hyperbaric oxygen treatment.[109]

Space-Occupying Lesion

Headache in the patient with history of malignancy can occur from a variety of causes, including the mass effect of the tumor itself or as a result of the therapy.[110] Although traditional teaching holds that a morning or nocturnal headache can be suggestive of intracranial malignancy, this pattern is actually uncommon in adult patients, with nausea, vomiting, and neurologic abnormalities being far more common.[110,111] Both primary and metastatic tumors are equally likely to cause headache at a rate of approximately 60%.[112] The most common primary sites for metastases to the brain are as follows: lung (19.9%), melanoma (6.9%), renal (6.5%), breast (5.1%), and colo-rectal (1.8%).[113] It is important to note that brain cancer rarely presents with headache as its sole presenting feature, occurring in only 2% to 8% of patients.[114] Most patients with primary or metastatic disease will demonstrate concomitant neurologic deficits, neuropsychiatric disorders, or seizures. Initial evaluation should include a complete physical examination to evaluate for signs of increased ICP, such as neurologic defi-cits, visual field defects, and optic disc edema. For most neurooncology applications, MRI is superior to CT imaging, as MRI provides better anatomic resolution.[115] Howev-er, in the ED, a CT has the advantage of speed and convenience and can be used to initially evaluate for signs of increased ICP or secondary hemorrhage from a brain tumor.

In addition to pain caused by the tumor itself, patients with intracranial malignancy are at risk for intracranial hemorrhage. Approximately 1% to 11% of intracranial hem-orrhage cases are secondary to malignancy, most commonly from metastatic solid tu-mors. Therefore, new headaches in patients with identified tumors should be further investigated via neuroimaging.[116] Finally, patients receiving chemotherapeutic agents or radiation therapy and those who have received a craniotomy can all present with the onset of a new type of headache. In such patients, the clinician should first evaluate the possibility of other more serious causes before attributing the symptoms to ther-apeutic interventions.

DISCLOSURE

The authors have nothing to disclose.

REFERENCES

1. Available at: https://www.cdc.gov/nchs/data/nhamcs/web_tables/2017_ed_web_tables-508.pdf. Accessed July 1, 2020.
2. Headache Classification Committee of the International Headache Society (IHS) The International Classification of Headache Disorders, 3rd edition. Cephalalgia 2018;38(1):1–211.
3. Morgenstern LB, Huber JC, Luna-Gonzales H, et al. Headache in the emer-gency department. Headache 2001;41(6):537–41.
4. Douglas AC, Wippold FJ 2nd, Broderick DF, et al. ACR appropriateness criteria headache. J Am Coll Radiol 2014;11(7):657–67.
5. American College of Emergency Physicians Clinical Policies Subcommittee (Writing Committee) on Acute Headache:, Godwin SA, Cherkas DS, Panagos PD, et al. Clinical policy: critical issues in the evaluation and manage-ment of adult patients presenting to the emergency department with acute headache. Ann Emerg Med 2019;74(4):e41–74.
6. Edlow JA, Panagos PD, Godwin SA, et al. American College of Emergency Phy-sicians. Clinical policy: critical issues in the evaluation and management of adult patients presenting to the emergency department with acute headache. Ann Emerg Med 2008;52(4):407–36.
7. Pope JV, Edlow JA. Favorable response to analgesics does not predict a benign etiology of headache. Headache 2008;48:944.
8. Pfadenhauer K, Schonsteiner T, Keller H. The risks of sumatriptan administration in patients with unrecognized subarachnoid haemorrhage (SAH). Cephalalgia 2006;26:320.
9. Lipton RB, Mazer C, Newman LC, et al. Sumatriptan relieves migraine-like head-aches associated with carbon monoxide exposure. Headache 1997;37:392.

10. Abisaab J, Nevadunsky N, Flomenbaum N. Emergency department presentation of bilateral carotid artery dissections in a postpartum patient. Ann Emerg Med 2004;44:484.
11. Leira EC, Cruz-Flores S, Leacock RO, et al. Sumatriptan can alleviate headaches due to carotid artery dissection. Headache 2001;41:590.
12. Prokhorov S, Khanna S, Alapati D, et al. Subcutaneous sumatriptan relieved migraine-like headache in two adolescents with aseptic meningitis. Headache 2008;48:1235.
13. Rosenberg JH, Silberstein SD. The headache of SAH responds to sumatriptan. Headache 2005;45:597.
14. Barclay CL, Shuaib A, Montoya D, et al. Response of non-migrainous headaches to chlorpromazine. Headache 1990;30:85.
15. Anderson C, Ni Mhurchu C, Scott D, et al. Australasian Cooperative Research on Subarachnoid Hemorrhage Study Group. Triggers of subarachnoid hemorrhage: role of physical exertion, smoking, and alcohol in the Australasian Cooperative Research on Subarachnoid Hemorrhage Study (ACROSS). Stroke 2003; 34(7):1771–6.
16. van Gijn J, Kerr RS, Rinkel GJ. Subarachnoid haemorrhage. Lancet 2007; 369(9558):306–18.
17. Edlow JA. Managing patients with nontraumatic, severe, rapid-onset headache. Ann Emerg Med 2018;71(3):400–8.
18. Carpenter CR, Hussain AM, Ward MJ, et al. Spontaneous subarachnoid hemorrhage: a systematic review and meta-analysis describing the diagnostic accuracy of history, physical examination, imaging, and lumbar puncture with an exploration of test thresholds. Acad Emerg Med 2016;23(9):963–1003.
19. Perry JJ, Stiell IG, Sivilotti ML, et al. Clinical decision rules to rule out subarachnoid hemorrhage for acute headache. JAMA 2013;310(12):1248–55.
20. Perry JJ, Sivilotti MLA, Sutherland J, et al. Validation of the Ottawa Subarachnoid Hemorrhage Rule in patients with acute headache. CMAJ 2017;189(45): E1379–85.
21. Perry JJ, Stiell IG, Sivilotti ML, et al. Sensitivity of computed tomography performed within six hours of onset of headache for diagnosis of subarachnoid haemorrhage: prospective cohort study. BMJ 2011;343:d4277.
22. Bellolio MF, Hess EP, Gilani WI, et al. External validation of the Ottawa subarachnoid hemorrhage clinical decision rule in patients with acute headache. Am J Emerg Med 2015;33(2):244–9.
23. Perry JJ, Sivilotti MLA, Émond M, et al. Prospective implementation of the Ottawa Subarachnoid Hemorrhage Rule and 6-Hour Computed Tomography Rule. Stroke 2020;51(2):424–30.
24. Dubosh NM, Bellolio MF, Rabinstein AA, et al. Sensitivity of early brain computed tomography to exclude aneurysmal subarachnoid hemorrhage: a systematic review and meta-analysis. Stroke 2016;47(3):750–5.
25. Blok KM, Rinkel GJ, Majoie CB, et al. CT within 6 hours of headache onset to rule out subarachnoid hemorrhage in nonacademic hospitals. Neurology 2015; 84(19):1927–32.
26. Backes D, Rinkel GJ, Kemperman H, et al. Time-dependent test characteristics of head computed tomography in patients suspected of nontraumatic subarachnoid hemorrhage. Stroke 2012;43(8):2115–9.
27. Perry JJ, Spacek A, Forbes M, et al. Is the combination of negative computed tomography result and negative lumbar puncture result sufficient to rule out subarachnoid hemorrhage? Ann Emerg Med 2008;51(6):707–13.

28. Meurer WJ, Walsh B, Vilke GM, et al. Clinical guidelines for the emergency department evaluation of subarachnoid hemorrhage. J Emerg Med 2016; 50(4):696–701.
29. Donmez H, Serifov E, Kahriman G, et al. Comparison of 16-row multislice CT angiography with conventional angiography for detection and evaluation of intracranial aneurysms. Eur J Radiol 2011;80(2):455–61.
30. Lu L, Zhang LJ, Poon CS, et al. Digital subtraction CT angiography for detection of intracranial aneurysms: comparison with three-dimensional digital subtraction angiography. Radiology 2012;262(2):605–12.
31. McCormack RF, Hutson A. Can computed tomography angiography of the brain replace lumbar puncture in the evaluation of acute-onset headache after a negative noncontrast cranial computed tomography scan? Acad Emerg Med 2010;17(4):444–51.
32. Carstairs SD, Tanen DA, Duncan TD, et al. Computed tomographic angiography for the evaluation of aneurysmal subarachnoid hemorrhage. Acad Emerg Med 2006;13(5):486–92.
33. Edlow JA. What are the unintended consequences of changing the diagnostic paradigm for subarachnoid hemorrhage after brain computed tomography to computed tomographic angiography in place of lumbar puncture? Acad Emerg Med 2010;17(9):991–5 [discussion: 996–7].
34. Nedeltchev K, der Maur TA, Georgiadis D, et al. Ischaemic stroke in young adults: predictors of outcome and recurrence. J Neurol Neurosurg Psychiatry 2005;76(2):191–5.
35. Putaala J, Metso AJ, Metso TM, et al. Analysis of 1008 consecutive patients aged 15 to 49 with first-ever ischemic stroke: the Helsinki young stroke registry. Stroke 2009;40(4):1195–203.
36. Schievink WI. Spontaneous dissection of the carotid and vertebral arteries. N Engl J Med 2001;344(12):898–906.
37. Engelter ST, Grond-Ginsbach C, Metso TM, et al. Cervical Artery Dissection and Ischemic Stroke Patients Study Group. Cervical artery dissection: trauma and other potential mechanical trigger events. Neurology 2013;80(21):1950–7.
38. Cassidy JD, Boyle E, Côté P, et al. Risk of carotid stroke after chiropractic care: a population-based case-crossover study. J Stroke Cerebrovasc Dis 2017; 26(4):842–50.
39. Silbert PL, Mokri B, Schievink WI. Headache and neck pain in spontaneous internal carotid and vertebral artery dissections. Neurology 1995;45(8):1517–22.
40. Debette S, Grond-Ginsbach C, Bodenant M, et al. Cervical Artery Dissection Ischemic Stroke Patients (CADISP) Group. Differential features of carotid and vertebral artery dissections: the CADISP study. Neurology 2011;77(12): 1174–81.
41. Saeed AB, Shuaib A, Al-Sulaiti G, et al. Vertebral artery dissection: warning symptoms, clinical features and prognosis in 26 patients. Can J Neurol Sci 2000;27(4):292–6.
42. Traenka C, Dougoud D, Simonetti BG, et al. Cervical artery dissection in patients ≥60 years: often painless, few mechanical triggers. Neurology 2017;88(14): 1313–20.
43. Winer JB, Plant G. Stuttering pituitary apoplexy resembling meningitis. J Neurol Neurosurg Psychiatry 1990;53:440.
44. Gottesman RF, Sharma P, Robinson KA, et al. Clinical characteristics of symptomatic vertebral artery dissection: a systematic review. Neurologist 2012; 18(5):245–54.

45. Sturzenegger M, Huber P. Cranial nerve palsies in spontaneous carotid artery dissection. J Neurol Neurosurg Psychiatry 1993;56(11):1191–9.
46. Provenzale JM, Sarikaya B. Comparison of test performance characteristics of MRI, MR angiography, and CT angiography in the diagnosis of carotid and vertebral artery dissection: a review of the medical literature. AJR Am J Roentgenol 2009;193(4):1167–74.
47. Hanning U, Sporns PB, Schmiedel M, et al. CT versus MR techniques in the detection of cervical artery dissection. J Neuroimaging 2017;27(6):607–12.
48. Benninger DH, Baumgartner RW. Ultrasound diagnosis of cervical artery dissection. Front Neurol Neurosci 2006;21:70–84.
49. Morris NA, Merkler AE, Gialdini G, et al. Timing of incident stroke risk after cervical artery dissection presenting without ischemia [published correction appears in Stroke. 2018;49(10):e308]. Stroke 2017;48(3):551–5.
50. González-Gay MA, García-Porrúa C. Epidemiology of the vasculitides. Rheum Dis Clin North Am 2001;27(4):729–49.
51. Gonzalez-Gay MA, Miranda-Filloy JA, Lopez-Diaz MJ, et al. Giant cell arteritis in northwestern Spain: a 25-year epidemiologic study. Medicine (Baltimore) 2007; 86(2):61–8.
52. Salvarani C, Crowson CS, O'Fallon WM, et al. Reappraisal of the epidemiology of giant cell arteritis in Olmsted County, Minnesota, over a fifty-year period. Arthritis Rheum 2004;51(2):264–8.
53. Liu NH, LaBree LD, Feldon SE, et al. The epidemiology of giant cell arteritis: a 12-year retrospective study. Ophthalmology 2001;108(6):1145–9.
54. Hunder GG, Bloch DA, Michel BA, et al. The American College of Rheumatology 1990 criteria for the classification of giant cell arteritis. Arthritis Rheum 1990; 33(8):1122–8.
55. Smetana GW, Shmerling RH. Does this patient have temporal arteritis? JAMA 2002;287(1):92–101.
56. Walvick MD, Walvick MP. Giant cell arteritis: laboratory predictors of a positive temporal artery biopsy. Ophthalmology 2011;118(6):1201–4.
57. Gonzalez-Gay MA, Vazquez-Rodriguez TR, Lopez-Diaz MJ, et al. Epidemiology of giant cell arteritis and polymyalgia rheumatica. Arthritis Rheum 2009;61(10): 1454–61.
58. Tal S, Guller V, Gurevich A, et al. Fever of unknown origin in the elderly. J Intern Med 2002;252(4):295–304.
59. Serling-Boyd N, Stone JH. Recent advances in the diagnosis and management of giant cell arteritis. Curr Opin Rheumatol 2020;32(3):201–7.
60. Duftner C, Dejaco C, Sepriano A, et al. Imaging in diagnosis, outcome prediction and monitoring of large vessel vasculitis: a systematic literature review and meta-analysis informing the EULAR recommendations. RMD Open 2018;4(1): e000612.
61. Hayreh SS, Podhajsky PA, Zimmerman B. Occult giant cell arteritis: ocular manifestations. Am J Ophthalmol 1998;125(4):521–6 [Erratum appears in Am J Ophthalmol 1998;125(6):893].
62. Achkar AA, Lie JT, Hunder GG, et al. How does previous corticosteroid treatment affect the biopsy findings in giant cell (temporal) arteritis? Ann Intern Med 1994;120(12):987–92.
63. Ferro JM, Canhão P, Stam J, et al, ISCVT Investigators. Prognosis of cerebral vein and dural sinus thrombosis: results of the International Study on Cerebral Vein and Dural Sinus Thrombosis (ISCVT). Stroke 2004;35(3):664–70.

64. Zuurbier SM, Arnold M, Middeldorp S, et al. Risk of cerebral venous thrombosis in obese women. JAMA Neurol 2016;73(5):579–84.
65. Zuurbier SM, Hiltunen S, Lindgren E, et al. Cerebral venous thrombosis in older patients. Stroke 2018;49(1):197–200.
66. Duman T, Uluduz D, Midi I, et al. A multicenter study of 1144 patients with cerebral venous thrombosis: the VENOST Study. J Stroke Cerebrovasc Dis 2017;26(8):1848–57.
67. Crassard I, Bousser MG. Headache in patients with cerebral venous thrombosis. Rev Neurol (Paris) 2005;161(6–7):706–8.
68. Cumurciuc R, Crassard I, Sarov M, et al. Headache as the only neurological sign of cerebral venous thrombosis: a series of 17 cases. J Neurol Neurosurg Psychiatry 2005;76(8):1084–7.
69. deBruijn SF, StamJ, Kappelle LJ. Thunderclap headache as first symptom of cerebral venous sinus thrombosis. CVST Study Group. Lancet 1996;348(9042): 1623–5.
70. Saposnik G, Barinagarrementeria F, Brown RD Jr, et al. American Heart Association Stroke Council and the Council on Epidemiology and Prevention. Diagnosis and management of cerebral venous thrombosis: a statement for healthcare professionals from the American Heart Association/American Stroke Association. Stroke 2011;42(4):1158–92.
71. Girot M, Ferro JM, Canhão P, et al. Predictors of outcome in patients with cerebral venous thrombosis and intracerebral hemorrhage. Stroke 2007;38(2): 337–42.
72. Ordieres-Ortega L, Demelo-Rodríguez P, Galeano-Valle F, et al. Predictive value of D-dimer testing for the diagnosis of venous thrombosis in unusual locations: a systematic review. Thromb Res 2020;189:5–12.
73. Dentali F, Squizzato A, Marchesi C, et al. D-dimer testing in the diagnosis of cerebral vein thrombosis: a systematic review and a meta-analysis of the literature. J Thromb Haemost 2012;10(4):582–9.
74. Khandelwal N, Agarwal A, Kochhar R, et al. Comparison of CT venography with MR venography in cerebral sinovenous thrombosis. AJR Am J Roentgenol 2006; 187(6):1637–43.
75. Friedman DI, Jacobson DM. Diagnostic criteria for idiopathic intracranial hypertension. Neurology 2002;59(10):1492–5.
76. Wall M, Kupersmith MJ, Kieburtz KD, et al. NORDIC Idiopathic Intracranial Hypertension Study Group. The idiopathic intracranial hypertension treatment trial: clinical profile at baseline. JAMA Neurol 2014;71(6):693–701.
77. Corbett JJ, Savino PJ, Thompson HS, et al. Visual loss in pseudotumor cerebri. Follow-up of 57 patients from five to 41 years and a profile of 14 patients with permanent severe visual loss. Arch Neurol 1982;39(8):461–74.
78. Giuseffi V, Wall M, Siegel PZ, et al. Symptoms and disease associations in idiopathic intracranial hypertension (pseudotumor cerebri): a case-control study. Neurology 1991;41(2 Pt 1):239–44.
79. Crassard I, Bousser MG. Cerebral venous thrombosis. J Neuroophthalmol 2004; 24(2):156–63.
80. Bonomi L, Marchini G, Marraffa M, et al. Epidemiology of angle-closure glaucoma: prevalence, clinical types, and association with peripheral anterior chamber depth in the Egna-Neumarkt Glaucoma Study. Ophthalmology 2000;107(5): 998–1003.
81. Saw SM, Gazzard G, Friedman DS. Interventions for angle-closure glaucoma: an evidence-based update. Ophthalmology 2003;110(10):1869–930.

82. Choong YF, Irfan S, Menage MJ. Acute angle closure glaucoma: an evaluation of a protocol for acute treatment. Eye (Lond) 1999;13(Pt 5):613–6.
83. Thigpen MC, Whitney CG, Messonnier NE, et al. Emerging Infections Programs Network. Bacterial meningitis in the United States, 1998-2007. N Engl J Med 2011;364(21):2016–25.
84. Van de Beek D, de Gans J, Spanjaard L, et al. Clinical features and prognostic factors in adults with bacterial meningitis. N Engl J Med 2004;351(18):1849–59.
85. Brouwer MC, Thwaites GE, Tunkel AR, et al. Dilemmas in the diagnosis of acute community-acquired bacterial meningitis. Lancet 2012;380(9854):1684–92.
86. Attia J, Hatala R, Cook DJ, et al. The rational clinical examination. Does this adult patient have acute meningitis? JAMA 1999;282(2):175–81.
87. Nakao JH, Jafri FN, Shah K, et al. Jolt accentuation of headache and other clinical signs: poor predictors of meningitis in adults. Am J Emerg Med 2014; 32(1):24–8.
88. Tunkel AR, Hartman BJ, Kaplan SL, et al. Practice guidelines for the management of bacterial meningitis. Clin Infect Dis 2004;39(9):1267–84.
89. Gopal AK, Whitehouse JD, Simel DL, et al. Cranial computed tomography before lumbar puncture: a prospective clinical evaluation. Arch Intern Med 1999;159(22):2681–5 [Erratum appears in Arch Intern Med 2000;160(21):3223].
90. Hasbun R, Abrahams J, Jekel J, et al. Computed tomography of the head before lumbar puncture in adults with suspected meningitis. N Engl J Med 2001; 345(24):1727–33.
91. Salazar L, Hasbun R. Cranial imaging before lumbar puncture in adults with community-acquired meningitis: clinical utility and adherence to the Infectious Diseases Society of America Guidelines. Clin Infect Dis 2017;64(12):1657–62.
92. Abalos E, Cuesta C, Grosso AL, et al. Global and regional estimates of pre-eclampsia and eclampsia: a systematic review. Eur J Obstet Gynecol Reprod Biol 2013;170(1):1–7.
93. American College of Obstetricians and Gynecologists, Task Force on Hypertension in Pregnancy. Hypertension in pregnancy. Report of the American College of Obstetricians and Gynecologists' task force on hypertension in pregnancy. Obstet Gynecol 2013;122(5):1122–31.
94. Schoen JC, Campbell RL, Sadosty AT. Headache in pregnancy: an approach to emergency department evaluation and management. West J Emerg Med 2015; 16(2):291–301.
95. Melhado EM, Maciel JA Jr, Guerreiro CA. Headache during gestation: evaluation of 1101 women. Can J Neurol Sci 2007;34(2):187–92.
96. Lubina A, Olchovsky D, Berezin M, et al. Management of pituitary apoplexy: clinical experience with 40 patients. Acta Neurochir (Wien) 2005;147(2):151–7 [discussion: 157].
97. Sibal L, Ball SG, Connolly V, et al. Pituitary apoplexy: a review of clinical presentation, management and outcome in 45 cases. Pituitary 2004;7(3):157–63.
98. Nawar RN, AbdelMannan D, Selman WR, et al. Pituitary tumor apoplexy: a review. J Intensive Care Med 2008;23(2):75–90.
99. Bahmani Kashkouli M, Khalatbari MR, Yahyavi ST, et al. Pituitary apoplexy presenting as acute painful isolated unilateral third cranial nerve palsy. Arch Iran Med 2008;11(4):466–8.
100. L'Huillier F, Combes C, Martin N, et al. MRI in the diagnosis of so-called pituitary apoplexy: seven cases. J Neuroradiol 1989;16(3):221–37.
101. Piotin M, Tampieri D, Rüfenacht DA, et al. The various MRI patterns of pituitary apoplexy. Eur Radiol 1999;9(5):918–23.

102. Hampson NB, Weaver LK. Carbon monoxide poisoning: a new incidence for an old disease. Undersea Hyperb Med 2007;34(3):163–8.
103. Weaver LK. Clinical practice. Carbon monoxide poisoning. N Engl J Med 2009; 360(12):1217–25.
104. Amitai Y, Zlotogorski Z, Golan-Katzav V, et al. Neuropsychological impairment from acute low-level exposure to carbon monoxide. Arch Neurol 1998;55(6): 845–8.
105. Heckerling PS, Leikin JB, Terzian CG, et al. Occult carbon monoxide poisoning in patients with neurologic illness. J Toxicol Clin Toxicol 1990;28(1):29–44.
106. Jasper BW, Hopkins RO, Duker HV, et al. Affective outcome following carbon monoxide poisoning: a prospective longitudinal study. Cogn Behav Neurol 2005;18(2):127–34.
107. Choi IS. Delayed neurologic sequelae in carbon monoxide intoxication. Arch Neurol 1983;40(7):433–5.
108. Bozeman WP, Myers RA, Barish RA. Confirmation of the pulse oximetry gap in carbon monoxide poisoning. Ann Emerg Med 1997;30(5):608–11.
109. Buckley NA, Juurlink DN, Isbister G, et al. Hyperbaric oxygen for carbon monoxide poisoning. Cochrane Database Syst Rev 2011;4:CD002041.
110. Kirby S, Purdy RA. Headache and brain tumors. Curr Neurol Neurosci Rep 2007;7(2):110–6.
111. Forsyth PA, Posner JB. Headaches in patients with brain tumors: a study of 111 patients. Neurology 1993;43(9):1678–83.
112. Schankin CJ, Ferrari U, Reinisch VM, et al. Characteristics of brain tumour-associated headache. Cephalalgia 2007;27(8):904–11.
113. Barnholtz-Sloan JS, Sloan AE, Davis FG, et al. Incidence proportions of brain metastases in patients diagnosed (1973 to 2001) in the Metropolitan Detroit Cancer Surveillance System. J Clin Oncol 2004;22(14):2865–72.
114. Kirby S, Purdy RA. Headaches and brain tumors. Neurol Clin 2014;32(2): 423–32.
115. O'Neill BE, Hochhalter CB, Carr C, et al. Advances in neuro-oncology imaging techniques. Ochsner J 2018;18(3):236–41.
116. Navi BB, Reichman JS, Berlin D, et al. Intracerebral and subarachnoid hemorrhage in patients with cancer. Neurology 2010;74(6):494–501.

Diagnosis and Initial Emergency Department Management of Subarachnoid Hemorrhage

Nicole M. Dubosh, MD*, Jonathan A. Edlow, MD

KEYWORDS

- Subarachnoid hemorrhage • Cerebral aneurysm • Lumbar puncture
- Brain computed tomography

KEY POINTS

- Ruptured aneurysms are the most common cause of atraumatic subarachnoid hemorrhage and there are excellent endovascular and surgical treatments.
- Misdiagnosis remains an important issue especially in well-appearing patients, for whom these treatments are the most effective.
- Noncontrast computed tomography scan sensitivity approaches 100% if done within 6 hours of the headache onset and read by an experienced radiologist.
- Beyond 6 hours, some other diagnostic testing is necessary and we recommend lumbar puncture.
- Once the diagnosis of nontraumatic subarachnoid hemorrhage is made, there is a short checklist of next steps related to defining the offending vascular lesion, consulting a neurosurgeon, and starting treatments.

INTRODUCTION

Nature of the Problem

Nontraumatic headache is the seventh most common complaint in patients presenting to the emergency department (ED).[1] Although many causes of headache are benign, subarachnoid hemorrhage (SAH) is one serious etiology and is a true medical emergency in that time-dependent diagnostic and management techniques exist.[2,3] The clinical presentation in patients with SAH is highly variable and the classic "textbook" illness script of thunderclap headache, neck stiffness, and altered mental status may not occur. Misdiagnosis occurs in 12% to 50% of patients and is more common in

Department of Emergency Medicine, Beth Israel Deaconess Medical Center and Harvard Medical School, One Deaconess Road, Rosenburg 2, Boston, MA 02115, USA
* Corresponding author.
E-mail address: ndubosh@bidmc.harvard.edu

Emerg Med Clin N Am 39 (2021) 87–99
https://doi.org/10.1016/j.emc.2020.09.005
0733-8627/21/© 2020 Elsevier Inc. All rights reserved.
emed.theclinics.com

patients with atypical presentations.[4,5] Misdiagnosis also accounts for a substantial proportion of return ED visits in patients discharged with a diagnosis of headache.[6] Therefore, deciding which patients to evaluate for SAH is a critical issue for emergency physicians. Recent data have emerged that has shifted the diagnostic approach since the last publication in this series. This article reviews the most recent literature and guideline revisions in the diagnosis and ED management of atraumatic SAH.

DISCUSSION
Epidemiology

Although trauma is the leading cause of SAH, the incidence of atraumatic SAH is estimated to range from 6 to 9 in 100,000.[3,7–9] These cases account for less than 1% of all ED patients with headache; however, the disease burden is high.[5] One-third of patients die within weeks of the hemorrhage and the majority of those who survive suffer from cognitive impairment or long-term complications.[10] Furthermore, one-half of patients who present with SAH are under age 55.[9] In recent years, the incidence has found to be decreasing slightly with better blood pressure treatment and decreasing smoking rates, although regional variation continues to exist.[7,11]

The most common cause of atraumatic SAH is a ruptured cerebral aneurysm, accounting for 85% of cases, followed by nonaneurysmal venous "perimesencephalic" hemorrhages and arteriovenous malformations.[2,3,12] In the general population, approximately 2% harbor cerebral aneurysms, yet the vast majority of these never rupture.[13] Other, less common causes of atraumatic SAH include amyloid angiopathy, hypertension, and reversible cerebral vasoconstriction syndrome. Risk factors for SAH owing to aneurysm rupture include smoking, hypertension, alcohol abuse, sympathomimetic drug use, having a first-degree relative with a cerebral aneurysm, female sex, and certain genetic conditions including type IV Ehlers–Danlos syndrome and polycystic kidney disease.[5,14]

Patterns of Hemorrhage

The location of the hemorrhage pattern on a computed tomography (CT) scan can be useful in predicting the presence of an aneurysm, location of the aneurysm, whether or not it was traumatic, and the likelihood of an angiogram-negative SAH. Approximately 70% of aneurysms occur in the anterior communicating artery, posterior communicating artery, and middle cerebral artery.[15] Blood from a ruptured aneurysm typically surrounds the basal cisterns. In traumatic SAH, the blood is typically located in areas of coup or contrecoup force, or higher up in the cerebral convexities.[2] This difference in location may be particularly helpful in patients with SAH who may have fallen from syncope and present with a headache. Finally, convexal SAH has been described in various case series and the etiologies are believed to be related to reversible cerebral vasoconstriction syndrome in younger patients or cerebral amyloid angiopathy as opposed to aneurysmal in origin.[16,17] Patterns of blood are displayed in **Fig. 1**.

Clinical Presentation

SAH has a wide variety of clinical presentations and, therefore, deciding which patients require evaluation is a critical issue for emergency physicians. Approximately 12% of patients die before reaching the hospital and up to 25% of patients die before admission to the hospital ward or intensive care unit.[5,12] For those presenting to the ED, one can consider the spectrum of presentation along a bell-shaped curve (**Fig. 2**). On 1 side of the curve are critically ill patients who come in altered and oftentimes comatose or with clear-cut focal neurologic deficits. Although the diagnosis may

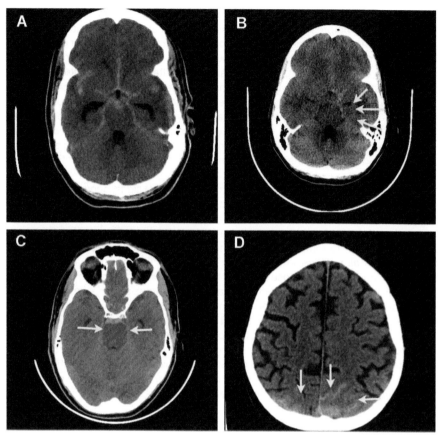

Fig. 1. Patterns of hemorrhage. (A) Obvious aneurysmal SAH. (B) More subtle SAH. (C) Peri-mesencephalic hemorrhage. (D) Convexal SAH. (*Courtesy of* J. Edlow, MD.)

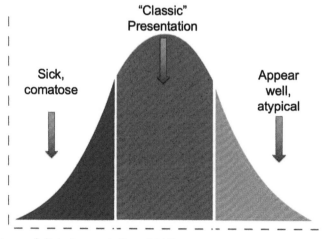

Fig. 2. Spectrum of clinical presentation of SAH.

not be clear cut initially, these patients will undergo an extensive workup. In the middle are the patients who present with the more classic symptoms with thunderclap headache, neck pain, and/or vomiting and syncope. Oftentimes the headache is exertional. The need for diagnostic workup in this group is clear. On the other side of the curve, however, are the less typical presentations. These patients will often describe symptoms of isolated neck pain, vomiting, sinusitis-type headache, headache with an elevated blood pressure, mildly altered level of consciousness, chest pain, or an abnormal electrocardiogram, all less classic symptoms but nevertheless well-described in the literature.[2–4,18,19] It is this group of patients who tend to be misdiagnosed or have a delay in diagnosis, which in turn leads to treatment delays and poorer outcomes. Understanding the full spectrum of presentations is important for avoiding misdiagnosis.

As always, the physical examination begins with the vital signs, general appearance, and assessment of airway, breathing, and circulation. A focused physical examination should be performed once the patient is stabilized that includes a relevant neurologic examination. In patients who cannot give a full history or are comatose, ophthalmoscopic examination looking for retinal hemorrhages, a finding observed in approximately 10% of all patients with SAH, can be helpful.[20] This finding may be the only clue to the diagnosis in comatose patients. In many cases, the neurologic examination is nonfocal and, therefore, less useful for making the diagnosis. Abnormal examination findings can sometimes suggest the location of an offending aneurysm. Meningismus is oftentimes a later finding and should not be relied on in excluding the diagnosis.

In a large, prospective population of ED patients presenting to 6 Canadian EDs with thunderclap headache (defined as reaching maximum intensity within 1 hour), Perry and colleagues[19] proposed the Ottawa Subarachnoid Rules. Of the 2000 patients included in this cohort, 130 (6.5%) had SAH, making the study population representative that seen in practice. The authors developed 3 clinical decision rules, all of which were 100% sensitive for SAH that would have decreased the rates of investigations from 83% (baseline) to between 64% and 74%. The rule can be applied in alert patients 15 years of age or older who have no recent head trauma, lack new neurologic deficits, and have no history of a prior aneurysm, brain tumor, or SAH. If 1 or more criteria are present, SAH cannot be ruled out and the patient requires a workup:

- Age greater than 40 years
- Complaint of neck pain or stiffness
- Witnessed loss of consciousness
- Onset with exertion
- Thunderclap headache
- Limited neck flexion on examination

The Ottawa Subarachnoid Rules have since been internally and externally validated and are highly sensitive for ruling out SAH.[21–23] It is important to remember that the differential diagnosis for thunderclap headache is broad and only 10% of these patients will have a SAH.[3,24] Emergency physicians must consider the differential diagnosis for this type of headache, which includes both serious and less serious etiologies, which in turn may require additional workup **Box 1** summarizes other causes of thunderclap headache.

Diagnostic Approach

In patients for whom SAH is suspected, the initial testing modality is brain imaging. This modality is most commonly a noncontrast CT scan, because it is most readily available in most EDs. MRI has extremely high sensitivity for hemorrhage, but the

---

Box 1
Differential diagnosis of thunderclap headache

"Cannot miss," emergent etiologies
  SAH
  Cervical or cranial artery dissection
  Cerebral venous sinus thrombosis
  Meningitis or encephalitis
  Hypertensive encephalopathy
  Idiopathic intracranial hypertension
  Temporal arteritis or central nervous system vasculitis
  Acute narrow angle closure glaucoma
  Spontaneous intracranial hypotension
  Reversible cerebral vasoconstriction syndrome
  Carbon monoxide poisoning
  Pituitary apoplexy
  Mass lesions, including
    Abscess
    Intracranial hemorrhage
    Tumor
    Colloid cyst

Benign etiologies
  Migraine
  Cluster headache
  Tension headache
  Exertional headache
  Sinusitis
  Coital headache

---

sensitivity early on is unknown[25] and is not often possible as an initial imaging modality in the ED. When performed in the first 24 hours of headache onset, the sensitivity of CT scan for detecting subarachnoid blood ranges from 90% to 100% and approaches 100% when performed within the first 6 hours.[26–31] The sensitivity decreases as time from onset to CT scan elapses owing to the dilution of blood by the normal flow of cerebrospinal fluid (CSF).[32] Other factors that decrease sensitivity include technical issues (ie, older CT scanners <32 slices or patient movement), interpretation error, small-volume bleeds, and anemia.[31,33–35]

There has been a growing body of literature demonstrating the sensitivity of CT scan approaches 100% when the patient is imaged within 6 hours of headache onset. In a 2016 meta-analysis of 8907 patients, the incidence of SAH on noncontrast brain CT performed within 6 hours and read by an attending radiologist in neurologically intact patients was 1.46 in 1000, with an overall sensitivity of 98.7%.[31] Perry and colleagues sought to validate both the Ottawa SAH Rules and the 6-hour CT scan rule in a prospective study at 6 Canadian EDs after implementing education on both of these approaches. In their analysis of 3672 patients, they found the Ottawa Rule was 100% sensitive (95% confidence interval, 98.1%–100%), and the 6-hour head CT scan rule was 95.5% sensitive (95% confidence interval, 89.8%–98.5%) for SAH. Furthermore, hospital admission rates were significantly decreased after this was implemented. The 5 missed SAH on the 6-hour head CT scan were owing to a radiology misread, 2 incidental aneurysms, 1 nonaneurysmal cause, and 1 profoundly anemic patient.[36] As a result of the growing body of evidence, the American College of Emergency Physicians 2019 Clinical Policy on the Evaluation and Management of Adult Patients presenting the ED with Acute Headache recommends that a noncontrast head CT scan performed within 6 hours of headache onset precludes the need for further diagnostic workup for SAH if the CT scan was performed with a modern generation scanner (Level B evidence).[37] Before this clinical policy update, lumbar puncture was recommend to definitively rule out SAH. The authors recommended that the decision to invoke the 6 hour rule and defer lumbar puncture takes into account the limitations of CT scans and applies this only to cases in which the patient is neurologically intact, the CT scan is read by an experienced radiologist, the scan was performed with modern CT scanner (third generation or higher), the CT scan is of strong technical quality, and the patient is not anemic.

In patients with a negative head CT scan more than 6 hours after the onset of headache, lumbar puncture to assess for the presence of red blood cells (RBCs) or xanthochromia will definitively rule out SAH. Both the number of RBCs and the presence of xanthochromia are a function of time from the bleed. Xanthochromia, or the yellowish hue resulting from the breakdown of hemoglobin, is detected by visual inspection (in most North American laboratories) or spectrophotometry and is highly sensitive for SAH.[38,39] As with CT scan, there are timing considerations one must consider with the lumbar puncture. RBCs appear very early in the course after the hemorrhage occurs, within the first few hours.[40] Xanthrochromia may take up to 12 hours to develop, but is present by 6 hours.[40–43] Thus, assessing the CSF for both RBCs and the presence of xanthochromia is recommended.

Emergency physicians must be aware of the possibility of a traumatic lumbar puncture when interpreting CSF results. These occur when blood from local trauma or a venous plexus contaminates the fluid and are estimated to happen in 16% to 31% of lumbar punctures.[44,45] There is no universally accepted method of evaluating RBC clearance to establish the likelihood of traumatic lumbar puncture versus SAH. On the surface, a commonly held belief has held that if there are fewer RBCs in tube 4 than tube 1, the likelihood of a traumatic lumbar puncture is high and the probability of SAH is lower. In a prospective analysis of 1739 patients with headache who underwent lumbar puncture to rule out SAH, the presence of fewer than 2000×10^6/L RBCs in addition to absence of xanthochromia excluded the diagnosis of aneurysmal SAH, with a sensitivity of 100%.[45] Smaller studies support a less conservative assumption that less than 500 RBCs in tube 4 along with a decrease from tube 1 rules out SAH.[41,46]

For patients in whom the CSF analysis is suggestive of SAH, the next steps in the workup and management include vascular imaging and neurosurgical consultation. In the past several decades, most commonly using CT angiography (CTA) has become the imaging modality of choice because it is noninvasive and highly sensitive for cerebral aneurysms.[47,48] If no source is visible on the CTA, then digital subtraction angiography should be considered. There are some advocates of a CT scan/CTA approach as opposed to lumbar puncture in those patients who present greater than 6 hours after ictus. Although this strategy avoids the potential diagnostic challenge of traumatic tap as well as other complications of the lumbar puncture, there is a lack of robust data to support the superiority of this method. The 2019 American College of Emergency Physicians Clinical Policy thus makes a Level C recommendation to perform either an lumbar puncture or CTA after a negative noncontrast brain CT scan in patients for whom SAH is still suspected.[38] If forgoing the lumbar puncture and opting for a CTA instead, it is important to understand the limitations and consequences of this path. For one, a CTA will not detect subarachnoid blood and may miss up to 15% of those cases that are not aneurysmal. Because of its extremely high sensitivity, CTA may detect incidental aneurysms that are not in fact the cause of the headache and commit the patient to further diagnostic workups and in turn health care costs. Additional and potentially unnecessary vascular imaging also exposes the patient to higher doses of radiation exposure and contrast, both of which can have downstream consequences. The authors recommend using this approach only in those patients in whom there is high concern for SAH and lumbar puncture is not feasible (ie, patient refusal, anticoagulation use and inability to administer a reversal agent). A suggested diagnostic algorithm is displayed in **Fig. 3**.

Emergency Department Management

Patients found to have a SAH require prompt neurosurgical or neurointerventional consultation. Most of these patients will require endovascular coiling or microsurgical clipping if the source is aneurysmal, and/or ventriculostomy for complications such as hydrocephalus.[9,49,50] In unstable patients for whom there is a high suspicion for SAH, neurosurgical referral or consultation should be obtained early, even in parallel with the ED workup. The most recent SAH guidelines recommend that low-volume hospitals should consider early transfer of patients with aneurysmal SAH to high-volume centers (ie, >35 aneurysmal SAH cases per year) with experienced cerebrovascular surgeons, endovascular specialists, and multidisciplinary neurointensive care services.[9] A 2014 meta-analysis of more than 36,000 patients showed a decrease in in-hospital mortality for patients treated in high-volume centers with an odds ratio of 0.77 (95% confidence interval, 0.60–0.97).[51]

As with any critically ill patient, the emergency physician should prioritize airway, breathing, and circulation. Although most patients with SAH do not require intubation, definitive airway control should be considered in those with a depressed mental status, inability to protect the airway, or high suspicion for impending clinical deterioration. For patients being transferred to another facility, it is important to consider possible need for intubation in the context of transfer time. Standard rapid sequence intubation is the preferred technique for those patients who do require intubation. Pain should be adequately controlled with analgesics and sedation should be optimized for intubated patients. Patients should be placed on cardiac monitoring because some patients with severe brain injury are at risk for neurocardiac stunning.[52] Furthermore, patients should have nothing by mouth in anticipation of the need for surgical intervention. Any sudden deterioration in clinical status in the ED should prompt an immediate repeat head CT scan to assess for worsening hemorrhage or reversible complication such as hydrocephalus.

Blood pressure control is another important consideration in patients with SAH, although the data regarding the optimal target are sparse. Clinicians must balance the risk of hypoperfusion to an already injured brain against the risk of hematoma expansion and rebleeding. The data on hypertension management and the effect on mortality are conflicting.[53–55] The American Heart Association recommends maintaining a systolic blood pressure less than 160 mm Hg,[9] although it is important to note that there is no conclusive evidence for this target and many neurosurgeons prefer a lower blood pressure based on their training and experience. In choosing an antihypertensive agent for these patients, the emergency physician should consider those that are titratable such as nicardipine, labetalol, clevidipine, and esmolol.

Anticoagulation reversal should be initiated as soon as possible in those patients on anticoagulant medications. Protocols for reversal vary by institution depending on available agents. For patients on vitamin K antagonists, 4-factor prothrombin concentrates are the preferred reversal agent owing to their rapid onset and rapid infusion ability, along with vitamin K.[56] If prothrombin concentrates are not available, fresh frozen plasma should be given. Patients on factor Xa inhibitors (apixaban, rivaroxaban) should be reversed with andexanet alpha, which has been recently approved by the US Food and Drug Administration. If this agent is not available, prothrombin

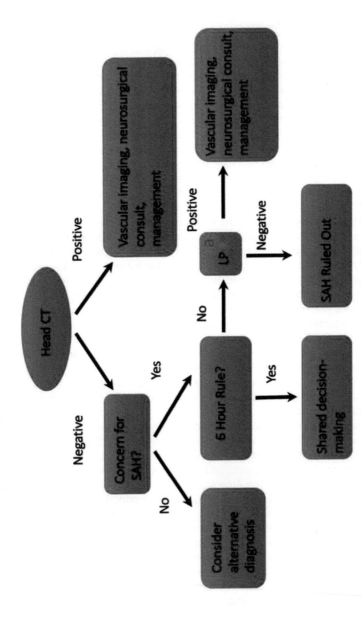

Fig. 3. Diagnostic algorithm for SAH. [a]CTA may also be considered if LP is not feasible. LP, lumbar puncture.

Box 2
Initial ED management considerations for SAH

Vascular imaging to identify the lesion

Neurosurgical consultation and/or transfer to a high-volume center

Airway protection if this is compromised or for expected worsening clinical course

Blood pressure control with a goal systolic blood pressure of less than 160 mm Hg

Analgesia and sedation administration as needed

Cardiac monitoring

Nimodipine for possible vasospasm

Consideration of seizure prophylaxis and treatment

Anticoagulation reversal if indicated

---

concentrates should be administered. Direct thrombin inhibitors (ie, dabigatran) should be reversed with idarucizaimab.

Cerebral vasospasm is a known complication in SAH in the first 2 weeks after bleeding, and peaks within 7 to 10 days, and can lead to increased neurologic deterioration and significant morbidity in these patients. Nimodipine, a calcium channel antagonist, has been shown to decrease cerebral ischemia (although the precise mechanism is likely not by reduction of vasospasm) and is the recommended agent for this complication.[9,57] Seizures occur in less than 20% of patients with SAH.[58] Although the evidence is sparse, antiepileptic administration should be used for actively seizing patients, for those with higher clinical grade hemorrhages, and should be considered for seizure prophylaxis.[9] A summary of ED management considerations is displayed in **Box 2**.

SUMMARY

Atraumatic SAH is a rare but serious cause of headache and a true medical emergency. The clinical presentation of SAH is broad and atypical presentations often lead to misdiagnosis. The initial diagnostic workup begins with a noncontrast brain CT scan followed by lumbar puncture and/or vascular imaging depending on the time of symptom onset. Emergency physicians must be aware of the limitations of various diagnostic tests and consider these in the ED workup. Once the diagnosis of SAH is established, these patients require prompt neurosurgical evaluation at a high-volume center. The emergency physician should consider initial management issues, including airway, blood pressure control, administration of analgesics, cardiac monitor, treatment of vasospasm, anticoagulation reversal, and seizure treatment in all of these patients.

CLINICS CARE POINTS

- Ruptured aneurysms are the most common cause of atraumatic SAH and there are excellent endovascular and surgical treatments.
- Misdiagnosis remains an important issue, especially in well-appearing patients, for whom these treatments are the most effective.
- Noncontrast CT scan sensitivity approaches 100% if done within 6 hours of the headache onset and read by an experienced radiologist.

- Beyond 6 hours, some other diagnostic test is necessary and we recommend lumbar puncture.
- Once the diagnosis of nontraumatic SAH is made in the ED, there is a short checklist of next steps related to defining the offending vascular lesion, consulting a neurosurgeon and starting treatments to decrease the likelihood of complications.

DISCLOSURE

The authors have no disclosures.

REFERENCES

1. Centers for Disease Control and Prevention. National Hospital Ambulatory Medical Care Survey: 2017 emergency department summary tables. Available at: https://www.cdc.gov/nchs/data/nhamcs/web_tables/2017_ed_web_tables-508.pdf. Accessed June 13, 2020.
2. Edlow JA, Caplan LR. Avoiding pitfalls in the diagnosis of subarachnoid hemorrhage. N Engl J Med 2000;342:29–36.
3. Edlow JA, Malek AM, Ogilvy CS. Aneurysmal subarachnoid hemorrhage: update for emergency physicians. J Emerg Med 2008;34:237–51.
4. Vermeulen MJ, Schull MJ. Missed diagnosis of subarachnoid hemorrhage in the emergency department. Stroke 2007;38:1216–21.
5. Aisiku I, Edlow J, Goldstein J, et al. An evidence-based approach to diagnosis and management of subarachnoid hemorrhage in the emergency department. Emerg Med Pract 2014;16:1–30.
6. Dubosh NM, Edlow JA, Goto T, et al. Missed serious neurological conditions in emergency department patients discharged with nonspecific diagnoses of headache or back pain. Ann Emerg Med 2019;74:549–61.
7. Etiman N, Chang H, Hackenberg K, et al. Worldwide incidence of aneurysmal subarachnoid hemorrhage according to region, time period, blood pressure and smoking prevalence in the population a systematic review and meta-analysis. JAMA Neurol 2019;76:588–97.
8. de Rooij NK, Linn FH, van der Plas JA, et al. Incidence of subarachnoid haemorrhage: a systematic review with emphasis on region, age, gender and time trends. J Neurol Neurosurg Psychiatry 2007;78:1365–72.
9. Connolly ES Jr, Rabinstein AA, Carhuapoma JR, et al. Guidelines for the management of aneurysmal subarachnoid hemorrhage: a guideline for healthcare professionals from the American Heart Association/American Stroke Association. Stroke 2012;43:1711–37.
10. Nieuwkamp DJ, Setz LE, Algra A, et al. Changes in case fatality of aneurysmal subarachnoid haemorrhage over time, according to age, sex, and region: a meta-analysis. Lancet Neurol 2009;8:635–42.
11. Korja M, Lehto H, Juvela S, et al. Incidence of subarachnoid hemorrhage is decreasing together with decreasing smoking rates. Neurology 2016;87:1118–23.
12. Schwedt TJ, Matharu MS, Dodick DW. Thunderclap headache. Lancet Neurol 2006;5:621–31.
13. Rinkel GJ, Djibuti M, Algra A, et al. Prevalence and risk of rupture of intracranial aneurysms: a systematic review. Stroke 1998;29:251–6.
14. Edlow JA. What are the unintended consequences of changing the diagnostic paradigm for subarachnoid hemorrhage after brain computed tomography to

computed tomographic angiography in place of lumbar puncture? Acad Emerg Med 2010;17:991–7.

15. Brisman JL, Song JK, Newell DW. Cerebral aneurysms. The New Engl J Med 2006;355:928–39.

16. Kumar S, Goddeau RP Jr, Selim MH, et al. Atraumatic convexal subarachnoid hemorrhage: clinical presentation, imaging patterns, and etiologies. Neurology 2010;74:893–9.

17. Mas J, Bouly S, Mourand I, et al. Focal convexal subarachnoid hemorrhage: clinical presentation, imaging patterns and etiologic findings in 23 patients. Rev Neurol (Paris) 2013;169:59–66.

18. Pope JV, Edlow JA. Avoiding misdiagnosis in patients with neurological emergencies. Emerg Med Int 2012;2012:949275.

19. Perry JJ, Stiell IG, Sivilotti ML, et al. High risk clinical characteristics for subarachnoid haemorrhage in patients with acute headache: prospective cohort study. BMJ 2010;341:c5204.

20. Fountas KN, Kapsalaki EZ, Lee GP, et al. Terson hemorrhage in patients suffering aneurysmal subarachnoid hemorrhage: predisposing factors and prognostic significance. J Neurosurg 2008;109:439–44.

21. Perry JJ, Stiell IG, Sivilotti ML, et al. Clinical decision rules to rule out subarachnoid hemorrhage for acute headache. JAMA 2013;310:1248–55.

22. Bellolio MF, Hess EP, Gilani WI, et al. External validation of the Ottawa subarachnoid hemorrhage clinical decision rule in patients with acute headache. Am J Emerg Med 2015;33:244–9.

23. Perry JJ, Sivilotti MLA, Sutherland J, et al. Validation of the Ottawa subarachnoid hemorrhage rule in patients with acute headache. CMAJ 2017;189:E1379–85.

24. Edlow JA. Managing patients with Nontraumatic, severe, rapid-onset headache. Ann Emerg Med 2018;71(3):400–8.

25. Verma RK, Kottke R, Andereggen L, et al. Detecting subarachnoid hemorrhage: comparison of combined FLAIR/SWI versus CT. Eur J Radiol 2013;82:1539–45.

26. Morgenstern LB, Luna-Gonzales H, Huber JC Jr, et al. Worst headache and subarachnoid hemorrhage: prospective, modern computed tomography and spinal fluid analysis. Ann Emerg Med 1998;32:297–304.

27. Perry JJ, Stiell IG, Sivilotti ML, et al. Sensitivity of computed tomography performed within six hours of onset of headache for diagnosis of subarachnoid haemorrhage: prospective cohort study. BMJ 2011;343:d4277.

28. Backes D, Rinkel GJ, Kemperman H, et al. Time-dependent test characteristics of head computed tomography in patients suspected of nontraumatic subarachnoid hemorrhage. Stroke 2012;43:2115–9.

29. Sidman R, Connolly E, Lemke T. Subarachnoid hemorrhage diagnosis: lumbar puncture is still needed when the computed tomography scan is normal. Acad Emerg Med 1996;3:827–31.

30. Dupont SA, Wijdicks EF, Manno EM, et al. Timing of computed tomography and prediction of vasospasm after aneurysmal subarachnoid hemorrhage. Neurocrit Care 2009;11:71–5.

31. Dubosh NM, Bellolio MF, Rabinstein AA, et al. Sensitivity of early brain computed tomography to exclude aneurysmal subarachnoid hemorrhage: a systematic review and meta-analysis. Stroke 2016;47:750–5.

32. Fishman RA. Cerebrospinal fluid in diseases of the nervous system. 2nd edition. Philadelphia: W.B. Saunders Company; 1992.

33. Oh SY, Lim YC, Shim YS, et al. Initial misdiagnosis of aneurysmal subarachnoid hemorrhage: associating factors and its prognosis. Acta Neurochir (Wien) 2018; 160:1105–13.

34. Bruni SG, Bartlett E, Yu E. Factors involved in discrepant preliminary radiology resident interpretations of neuroradiological imaging studies: a retrospective analysis. AJR Am J Roentgenol 2012;198:1367–74.

35. Dubosh NM, Edlow JA, Lefton M, et al. Types of diagnostic errors in neurological emergencies in the emergency department. Diagnosis (Berl) 2015;2:21–8.

36. Perry JJ, Sivilotti MLA, Émond M, et al. Prospective Implementation of the Ottawa subarachnoid hemorrhage rule and 6-hour computed tomography rule. Stroke 2020;51(2):424–30.

37. American College of Emergency Physicians Clinical Policies Subcommittee (Writing Committee) on Acute Headache, Godwin SA, Cherkas DS, et al. Clinical policy: critical issues in the evaluation and management of adult patients presenting to the emergency department with acute headache. Ann Emerg Med 2019; 74:e41–74.

38. Dupont SA, Wijdicks EF, Manno EM, et al. Thunderclap headache and normal computed tomographic results: value of cerebrospinal fluid analysis. Mayo Clin Proc 2008;83:1326–31.

39. Perry JJ, Sivilotti ML, Stiell IG, et al. Should spectrophotometry be used to identify xanthrochromia in the cerebrospinal fluid of alert patients suspected of having subarachnoid hemorrhage? Stroke 2016;37:2467–72.

40. Walton J. Subarachnoid hemorrhage. Edinburgh: E & S Livingstone, Ltd; 1956.

41. Marcolini E, Hine J. Approach to the diagnosis and management of subarachnoid hemorrhage. West J Emerg Med 2019;20:203–11.

42. Carpenter CR, Hussain AM, Ward MJ, et al. Spontaneous subarachnoid hemorrhage: a systematic review and meta-analysis describing the diagnostic accuracy of history, physical examination, imaging, and lumbar puncture with an exploration of test thresholds. Acad Emerg Med 2016;23:963–1003.

43. Czuczman AD, Thomas LE, Boulanger AB, et al. Interpreting red blood cells in lumbar puncture: distinguishing true subarachnoid hemorrhage from traumatic tap. Acad Emerg Med 2013;20:247–56.

44. Shah KH, Richard KM, Nicholas S, et al. Incidence of traumatic lumbar puncture. Acad Emerg Med 2003;10:151–4.

45. Perry JJ, Alyahya B, Sivilotti ML, et al. Differentiation between traumatic tap and aneurysmal subarachnoid hemorrhage: prospective cohort study. BMJ 2015;350: h568.

46. Gorchynski J, Oman J, Newton T. Interpretation of traumatic lumbar punctures in the setting of possible subarachnoid hemorrhage: who can be safely discharged? Cal J Emerg Med 2007;8:3–7.

47. McCormack RF, Hutson A. Can computed tomography angiography of the brain replace lumbar puncture in the evaluation of acute-onset headache after a negative noncontrast cranial computed tomography scan? Acad Emerg Med 2010;17: 444–51.

48. Menke J, Larsen J, Kallenberg K. Diagnosing cerebral aneurysms by computed tomographic angiography: meta-analysis. Ann Neurol 2011;69:646–54.

49. Molyneux A, Kerr R, Stratton I, et al. International Subarachnoid Aneurysm Trial (ISAT) of neurosurgical clipping versus endovascular coiling in 2143 patients with ruptured intracranial aneurysms: a randomised trial. Lancet 2002;360: 1267–74.

50. Bederson JB, Connolly ES, Batjer HH, et al. Guidelines for the management of aneurysmal subarachnoid hemorrhage: a statement for healthcare professionals from a special writing group of the Stroke Council, American Heart Association. Stroke 2009;40:994–1025.
51. Boogaarts HD, van Amerongen MJ, de Vries J, et al. Caseload as a factor for outcome in aneurysmal subarachnoid hemorrhage: a systematic review and meta-analysis. J Neurosurg 2014;120:605–11.
52. Wybraniec MT, Mizia-Stec K, Krzych L. Neurocardiogenic injury in subarachnoid hemorrhage: a wide spectrum of catecholamine-mediated brain-heart interactions. Cardiol J 2014;2:220–8.
53. Ohkuma H, Tsurutani H, Suzuki S. Incidence and significance of early aneurysmal rebleeding before neurosurgical or neurological management. Stroke 2001;32:1176–80.
54. Naidech AM, Janjua N, Kreiter KT, et al. Predictors and impact of aneurysm rebleeding after subarachnoid hemorrhage. Arch Neurol 2005;62:410–6.
55. Woodfield J, Rane N, Cudlip S, et al. Value of delayed MRI in angiogram-negative subarachnoid haemorrhage. Clin Radiol 2014;69:350–6.
56. Christos S, Naples R. Anticoagulation reversal and treatment strategies in major bleeding: update 2016. West J Emerg Med 2016;17:264–70.
57. Dorhout Mees SM, Rinkel GJ, Feigin VL, et al. Calcium antagonists for aneurysmal subarachnoid haemorrhage. Cochrane Database Syst Rev 2007;CD000277.
58. Lin CL, Dumont AS, Lieu AS, et al. Characterization of perioperative seizures and epilepsy following aneurysmal subarachnoid hemorrhage. J Neurosurg 2003;99:978–85.

Central Nervous System Infections in the Immunocompromised Adult Presenting to the Emergency Department

Robert J. Stephens, MD, MSCI[a],*, Stephen Y. Liang, MD, MPHS[b,c]

KEYWORDS

- Immunocompromise • CNS infection • Meningitis • HIV • Transplant

KEY POINTS

- Emergency physicians should maintain a high index of suspicion for central nervous system infection in immunocompromised patients.
- The diagnostic approach to central nervous system infection in immunocompromised patients should include neuroimaging, lumbar puncture for cerebrospinal fluid sampling when appropriate, and pathogen-directed testing based on the differential diagnosis.
- Early empiric antimicrobial therapy should include coverage for community-acquired bacteria (eg, *Streptococcus pneumoniae*), *Listeria monocytogenes*, and herpes simplex virus.
- Infectious disease, oncology, hematology, transplant, and other subspecialists should be consulted early in the management of immunocompromised patients with central nervous system infection.

The population of immunocompromised patients in the United States is increasing. More than 650,000 patients with cancer receive cytotoxic chemotherapy annually and this population is expected to rise in the coming years. In 2012, more than 90,000 patients with cancer were hospitalized for neutropenic fever owing to chemotherapy and subsequent immunosuppression.[1] The number of solid organ transplants (SOT) performed annually has more than tripled since the Organ Procurement and Transplant Network began data collection in 1987 as advances in immunosuppression

---

[a] Department of Emergency Medicine, Washington University School of Medicine, 660 South Euclid Avenue, St Louis, MO 63110, USA; [b] Department of Emergency Medicine, Washington University School of Medicine, 660 South Euclid Avenue, St Louis, MO 63110, USA; [c] Department of Internal Medicine, Division of Infectious Disease, Washington University School of Medicine, 660 South Euclid Avenue, St Louis, MO 63110, USA
* Corresponding author:
E-mail address: stephensr@wustl.edu

Emerg Med Clin N Am 39 (2021) 101–121
https://doi.org/10.1016/j.emc.2020.09.006
0733-8627/21/© 2020 Elsevier Inc. All rights reserved.

to prevent rejection have improved long-term survival.[2] More than 20,000 hematopoietic stem cell transplants (HSCT) are performed annually in the United States, and it is estimated there will be more than 500,000 HSCT survivors by 2030, many of whom will require immunosuppression to prevent graft-versus-host disease.[3] More than 37,000 cases of human immunodeficiency virus (HIV) infection were newly diagnosed in the United States every year from 2013 to 2018 and there are more than 1 million people living with HIV infection in the United States today.[4,5] The advent of novel immunomodulating drugs such as complement and check point inhibitors have also contributed to the expanding population of immunocompromised patients presenting for acute care in the emergency department (ED).[6,7] Although antimicrobial prophylaxis has greatly decreased the risk of opportunistic infection, immunocompromised patients remain significantly more vulnerable to infection compared to the general population.[8–10]

Central nervous system (CNS) infections are relatively rare in the developed world. Meningitis accounts only for 66,000 ED visits each year in the United States.[11] However, the risk for CNS infections is high among the immunocompromised, ranging from an 8-fold increase in HIV to a 30-fold increase in risk in allogenic HSCT recipients.[8–10] In an early case series from San Francisco from the 1980s, up to 60% of patients with AIDS developed a CNS infection, often diagnosed on initial presentation to care.[12] In another series, 3% of cardiac transplant patients developed a CNS infection within the first 4 years after transplant.[13] Among allogenic HSCT, 4% had a CNS infection during the first year and this factor was significantly associated with mortality.[14] Immunocompromised patients are more likely to present atypically with subtle signs and symptoms.[15] A high index of suspicion is necessary to avoid missing a diagnosis of a CNS infection in this challenging patient population.

In this review, we discuss an approach to CNS infections in immunocompromised patients. We address common pathogens, clinical presentations, laboratory findings, and imaging correlates, and provide a basic framework for the initial evaluation and empiric management of suspected CNS infection in immunocompromised patients presenting to the ED.

COMMON CLINICAL SYNDROMES

Inflammation of the meninges, termed meningitis, can be bacterial, viral, fungal, or parasitic in etiology. Classically, these patients present with altered mental status, nuchal rigidity, and fever, but this triad is seen in only a minority of patients. Other symptoms may include rash, headache, cranial nerve abnormalities, nausea, emesis, and seizures. Clinical examination is not sensitive and cannot be used to exclude meningitis.[16]

Parenchymal inflammation of the brain constitutes encephalitis. As with meningitis, patients with encephalitis may present with headache and fever but are more likely to have focal neurologic deficits and seizures. Deficits will correspond to the region of inflammation. Herpes simplex virus (HSV) encephalitis, for example, classically affects the temporal lobes, resulting in disinhibition and psychotic behavior, and is often confused with acute psychiatric illness.[17]

Brain abscesses, collections of purulent material in the brain parenchyma, are commonly caused by hematogenous or contiguous spread of a bacterial infection.[18] Although rare in the general population, brain abscesses are more common among the immunocompromised.[19] Clinical presentations are variable and often subacute in nature. Although new-onset seizures are a relatively common presenting symptom, fever occurs in less than one-half of patients.[18] More subtle signs include ataxia and cranial nerve palsies. Other associated symptoms such as nausea and headache can arise from mass effect and increased intracranial pressure.[18]

CNS infections in the immunocompromised can result in the development of inflammatory or malignant space-occupying intracranial lesions.[20] As with brain abscesses, presentations may vary based on the location and size of the lesion and may reflect signs of increased intracranial pressure. Symptoms can be subacute because these lesions are often slow growing.[20]

APPROACH TO CENTRAL NERVOUS SYSTEM INFECTION IN THE EMERGENCY DEPARTMENT

Initial evaluation with neuroimaging in the ED helps to inform decision making regarding the safety of lumbar puncture (LP) in cases of suspected meningitis or encephalitis through exclusion of intracranial mass lesions with the potential to promote intracranial herniation.[21,22] In the case of a brain abscess, neuroimaging helps establish the diagnosis. Given the time-sensitive nature of many CNS infections, computed tomography (CT) scan of the brain with and without contrast is the preferred initial imaging modality in the ED. MRI is time consuming but more sensitive than a CT scan in its ability to differentiate multiple lesions.[23] The presence of an intracranial mass lesion with evidence of mass effect and/or herniation on neuroimaging necessitates emergent neurosurgical consultation.[24]

LP to obtain cerebrospinal fluid (CSF) for diagnostic testing is warranted if there is clinical suspicion of meningitis or encephalitis. Adherence to aseptic technique is important, both for patient safety and to avoid specimen contamination. Because this procedure can be technically complicated in some patients, it is vital to collect adequate volumes of CSF to evaluate for a wide range of probable and serious pathogens. The International Encephalitis Consortium recommends that at least 20 mL of CSF be collected in adults; any unused CSF should be saved for future testing.[25] At a minimum, CSF studies should include measuring an opening pressure and obtaining CSF glucose, protein, white blood cell count with differential, and bacterial culture. Additional CSF testing should hinge on an assessment of the patient's immunocompromised state and further consideration of the differential diagnosis of CNS infections possible.

Time-to-antibiotics remains one of the most important predictors of outcome in CNS infection. Therefore, neuroimaging and LP, if indicated, should take high priority with the objective of initiating empiric broad-spectrum antibiotic therapy within the first 2 hours of ED presentation.[26,27] However, if the patient is clinically unstable or delays in obtaining these studies are anticipated, it is reasonable to start empiric antibiotics immediately. Although data are limited to the immunocompetent pediatric population, time to sterilization of the CSF by antibiotics occurs within hours and, in some cases, in as little as 15 minutes.[28] There is evidence to suggest that *Neisseria meningiditis* present in CSF is likely to be killed within 2 hours of antibiotic treatment, whereas *Streptococcus pneumoniae* may require more than 4 hours.[28] Empiric antibiotics should be held until after LP whenever safe and feasible to maximize the yield of CSF cultures. Our recommended diagnostic and treatment approach to CNS infection in the immunocompromised is outlined in **Fig. 1**.

Early involvement of an infectious disease specialist can aid in diagnostic planning and has been associated with improved patient outcomes.[29] Consultation with members of the patient's care team (eg, oncologists, hematologists, transplant specialists) familiar with their history and immunosuppression regimen also promotes high-quality, patient-centered care in the ED.

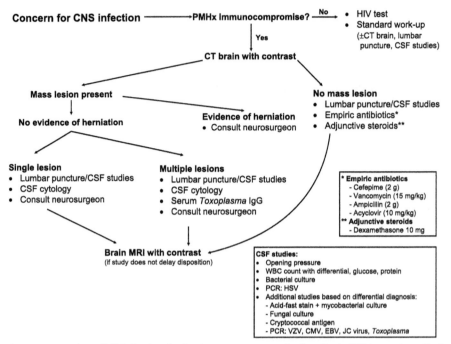

Fig 1. Approach to CNS infection in the immunocompromised patient. PMHx, past medical history. (*Modified from* Tan IL, Smith BR, von Geldern G, et al. *Lancet Neurol* 2012;11(7):605–17.)

A DIFFERENTIAL DIAGNOSIS OF A CENTRAL NERVOUS SYSTEM INFECTION IN IMMUNOCOMPROMISED PATIENTS

Immunocompromised states owing to cancer-related chemotherapy, immunosuppression to prevent rejection after SOT or HSCT, HIV infection, and immunomodulatory therapies render patients susceptible to distinct spectrums of CNS infection.

Among patients who have recently undergone cytotoxic chemotherapy, the degree and duration of neutropenia are important to know.[30] Neutrophils play an integral role in the immune response to infection owing to bacteria and fungi, particularly at mucosal surfaces.[30] Classically, the nadir of neutropenia occurs 7 to 12 days after chemotherapy, but may vary by regimen. Neutropenia can still be present even after patients receive recombinant granulocyte colony-stimulating factors.[31] Patients receiving chemotherapy should be considered neutropenic until their absolute neutrophil count can be determined.

In patients receiving maintenance immunosuppression after SOT or HSCT, the risk for and spectrum of CNS infection is determined by a patient's net state of immunosuppression.[32] Dose, duration, and combination of immunosuppressants are key determinants. Immunosuppression is driven by lymphocyte dysfunction; therefore, fungi and viruses are predominant pathogens. Time from initiation of post-transplantation immunosuppression is also an important factor. In the month immediately after transplantation, immunosuppression has not yet fully taken effect; therefore, most infections are associated with health care (eg, surgery, hospitalization) and opportunistic infections are rare. The highest risk period for opportunistic infection owing to fungi and viruses is between 1 and 6 months after transplantation. After 6 months, community-acquired pathogens become more common as immunosuppression is tapered. Regardless of the time after transplant, most patients remain at substantially higher risk of CNS infection compared with the general population.[32]

HIV primarily targets CD4 T lymphocytes, leading to immunosuppression and impaired cell-mediated immunity.[33] Consequently, opportunistic viruses and fungi are common causes of CNS infection in patients with AIDS.[34] In persons living with HIV, the CD4 count is an important predictor of which pathogens should be considered in the differential diagnosis for CNS infection. Unless laboratory data are available from the past 3 months, a CD4 count and HIV viral load should be obtained in all patients with HIV presenting to the ED the for evaluation of CNS infection.

Novel immunotherapies used in the treatment of hematologic malignancies, including check point inhibitors and chimeric antigen receptor T-cell therapy, do not behave like typical immunosuppressive chemotherapy agents. Patients receiving these therapies will not usually present with neutropenia. The most serious side effects of these drugs are often autoimmune or cytokine mediated. Neurotoxicity is among the most common adverse effects of chimeric antigen receptor T-cell therapy and serious neurologic adverse events such as encephalitis, seizures, and altered mental status occur, albeit rarely.[7] These adverse reactions are indistinguishable from an infectious process.[35] However, neurologic symptoms should not be attributed to an adverse drug reaction until a CNS infection has been ruled out.

The complement system plays a vital role in the immune response to encapsulated organisms, in particular *N meningiditis*. Patients with complement deficiencies are at marked increased risk of developing *N meningiditis* infection. Recently, the complement-inhibiting drugs ravulizumab and eculizumab have been used to treat atypical hemolytic uremic syndrome and paroxysmal nocturnal hemoglobinuria. Despite meningococcal vaccination, patients receiving these drugs remain at an increased risk of developing meningococcal disease.[6]

ADDITIONAL CONSIDERATIONS

Immunocompromised patients engaged in care are frequently prescribed antimicrobial prophylaxis to prevent opportunistic infections. An accurate medication list and history regarding compliance are important in informing the differential diagnosis of CNS infection. Prophylaxis against cytomegalovirus (CMV) infection significantly reduces the risk of reactivation with CMV, but also with HSV and varicella zoster virus (VZV).[36,37] Yet, antimicrobial dosing for prophylaxis against some infections may not be adequate to prevent others. For example, *Pneumocystis jirovecii* prophylaxis dosing for trimethoprim-sulfamethoxazole (TMP-SMX) adequately prevents toxoplasmosis, but not nocardiosis.[38,39] Furthermore, although prophylactic antimicrobials decrease the risk of opportunistic infections, clinically significant "breakthrough" infections can still occur. Current prophylactic antimicrobial use should be elicited for each patient, but this information should not obviate a diagnostic workup or the initiation of empiric antimicrobial treatment if clinical suspicion for an opportunistic infection remains high.

Immunization has proven vital in preventing bacterial meningitis among immunocompromised patients. Vaccination against *Haemophilus influenzae, S pneumoniae,* and *N meningiditis* have decreased the rates of bacterial meningitis in the United States, but mortality among those infected remains stubbornly unchanged.[40,41] Meningococcal meningitis rates have dropped so precipitously that they now match rates of nosocomial CNS infections owing to *Staphylococcus spp* and Gram-negative bacilli. Immunization can be less protective in the immunocompromised.[32] Although immunization against *H influenzae*, *S pneumoniae*, and *N meningiditis* may render these pathogens lower on the differential diagnosis for CNS infection, empiric antimicrobial coverage including these organisms is still recommended until an alternative etiology has been identified, given the devastating nature of these infections.

Recent neurosurgical procedures (eg, shunt placement, intrathecal chemotherapy) are also vital pieces of the history that can guide diagnostic evaluation and empiric antibiotic therapy for CNS infection. Postsurgical patients are at increased risk of CNS infection secondary to skin flora such as coagulase-negative *Staphylococci*, *Staphylococcus aureus*, and Gram-negative bacilli.[42] Early neurosurgical consultation is advised in these instances.

BACTERIAL CENTRAL NERVOUS SYSTEM INFECTIONS

Bacterial pathogens frequently associated with CNS infection in the immunocompromised are summarized in **Table 1**.

Common Acquired Bacteria

Bacteria can gain entry to the CNS through contiguous spread from sinus or dental infections or hematogenous seeding. Rarely, neurosurgical procedures or traumatic communication with the subarachnoid space can also inoculate the CNS with bacteria. *S pneumoniae*, *H influenzae*, and *N meningiditis* remain the most common pathogens associated with bacterial meningitis.[40] Morbidity and mortality rates are especially high among immunocompromised patients.[8,10] Less common, pyogenic brain abscesses are often polymicrobial or owing to *Streptococcus* or *Staphylococcus* species; gram-negative bacteria are implicated in up to 15% of cases.[18]

Table 1
Bacterial pathogens implicated in CNS disease in immunocompromised patients and associated clinical findings

Pathogen	Typical CNS Syndrome	Typical Computed Tomographic Findings	Typical/Important CSF Findings
S pneumonia *H influenzae* *N meningiditis*	Meningitis	Unremarkable	Protein high, glucose low Neutrophilic pleocytosis Gram stain can be informative (*S pneumoniae/H influenzae/N meningiditis*)
L monocytogenes	Meningoencephalitis	Unremarkable	Protein high, glucose low Lymphocytic pleocytosis Gram stain may be negative
Nocardia spp.	Brain abscess	May show abscess	Protein high, glucose low Neutrophilic pleocytosis
M tuberculosis	Three phases: 1. Subacute mental status change 2. Meningitis 3. Paralytic	Variable	Protein high, glucose low Lymphocytic pleocytosis Acid-fast stain and mycobacterial culture poorly sensitive Multiple cultures often necessary

CSF findings of elevated protein, decreased glucose, and increased white blood cell (WBC) count with neutrophilic predominance are typical of bacterial meningitis, although up to 10% of cases may have a WBC count with lymphocytic predominance.[42] The diagnostic yield of a Gram stain is highest for S pneumoniae and H influenzae.[42] Nucleic acid amplification tests are not routinely used for bacterial pathogens owing to the high combined diagnostic yield of Gram stain and bacterial culture, although this is standard of care in the United Kingdom.[42,43]

Third- and fourth-generation cephalosporins (eg, ceftriaxone, cefepime) are generally recommended for the treatment of community-acquired bacterial meningitis.[44] In countries including the United States, where penicillin-resistant strains of S pneumoniae are prevalent, vancomycin should be empirically added pending CSF culture and antibiotic susceptibility testing.[43] Adjunctive dexamethasone has been supported to decreased mortality associated with bacterial meningitis, with a benefit demonstrated in the setting of infection owing to S pneumoniae.[45] Corticosteroid therapy for meningitis in immunosuppressed patients has not been subjected to rigorous investigation.

Listeria

Listeria monocytogenes can be a serious CNS pathogen in the immunocompromised. Almost 90% of neurolisteriosis cases are associated with immunosuppression, with solid organ malignancy being the most common comorbidity. Active cancer and monocytopenias are significantly associated with mortality. The mortality rate for neurolisteriosis is nearly 30%; only 40% of survivors make a full recovery and one-half experience long-term neurologic sequelae.[46]

Meningoencephalitis is the most common presentation, although isolated meningitis and encephalitis can also occur. Encephalitis is an independent risk factor for death.[46] Rhomboencephalitis (brainstem or cerebellar involvement) comprises less than 20% of cases, manifesting with headache, fever, and vomiting, but also brainstem-specific symptoms such as cranial nerve palsies, cerebellar dysfunction, and motor and sensory deficits. Brain abscess is a rare complication marked by focal neurologic deficits determined by the location of the abscess.[46] Fever is present in approximately 90% of patients with neurolisteriosis and most patients have altered mental status.[46]

CSF findings in neurolisteriosis are variable. L monocytogenes is one of the few bacteria that can present with lymphocytic predominance on CSF WBC count. Gram stain is positive in only one-third of cases, although CSF culture is usually positive.[42,46–48] Neuroimaging may show abscess, small intracranial hemorrhage, or periventricular enhancement, none of which is specific.[49]

Cephalosporins commonly used to cover typical community-acquired bacteria associated with CNS infection are ineffective against neurolisteriosis.[50] Failure to initiate appropriate empiric antibiotic therapy is associated with significantly worse outcome.[46,50] Aminopenicillins (eg, ampicillin) are first-line agents for neurolisteriosis; meropenem and TMP-SMX can also be used. A secondary analysis of data demonstrated a trend toward improved outcomes with the addition of an aminoglycoside, but was not statistically significant.[50] Finally, corticosteroid therapy may significantly worsen survival, although confounding by indication was possible in a subgroup analysis.[46]

Nocardia

Infection with Nocardia spp. is rare, even among immunocompromised patients.[38,39] In a series of 1050 cases of nocardiosis, CNS involvement was present in 22% and systemic infection in 44%.[51] Glucocorticoid and calcineurin inhibitor use are among the most important risk factors for developing nocardiosis.[39] In a series of patients with HIV/AIDS with nocardiosis, all had a CD4 count of less than 200 cells/μL and a 75% had a CD4 count of less than 100 cells/μL.[52] CNS nocardiosis can manifest as a single or multiple brain abscesses, with symptoms ranging from acute focal neurologic deficits to altered mental status.[51]

Nocardia will grow in aerobic bacterial culture media, as well as fungal and acid-fast bacilli media.[53] There are no widely available serologic or molecular testing methods. Several case reports of CNS nocardiosis demonstrate CSF with neutrophilic pleocytosis, elevated protein, and decreased glucose levels consistent with bacterial meningitis, although this remains poorly characterized in the literature.[54]

CNS nocardiosis is treated with either a sulfonamide (most commonly high-dose TMP-SMX) or amikacin in combination with imipenem.[55] Sulfonamides should be considered even in patients with known intolerance or allergy provided appropriate desensitization can be achieved. Resistance to TMP-SMX is rare.[56] It is important to note that typical doses of TMP-SMX used for *P jirovecii* prophylaxis do not prevent *Nocardia* infection.[38,39]

Empiric Antibacterial Therapy for Central Nervous System Infection in the Immunocompromised Patient

Initial empiric antibiotic therapy for immunocompromised patients presenting to the ED with suspected CNS infection should include coverage of community-acquired bacteria (namely, *S pneumoniae*) and *L monocytogenes*. Expanded gram-negative coverage for *Pseudomonas aeruginosa* is also generally recommended in immunocompromised patients presenting with severe infection. Given these considerations, broad-spectrum antibacterial coverage for CNS infection in the ED can be achieved with a combination of vancomycin, cefepime, and ampicillin. Empiric therapy for CNS nocardiosis is seldom indicated in the ED, but may be considered in consultation with an infectious disease specialist in the appropriate clinical context.

VIRAL INFECTION

Viral pathogens often implicated in CNS infection in the immunocompromised are summarized in **Table 2**.

Herpes Simplex Virus

HSV is the most common cause of clinically significant viral encephalitis.[57] Rates of CNS infection owing to HSV are surprisingly similar between immunocompromised and immunocompetent patients.[58] Encephalitis owing to HSV-1 is more common than HSV-2, although significant overlap in clinical syndromes exists between both virus types.[59] Temporal lobe tropism is classically described in HSV encephalitis with focal seizure and behavioral changes (eg, hypomania, hypersexuality, hyperorality) commonly reported.[60,61] The mortality rate for HSV encephalitis can approach 70% if untreated versus 20% when treated and up to one-half of patients can have prolonged neurologic sequelae.[62] Early antiviral therapy is critical in decreasing mortality.[63]

Initial neuroimaging obtained in the ED, particularly CT scan, can be normal in patients with HSV encephalitis. Subtle hypodensities seen in the temporal lobes and insular cortex can progress later to hemorrhage.[64] Characteristic contrast enhancement in the temporal lobes is best seen on MRI.[62] The CSF is typically notable for a lymphocytic pleocytosis with elevated protein and normal glucose. Red blood cells are present in up to 85% of cases.[58] CSF HSV polymerase chain reaction (PCR) is

Table 2
Viral pathogens implicated in CNS disease in immunocompromised patients and associated clinical findings

Viral Pathogens	Typical CNS Syndrome	Typical Computed Tomographic Findings	Typical/Important CSF Findings
HSV	HSV-1: encephalitis HSV-2: meningitis	Unremarkable May have subtle changes in temporal lobe	Protein high, glucose normal Lymphocytic pleocytosis May have RBCs HSV PCR positive
VZV	Encephalitis	Unremarkable	Protein high, glucose normal Lymphocytic pleocytosis VZV PCR positive
CMV	Encephalitis Ventriculoencephalitis	Unremarkable Periventricular enhancement may be seen in ventriculoencephalitis	Protein high, glucose normal Lymphocytic pleocytosis CMV PCR positive
Epstein–Barr virus	PCNSL Focal neurologic deficits	Solitary contrast-enhancing hyperdensity	Unremarkable Epstein–Barr virus PCR may be positive.

highly sensitive and specific for the diagnosis of HSV encephalitis.[62] Given the severe morbidity and mortality associated with this disease, early empiric intravenous acyclovir should be administered to all immunocompromised patients presenting with symptoms compatible with viral encephalitis.

Varicella Zoster Virus

VZV reactivation, or herpes zoster, is common in the immunocompetent population and rarely causes disseminated disease. In contrast, immunocompromised patients are more likely to experience CNS disease and with greater illness severity. In the developed world, VZV is the second most common cause of viral encephalitis.[57] HIV infection remains an independent risk factor for herpes zoster even despite adequate viral suppression with antiretroviral therapy (ART); however, a stepwise increase in susceptibility occurs as CD4 counts decrease.[34] CNS infection owing to VZV reactivation in SOT recipients has been described in the literature, but remains rare. The intensity of immunosuppression after transplantation likely plays a role in susceptibility.[65] HSCT is also considered a risk factor for VZV reactivation, although disseminated disease with CNS involvement remains uncommon.[66]

CNS infection often occurs in the setting of disseminated herpes zoster and can take the form of encephalitis, aseptic meningitis, cerebellitis, myelitis, and even stroke-like syndromes.[57,67] The classic herpetic rash associated with disseminated VZV may not always be evident.[67] CSF findings include an elevated WBC count with lymphocytic predominance, elevated protein, and a normal glucose.[57] CT imaging is often unremarkable, although MRI may demonstrate ischemic or hemorrhagic lesions. CSF VZV PCR testing should be obtained and is highly sensitive and specific for the diagnosis.[57,65] It is important to note that VZV is highly contagious. Patients with suspicion for disseminated and/or CNS VZV infection should be placed immediately on airborne and contact precautions to protect health care personnel. VZV encephalitis is treated with intravenous acyclovir.

Cytomegalovirus

HIV infection is the most common epidemiologic risk factor for CMV CNS disease, particularly at CD4 counts of less than 50 cells/mm.[3] CMV infection can also be a concern in transplant recipients.[68]

CMV can cause a wide range of neurologic manifestations, including encephalitis, ventriculoencephalitis, retinitis, and polyradiculomyelopathy. The most common signs and symptoms of CNS infection, including lethargy, confusion, and coma, are not specific to CMV encephalitis. Copresentation with non-neurologic CMV disease, such as pneumonitis and colitis, occurs, but is uncommon. In CMV encephalitis, CSF findings may include lymphocytic pleocytosis, normal or slightly elevated protein, and a normal or slightly decreased glucose. CSF PCR for CMV is highly sensitive; in contrast, blood PCR has poor positive and negative predictive values and should not be used to diagnose CNS infection.[34,69] CT scan is often unremarkable in CMV encephalitis and MRI findings are similar to that of other viral encephalitides. However, in ventriculoencephalitis, imaging may show periventricular enhancement suggestive of but not definitive for CMV.[70] The treatment for CMV encephalitis is ganciclovir and/or foscarnet.

Epstein–Barr Virus

Immunocompromised patients are at increased risk of primary CNS lymphoma (PCNSL) associated with Epstein–Barr virus, the same virus responsible for infectious mononucleosis.[71] AIDS is the most important risk factor for PCNSL, particularly when the CD4 count is less than 50 cells/mm.[3,71] PCNSL is seen in SOT patients, although less commonly than in AIDS. As the duration of survival after SOT continues to improve, the annual case numbers for PCNSL are expected to increase.[72] In 1 cases series, 70% of patients with PCNSL presented to care with a focal neurologic deficit, 43% with neuropsychiatric symptoms, 33% with signs of increased intracranial pressure, and 14% with seizures.[73]

On neuroimaging, PCNSL is typically a solitary lesion, but can be multifocal in up to 15% of cases.[73] CT imaging most typically shows a single hyperdense, supratentorial mass that enhances with contrast.[74] However, CT scan, even with contrast, is only 85% sensitive.[75] CSF cell count, protein, and glucose levels are not clinically useful in establishing the diagnosis. CSF PCR for Epstein–Barr virus is approximately 80% specific for PCNSL, but only has a 30% positive predictive value.[76] CSF cytology can be helpful because it is specific but not sensitive for PCNSL.[75] The gold standard diagnostic modality for PCNSL is brain biopsy, so neurosurgical consultation is necessary in these patients.[75] The treatment of PCNSL entails chemotherapy with or without radiation and ART to treat underlying HIV infection when appropriate.

JC Virus

The overwhelming majority of human infections with JC virus occur during childhood followed by latency in the kidneys and lymphoid organs.[77] When a patient is immunosuppressed, reactivation of JC virus can lead to progressive multifocal leukoencephalopathy (PML), a demyelinating disease. Hematologic malignancies (leukemia) and lymphoma are the most common risk factors associated with PML.[78,79] In patients living with HIV, PML occurs most commonly in patients with CD4 counts of less than 200 cells/mm[3].[80,81] For those starting ART, rapid HIV viral suppression accompanied by CD4 lymphocyte recovery can result in immune reconstitution inflammatory syndrome weeks to months later with paradoxic worsening of preexisting infections, including JC virus, resulting in PML as well.

PML classically presents with a variable, subacute decrease in neurologic function accompanied by mixed focal deficits.[82] CT imaging may demonstrate areas of hypo-attenuation in the periventricular and subcortical white matter; MRI will show multi-focal white matter lesions in the same regions with little or no mass effect. CSF findings are characterized by elevated protein levels with normal glucose and WBC count.[82] CSF PCR for JC virus is the preferred test to confirm the diagnosis. In the ED, PML is a diagnosis of exclusion. The management of PML is centered on treating the underlying immunocompromised state from HIV infection with ART and decreasing or discontinuing existing immunosuppressive therapies a patient may be receiving.

Empiric Antiviral Therapy for Central Nervous System Infection in the Immunocompromised Patient

Initial empiric antiviral therapy for immunocompromised patients presenting to the ED with suspected viral CNS infection should cover HSV encephalitis. Intravenous acyclovir is therefore recommended in combination with broad-spectrum antibacterial therapy described previously.

FUNGAL INFECTION

Fungal pathogens frequently associated with CNS infection in the immunocompromised are summarized in **Table 3**.

Cryptococcus

Cryptococcus neoformans is one of the most common causes of opportunistic CNS infection in patients with HIV, particularly when the CD4 count is less than 100 cells/mm^3 and in the setting of immune reconstitution inflammatory syndrome after the initiation of ART. Up to 3% of SOT recipients develop cryptococcal disease, of which 52% to 61% have CNS involvement.[83] Approximately 70% of cases occur more than 1 year after transplantation. Other risk factors for cryptococcal disease include immunosuppression with calcineurin-inhibiting agents and glucocorticoids.

The classic presentation of cryptococcal infection is a subacute meningoencephalitis with slowly progressive fever, headache, and fatigue. Some patients experience meningismus and photophobia. Approximately 47% of patients will have a normal head CT scan, although a subset of patients may exhibit infectious granulomas (cryptococcomas) with mass effect. MRI may reveal leptomeningeal enhancement and pseudocyst.[84] CSF findings are often only mildly abnormal with subtle changes. Opening pressure is elevated above 25 cm H_2O in 60% to 80% of patients and is associated with more severe neurologic symptoms and a greater fungal burden.[85,86] This increased intracranial pressure is due to obstruction of the arachnoid villi by fungal polysaccharide. Cryptococcal polysaccharide serum antigen testing is extremely sensitive and should be obtained in these patients; CSF antigen testing is both sensitive and specific.[83] Initial induction therapy to treat cryptococcal meningoencephalitis begins with a combination of liposomal amphotericin B and flucytosine to rapidly sterilize the CSF, to be followed by consolidation with other antifungal agents.

Endemic Mycoses

Histoplasma capsulatum and *Coccidioides immitis* typically present as pulmonary disease, but can also cause CNS infection in immunocompromised patients. In patients

Table 3
Fungal pathogens and parasites implicated in CNS disease in immunocompromised patients and associated clinical findings

Pathogen	Typical CNS Syndrome	Typical CT Findings	Typical/Important CSF Findings
Fungal			
Endemic mycoses H capsulatum C immitis	Meningitis	Unremarkable	Protein high, glucose low Lymphocytic pleocytosis Slow growing in culture (weeks) Urine antigen highly sensitive
Candida spp.	Encephalopathy (microabscesses) Meningitis Brain abscess	Unremarkable (except in the case of brain abscess)	Unremarkable
Cryptococcus spp.	Meningoencephalitis	Unremarkable Cryptococcomas (less common)	Elevated opening pressure Elevated protein, glucose decreased Lymphocytic pleocytosis Positive cryptococcal antigen
Aspergillus spp.	Focal neurologic deficit Stroke-like symptoms	Brain abscess	Poorly described in the literature
Parasites			
Toxoplasma gondii	Focal encephalitis	Multiple contrast-enhancing lesions	CSF T gondii PCR is nonsensitive
Strongyloides stercoralis	Meningitis	Limited (may demonstrate abscesses or meningeal enhancement)	Lymphocytic pleocytosis Elevated protein, normal glucose

with HIV infection, CNS histoplasmosis is more common when the CD4 count is less than 150 cells/mm³; coccidioidomycosis with CNS involvement typically manifests at CD4 counts of less than 250 cells/mm³.[34] In SOT patients, CNS infection owing to endemic mycoses occurs in approximately 0.2% of patients, with a median time to onset of 12 months after transplantation.[87]

CNS disease stemming from endemic mycoses present as meningitis and may be challenging to distinguish from bacterial meningitis. Common symptoms include fever, headache, focal neurologic deficits, and altered mental status. Concomitant pulmonary disease may also be present.[34] CT imaging is often unrevealing. CSF studies include a WBC count with a lymphocytic predominance, elevated protein, and low glucose.[88] Cultures are positive in less than 40% of cases of cases.[89] A urine *Histoplasma* antigen assay has been shown to be highly sensitive for the diagnosis of disseminated histoplasmosis, although its sensitivity is less clear in more limited disease.[90] Liposomal amphotericin B is recommended for the treatment of CNS histoplasmosis. Fluconazole is the treatment of choice for coccidioidal meningitis.

Candida

Candida spp rarely cause invasive disease of the CNS. HSCT recipients are particularly at high risk for developing CNS candidiasis, as are patients with prolonged indwelling venous catheters. Patients with AIDS, despite frequently having oropharyngeal candidiasis, rarely develop invasive disease. *Candida* endocarditis, more common in the setting injection drug use, can result in septic embolization to the CNS leading to abscess formation.[91]

The most common presentation of CNS candidiasis is a nonspecific encephalopathy without focal findings secondary to multiple cerebral microabscesess. CSF and neuroimaging are typically not contributory. This form is often mistaken for other causes of encephalopathy with a diagnosis made at autopsy. Another subset of patients presents with meningitis, characterized by subacute onset of headache and fever. CSF classically demonstrates a lymphocyte predominance with elevated protein and low glucose; *Candida* is readily isolated in fungal culture in 80% of cases.[91] Less commonly, CNS candidiasis can take the form of cerebral macroabscesses identified on neuroimaging. Finally, *Candida* septic embolization can lead to vascular complications, including stroke, intracranial hemorrhage, and mycotic aneurysms, accounting for up to 23% of patients with CNS candidiasis.[91] CNS candidiasis is best treated initially with liposomal amphotericin B with or without flucytosine. Echinocandins (eg, micafungin) do not penetrate the CNS adequately and should not be used to treat CNS candidiasis.

Aspergillus

Invasive *Aspergillus* of the CNS has devastatingly poor outcomes, with a 99% mortality rate reported in the literature.[92] Patients with hematologic malignancy and bone marrow transplant account for approximately 45% and 25% of all aspergillosis cases, respectively.[93] SOT of the cardiopulmonary system are associated with significantly greater risk of aspergillosis than liver or kidney transplant; HIV/AIDS accounts for only about 4% of cases.[93]

Aspergillus usually invades the CNS directly from sinuses or the middle ear, leading to abscesses of the frontal or temporal lobe. This condition can present with either focal neurologic deficits or seizures. Hematogenous seeding of the CNS can lead to multifocal disease at the gray–white matter junction or angioinvasive disease, leading to stroke and intracranial hemorrhage.[94] In invasive aspergillosis, treatment with voriconazole is associated with improved survival and fewer adverse events than amphotericin.[95]

Empiric Antifungal Therapy for Central Nervous System Infection in the Immunocompromised Patient

The decision to start empiric antifungal therapy in the ED for CNS infection in an immunocompromised patient should be based on the level of concern for cryptococcal meningitis or endemic mycoses. If the suspicion is high for either, initiation of liposomal amphotericin B and flucytosine is reasonable. Liposomal amphotericin B is preferred over other amphotericin B formulations because it achieves superior concentrations in brain tissue.[96]

PARASITIC INFECTIONS

Parasites that can cause CNS infection in the immunocompromised are summarized in **Table 3**.

Toxoplasma gondii

Reactivation of latent *Toxoplasma gondii* can lead to CNS disease in immunocompromised patients previously infected with the parasite, usually from exposure to oocysts in cat litter or undercooked meat.[97,98] In patients living with HIV but not receiving appropriate prophylaxis, neurotoxoplasmosis is most commonly seen at CD4 counts of less than 100 cells/mm^3. Seronegative SOT recipients are at an increased risk for infection because *T gondii* can be transmitted in solid organs from donor to recipient, particularly with heart transplants.[99] Seropositive HSCT recipients approximately 2 to 4 months after transplant and those with graft-versus-host disease carry a higher risk of reactivation disease in the setting of profound immunosuppression.[99,100]

Neurotoxoplasmosis in immunocompromised patients typically manifests as encephalitis, characterized by fever, headache, focal neurologic deficits, altered mental status, and seizures.[101–103] CT imaging most typically shows multiple gray matter lesions, although single lesions or encephalitis without a discrete lesion can occur as well.[104] There is often significant vasogenic edema surrounding these lesions. MRI is more sensitive than CT scan, but is not recommended as a primary diagnostic tool in the ED.[105] CSF PCR for *T gondii* should be obtained but is considered a nonsensitive test and cannot be used to rule out disease.[106,107] Serum IgG antibodies are present in nearly all patients with cerebral toxoplasmosis.[86] Brain biopsy may be required to achieve a definitive diagnosis. Clinically, neurotoxoplasmosis can also resemble PML, PCNSL, or *Mycobacterium tuberculosis* (MTB) infection. Therefore, CSF JC virus PCR, Epstein–Barr virus PCR, cytology, and mycobacterial cultures should also be obtained as part of the evaluation.[108]

The initial antimicrobial therapy for neurotoxoplasmosis is a combination of pyrimethamine, sulfadiazine, and leucovorin. Initiation of this therapy in the ED should be made in consultation with an infectious disease specialist. Steroids can be administered in select patients with edema or mass effect on neuroimaging, although evidence to support this practice is weak and the decision should be considered in coordination with a neurosurgeon. Antiepileptics should be administered in patients presenting with seizure, but are not indicated as prophylaxis.[34]

Strongyloides stercoralis

Infection with the nematode *Strongyloides stercoralis* is common and often asymptomatic and chronic among immunocompetent individuals. Hyperinfection in the setting of immunosuppression can lead to the dissemination of S stercoralis larvae from sites of chronic infection in the lungs and gastrointestinal tract to other organs including the CNS, resulting in meningitis. Although corticosteroid therapy is a key risk factor for disseminated infection, cytotoxic drugs and immunosuppression for SOT and HSCT also pose a significant risk. Although S stercoralis hyperinfection was previously considered an AIDS-defining condition, cases described in the literature largely occurred in the setting of initiation of ART and subsequent immune reconstitution. As such, HIV is likely a less important risk factor.[109] Neuroimaging may demonstrate abscesses and meningeal enhancement.[110] CSF findings include lymphocytic pleocytosis, elevated protein, and normal glucose.[109] Although disseminated strongyloidiasis is treated with ivermectin, empiric therapy in the ED is not recommended without the involvement of an infectious disease specialist.

MYCOBACTERIAL INFECTIONS
Mycobacterium tuberculosis

MTB is a highly comorbid pathogen with HIV infection. Meningitis owing to MTB presents initially with nonspecific headache, fevers, and malaise; progresses to meningismus, lethargy, and confusion; and culminates in a paralytic phase with coma, seizures, and death.[111] Decisions to send CSF specimens for acid-fast bacillus smear and mycobacterial culture from the ED should be based on an assessment of traditional patient risk factors for MTB (eg, close contact with a known MTB case, prolonged exposure in an endemic region, institutional living situation, immunosuppression) and consultation with an infectious disease specialist. CSF findings are variable and mycobacterial culture has poor sensitivity. Current CSF nucleic acid amplification tests for MTB are not approved by the US Food and Drug Administration and are not readily available, despite high specificity and negative predictive value.[112] A diagnosis of MTB meningitis is likely to require inpatient admission; empiric MTB treatment in the ED is generally not recommended or warranted given the subacute nature of this infection.

SUMMARY

Immunocompromised patients with CNS infection presenting to ED care require a broad diagnostic workup, with a low threshold to perform neuroimaging and LP for CSF testing. A greater understanding of the differential diagnosis for CNS infection unique to specific patient populations can help inform ED evaluation for bacterial, viral, fungal, parasitic, and mycobacterial pathogens. Empiric broad-spectrum antibiotic therapy in the ED should include coverage of common bacterial pathogens (S pneumoniae, N meningitidis, and H influenzae) and L monocytogenes. If encephalitis is a concern, the addition of empiric antiviral therapy to cover HSV is recommended. Early involvement of an infectious disease consultant and other specialists familiar with the patient's immunocompromised state can further guide care and inform assessment and treatment for less common CNS infections owing to fungi, parasites, and mycobacteria.

DISCLOSURE

R.J. Stephens and S.Y. Liang have no conflicts of interest to disclose. S.Y. Liang received support through the Foundation for Barnes-Jewish Hospital and the Washington University Institute of Clinical and Translational Sciences which is, in part, supported by the NIH/National Center for Advancing Translational Sciences (NCATS), Clinical and Translational Science Award (CTSA) program (UL1TR002345).

REFERENCES

1. Tai E, Guy GP, Dunbar A, et al. Cost of cancer-related neutropenia or fever hospitalizations, United States, 2012. J Oncol Pract 2017;13(6):e552–61.
2. Fishman JA. Infection in organ transplantation. Am J Transpl 2017;17(4):856–79.
3. Majhail NS, Tao L, Bredeson C, et al. Prevalence of hematopoietic cell transplant survivors in the United States. Biol Blood Marrow Transpl 2013;19(10):1498–501.
4. Harris NS, Johnson AS, Huang YA, et al. Vital signs: status of human immunodeficiency virus testing, viral suppression, and HIV preexposure prophylaxis - United States, 2013-2018. MMWR Morb Mortal Wkly Rep 2019;68(48):1117–23.
5. Estimated HIV incidence and prevalence in the United States, 2014–2018. HIV Surveill Supplemental Rep 2020;25(1):1–77.
6. McNamara LA, Topaz N, Wang X, et al. High risk for invasive meningococcal disease among patients receiving eculizumab (Soliris) despite receipt of meningococcal vaccine. MMWR Morb Mortal Wkly Rep 2017;66(27):734–7.
7. Cuzzubbo S, Javeri F, Tissier M, et al. Neurological adverse events associated with immune checkpoint inhibitors: review of the literature. Eur J Cancer 2017;73:1–8.
8. van Veen KE, Brouwer MC, van der Ende A, et al. Bacterial meningitis in hematopoietic stem cell transplant recipients: a population-based prospective study. Bone Marrow Transpl 2016;51(11):1490–5.
9. van Veen KE, Brouwer MC, van der Ende A, et al. Bacterial meningitis in patients with HIV: a population-based prospective study. J Infect 2016;72(3):362–8.
10. van Veen KE, Brouwer MC, van der Ende A, et al. Bacterial meningitis in solid organ transplant recipients: a population-based prospective study. Transpl Infect Dis 2016;18(5):674–80.
11. Takhar SS, Ting SA, Camargo CA Jr, et al. U.S. emergency department visits for meningitis, 1993-2008. Acad Emerg Med 2012;19(6):632–9.
12. Levy RM, Bredesen DE, Rosenblum ML. Neurological manifestations of the acquired immunodeficiency syndrome (AIDS): experience at UCSF and review of the literature. J Neurosurg 1985;62(4):475–95.
13. van de Beek D, Patel R, Daly RC, et al. Central nervous system infections in heart transplant recipients. Arch Neurol 2007;64(12):1715–20.
14. Hanajiri R, Kobayashi T, Yoshioka K, et al. Central nervous system infection following allogeneic hematopoietic stem cell transplantation. Hematol Oncol Stem Cell Ther 2017;10(1):22–8.
15. Khatib U, van de Beek D, Lees JA, et al. Adults with suspected central nervous system infection: a prospective study of diagnostic accuracy. J Infect 2017;74(1):1–9.
16. Waghdhare S, Kalantri A, Joshi R, et al. Accuracy of physical signs for detecting meningitis: a hospital-based diagnostic accuracy study. Clin Neurol Neurosurg 2010;112(9):752–7.
17. Dorsett M, Liang SY. Diagnosis and treatment of central nervous system infections in the emergency department. Emerg Med Clin North Am 2016;34(4):917–42.

18. Brouwer MC, Coutinho JM, van de Beek D. Clinical characteristics and outcome of brain abscess: systematic review and meta-analysis. Neurology 2014;82(9): 806–13.

19. Nicolosi A, Hauser WA, Musicco M, et al. Incidence and prognosis of brain abscess in a defined population: Olmsted County, Minnesota, 1935-1981. Neuroepidemiology 1991;10(3):122–31.

20. Santosh V, Mahadevan A, Chickabasaviah YT, et al. Infectious lesions mimicking central nervous system neoplasms. Semin Diagn Pathol 2010;27(2):122–35.

21. Gopal AK, Whitehouse JD, Simel DL, et al. Cranial computed tomography before lumbar puncture: a prospective clinical evaluation. Arch Intern Med 1999;159(22):2681–5.

22. Hasbun R, Abrahams J, Jekel J, et al. Computed tomography of the head before lumbar puncture in adults with suspected meningitis. N Engl J Med 2001; 345(24):1727–33.

23. Skiest DJ. Focal neurological disease in patients with acquired immunodeficiency syndrome. Clin Infect Dis 2002;34(1):103–15.

24. Tan IL, Smith BR, von Geldern G, et al. HIV-associated opportunistic infections of the CNS. Lancet Neurol 2012;11(7):605–17.

25. Venkatesan A, Tunkel AR, Bloch KC, et al. Case definitions, diagnostic algorithms, and priorities in encephalitis: consensus statement of the international encephalitis consortium. Clin Infect Dis 2013;57(8):1114–28.

26. Koster-Rasmussen R, Korshin A, Meyer CN. Antibiotic treatment delay and outcome in acute bacterial meningitis. J Infect 2008;57(6):449–54.

27. Bodilsen J, Dalager-Pedersen M, Schonheyder HC, et al. Time to antibiotic therapy and outcome in bacterial meningitis: a Danish population-based cohort study. BMC Infect Dis 2016;16:392.

28. Kanegaye JT, Soliemanzadeh P, Bradley JS. Lumbar puncture in pediatric bacterial meningitis: defining the time interval for recovery of cerebrospinal fluid pathogens after parenteral antibiotic pretreatment. Pediatrics 2001;108(5): 1169–74.

29. Grindborg O, Naucler P, Sjolin J, et al. Adult bacterial meningitis-a quality registry study: earlier treatment and favourable outcome if initial management by infectious diseases physicians. Clin Microbiol Infect 2015;21(6):560–6.

30. Crawford J, Dale DC, Lyman GH. Chemotherapy-induced neutropenia: risks, consequences, and new directions for its management. Cancer 2004;100(2): 228–37.

31. Li Y, Klippel Z, Shih X, et al. Trajectory of absolute neutrophil counts in patients treated with pegfilgrastim on the day of chemotherapy versus the day after chemotherapy. Cancer Chemother Pharmacol 2016;77(4):703–12.

32. Fishman JA. Infection in solid-organ transplant recipients. N Engl J Med 2007; 357(25):2601–14.

33. Maartens G, Celum C, Lewin SR. HIV infection: epidemiology, pathogenesis, treatment, and prevention. Lancet 2014;384(9939):258–71.

34. Masur H, Brooks JT, Benson CA, et al. Prevention and treatment of opportunistic infections in HIV-infected adults and adolescents: updated guidelines from the Centers for Disease Control and Prevention, National Institutes of Health, and HIV Medicine Association of the Infectious Diseases Society of America. Clin Infect Dis 2014;58(9):1308–11.

35. Lee DW, Gardner R, Porter DL, et al. Current concepts in the diagnosis and management of cytokine release syndrome. Blood 2014;124(2):188–95.

36. Gane E, Saliba F, Valdecasas GJ, et al. Randomised trial of efficacy and safety of oral ganciclovir in the prevention of cytomegalovirus disease in liver-transplant recipients. The Oral Ganciclovir International Transplantation Study Group [corrected]. Lancet 1997;350(9093):1729-33.

37. Lowance D, Neumayer HH, Legendre CM, et al. Valacyclovir for the prevention of cytomegalovirus disease after renal transplantation. International Valacyclovir Cytomegalovirus Prophylaxis Transplantation Study Group. N Engl J Med 1999; 340(19):1462-70.

38. Peleg AY, Husain S, Qureshi ZA, et al. Risk factors, clinical characteristics, and outcome of Nocardia infection in organ transplant recipients: a matched case-control study. Clin Infect Dis 2007;44(10):1307-14.

39. Coussement J, Lebeaux D, van Delden C, et al. Nocardia infection in solid organ transplant recipients: a multicenter European case-control study. Clin Infect Dis 2016;63(3):338-45.

40. Thigpen MC, Whitney CG, Messonnier NE, et al. Bacterial meningitis in the United States, 1998-2007. N Engl J Med 2011;364(21):2016-25.

41. Castelblanco RL, Lee M, Hasbun R. Epidemiology of bacterial meningitis in the USA from 1997 to 2010: a population-based observational study. Lancet Infect Dis 2014;14(9):813-9.

42. Tunkel AR, Hartman BJ, Kaplan SL, et al. Practice guidelines for the management of bacterial meningitis. Clin Infect Dis 2004;39(9):1267-84.

43. McGill F, Heyderman RS, Michael BD, et al. The UK joint specialist societies guideline on the diagnosis and management of acute meningitis and meningococcal sepsis in immunocompetent adults. J Infect 2016;72(4):405-38.

44. Tunkel AR, Hasbun R, Bhimraj A, et al. 2017 Infectious Diseases Society of America's Clinical Practice Guidelines for healthcare-associated ventriculitis and meningitis. Clin Infect Dis 2017;64(6):e34-65.

45. de Gans J, van de Beek D. European dexamethasone in adulthood bacterial meningitis study I. Dexamethasone in adults with bacterial meningitis. N Engl J Med 2002;347(20):1549-56.

46. Charlier C, Perrodeau E, Leclercq A, et al. Clinical features and prognostic factors of listeriosis: the MONALISA national prospective cohort study. Lancet Infect Dis 2017;17(5):510-9.

47. Brouwer MC, van de Beek D, Heckenberg SG, et al. Community-acquired Listeria monocytogenes meningitis in adults. Clin Infect Dis 2006;43(10):1233-8.

48. Mylonakis E, Hohmann EL, Calderwood SB. Central nervous system infection with Listeria monocytogenes. 33 years' experience at a general hospital and review of 776 episodes from the literature. Medicine (Baltimore) 1998;77(5): 313-36.

49. Charlier C, Poiree S, Delavaud C, et al. Imaging of human neurolisteriosis: a prospective study of 71 cases. Clin Infect Dis 2018;67(9):1419-26.

50. Thonnings S, Knudsen JD, Schonheyder HC, et al. Antibiotic treatment and mortality in patients with Listeria monocytogenes meningitis or bacteraemia. Clin Microbiol Infect 2016;22(8):725-30.

51. Beaman BL, Beaman L. Nocardia species: host-parasite relationships. Clin Microbiol Rev 1994;7(2):213-64.

52. Nwuba CO, Kogo G, Ogbu N, et al. Nocardiosis - an emerging complication in the clinical management of HIV infected patients. Retrovirology 2012;9(Suppl 1): P134.

53. McNeil MM, Brown JM. The medically important aerobic actinomycetes: epidemiology and microbiology. Clin Microbiol Rev 1994;7(3):357-417.

54. Chow FC, Marson A, Liu C. Successful medical management of a Nocardia far-cinica multiloculated pontine abscess. BMJ Case Rep 2013;2013. bcr2013201308.
55. Restrepo A, Clark NM, Infectious Diseases Community of Practice of the American Society of Transplantation. Nocardia infections in solid organ transplantation: guidelines from the Infectious Diseases Community of Practice of the American Society of Transplantation. Clin Transpl 2019;33(9):e13509.
56. Brown-Elliott BA, Biehle J, Conville PS, et al. Sulfonamide resistance in isolates of Nocardia spp. from a US multicenter survey. J Clin Microbiol 2012;50(3): 670–2.
57. Grahn A, Studahl M. Varicella-zoster virus infections of the central nervous system - prognosis, diagnostics and treatment. J Infect 2015;71(3):281–93.
58. Levitz RE. Herpes simplex encephalitis: a review. Heart Lung 1998;27(3): 209–12.
59. Noska A, Kyrillos R, Hansen G, et al. The role of antiviral therapy in immunocompromised patients with herpes simplex virus meningitis. Clin Infect Dis 2015; 60(2):237–42.
60. Fisher CM. Hypomanic symptoms caused by herpes simplex encephalitis. Neurology 1996;47(6):1374–8.
61. Marlowe WB, Mancall EL, Thomas JJ. Complete Kluver-Bucy syndrome in man. Cortex 1975;11(1):53–9.
62. Tyler KL. Herpes simplex virus infections of the central nervous system: encephalitis and meningitis, including Mollaret's. Herpes 2004;11(Suppl 2):57A–64A.
63. Tunkel AR, Glaser CA, Bloch KC, et al. The management of encephalitis: clinical practice guidelines by the Infectious Diseases Society of America. Clin Infect Dis 2008;47(3):303–27.
64. Zimmerman RD, Russell EJ, Leeds NE, et al. CT in the early diagnosis of herpes simplex encephalitis. AJR Am J Roentgenol 1980;134(1):61–6.
65. Kang M, Aslam S. Varicella zoster virus encephalitis in solid organ transplant recipients: case series and review of literature. Transpl Infect Dis 2019;21(2): e13038.
66. Koc Y, Miller KB, Schenkein DP, et al. Varicella zoster virus infections following allogeneic bone marrow transplantation: frequency, risk factors, and clinical outcome. Biol Blood Marrow Transpl 2000;6(1):44–9.
67. Pahud BA, Glaser CA, Dekker CL, et al. Varicella zoster disease of the central nervous system: epidemiological, clinical, and laboratory features 10 years after the introduction of the varicella vaccine. J Infect Dis 2011;203(3):316–23.
68. Maschke M, Dietrich U, Prumbaum M, et al. Opportunistic CNS infection after bone marrow transplantation. Bone Marrow Transpl 1999;23(11):1167–76.
69. Arribas JR, Clifford DB, Fichtenbaum CJ, et al. Level of cytomegalovirus (CMV) DNA in cerebrospinal fluid of subjects with AIDS and CMV infection of the central nervous system. J Infect Dis 1995;172(2):527–31.
70. Brooks JT, Kaplan JE, Masur H. What's new in the 2009 US guidelines for prevention and treatment of opportunistic infections among adults and adolescents with HIV? Top HIV Med 2009;17(3):109–14.
71. Pluda JM, Venzon DJ, Tosato G, et al. Parameters affecting the development of non-Hodgkin's lymphoma in patients with severe human immunodeficiency virus infection receiving antiretroviral therapy. J Clin Oncol 1993;11(6):1099–107.
72. Chou AP, Lalezari S, Fong BM, et al. Post-transplantation primary central nervous system lymphoma: a case report and review of the literature. Surg Neurol Int 2011;2:130.

73. Bataille B, Delwail V, Menet E, et al. Primary intracerebral malignant lymphoma: report of 248 cases. J Neurosurg 2000;92(2):261–6.
74. Schwaighofer BW, Hesselink JR, Press GA, et al. Primary intracranial CNS lymphoma: MR manifestations. AJNR Am J Neuroradiol 1989;10(4):725–9.
75. Scott BJ, Douglas VC, Tihan T, et al. A systematic approach to the diagnosis of suspected central nervous system lymphoma. JAMA Neurol 2013;70(3):311–9.
76. Ivers LC, Kim AY, Sax PE. Predictive value of polymerase chain reaction of cerebrospinal fluid for detection of Epstein-Barr virus to establish the diagnosis of HIV-related primary central nervous system lymphoma. Clin Infect Dis 2004; 38(11):1629–32.
77. Weber T, Trebst C, Frye S, et al. Analysis of the systemic and intrathecal humoral immune response in progressive multifocal leukoencephalopathy. J Infect Dis 1997;176(1):250–4.
78. Sipila JOT, Soilu-Hanninen M, Rautava P, et al. Progressive multifocal leukoencephalopathy in Finland: a cross-sectional registry study. J Neurol 2019; 266(2):515–21.
79. Iacobaeus E, Burkill S, Bahmanyar S, et al. The national incidence of PML in Sweden, 1988-2013. Neurology 2018;90(6):e498–506.
80. Fong IW, Britton CB, Luinstra KE, et al. Diagnostic value of detecting JC virus DNA in cerebrospinal fluid of patients with progressive multifocal leukoencephalopathy. J Clin Microbiol 1995;33(2):484–6.
81. Berger JR, Pall L, Lanska D, et al. Progressive multifocal leukoencephalopathy in patients with HIV infection. J Neurovirol 1998;4(1):59–68.
82. Berger JR, Aksamit AJ, Clifford DB, et al. PML diagnostic criteria: consensus statement from the AAN Neuroinfectious Disease Section. Neurology 2013; 80(15):1430–8.
83. Perfect JR, Dismukes WE, Dromer F, et al. Clinical practice guidelines for the management of cryptococcal disease: 2010 update by the Infectious Diseases Society of America. Clin Infect Dis 2010;50(3):291–322.
84. Xia S, Li X, Shi Y, et al. A retrospective cohort study of lesion distribution of HIV-1 infection patients with cryptococcal meningoencephalitis on MRI: correlation with immunity and immune reconstitution. Medicine (Baltimore) 2016;95(6): e2654.
85. Graybill JR, Sobel J, Saag M, et al. Diagnosis and management of increased intracranial pressure in patients with AIDS and cryptococcal meningitis. The NIAID Mycoses Study Group and AIDS Cooperative Treatment Groups. Clin Infect Dis 2000;30(1):47–54.
86. Kaplan JE, Benson C, Holmes KK, et al. Guidelines for prevention and treatment of opportunistic infections in HIV-infected adults and adolescents: recommendations from CDC, the National Institutes of Health, and the HIV Medicine Association of the Infectious Diseases Society of America. MMWR Recomm Rep 2009;58(RR-4):1–207, quiz CE 1–4.
87. Wright AJ, Fishman JA. Central nervous system syndromes in solid organ transplant recipients. Clin Infect Dis 2014;59(7):1001–11.
88. Wheat LJ, Musial CE, Jenny-Avital E. Diagnosis and management of central nervous system histoplasmosis. Clin Infect Dis 2005;40(6):844–52.
89. Wheat J, Myint T, Guo Y, et al. Central nervous system histoplasmosis: multicenter retrospective study on clinical features, diagnostic approach and outcome of treatment. Medicine (Baltimore) 2018;97(13):e0245.
90. Wheat LJ. Approach to the diagnosis of the endemic mycoses. Clin Chest Med 2009;30(2):379–89, viii.

91. Sanchez-Portocarrero J, Perez-Cecilia E, Corral O, et al. The central nervous system and infection by Candida species. Diagn Microbiol Infect Dis 2000; 37(3):169–79.
92. Denning DW. Therapeutic outcome in invasive aspergillosis. Clin Infect Dis 1996;23(3):608–15.
93. Lin SJ, Schranz J, Teutsch SM. Aspergillosis case-fatality rate: systematic review of the literature. Clin Infect Dis 2001;32(3):358–66.
94. Patterson TF, Thompson GR 3rd, Denning DW, et al. Practice guidelines for the diagnosis and management of aspergillosis: 2016 update by the Infectious Diseases Society of America. Clin Infect Dis 2016;63(4):e1–60.
95. Herbrecht R, Denning DW, Patterson TF, et al. Voriconazole versus amphotericin B for primary therapy of invasive aspergillosis. N Engl J Med 2002;347(6):408–15.
96. Groll AH, Giri N, Petraitis V, et al. Comparative efficacy and distribution of lipid formulations of amphotericin B in experimental Candida albicans infection of the central nervous system. J Infect Dis 2000;182(1):274–82.
97. Jones JL, Dargelas V, Roberts J, et al. Risk factors for Toxoplasma gondii infection in the United States. Clin Infect Dis 2009;49(6):878–84.
98. Boyer KM, Holfels E, Roizen N, et al. Risk factors for Toxoplasma gondii infection in mothers of infants with congenital toxoplasmosis: implications for prenatal management and screening. Am J Obstet Gynecol 2005;192(2):564–71.
99. Derouin F, Pelloux H, Parasitology ESGoC. Prevention of toxoplasmosis in transplant patients. Clin Microbiol Infect 2008;14(12):1089–101.
100. Martino R, Maertens J, Bretagne S, et al. Toxoplasmosis after hematopoietic stem cell transplantation. Clin Infect Dis 2000;31(5):1188–95.
101. Luft BJ, Conley F, Remington JS, et al. Outbreak of central-nervous-system toxoplasmosis in Western Europe and North America. Lancet 1983;1(8328):781–4.
102. Luft BJ, Brooks RG, Conley FK, et al. Toxoplasmic encephalitis in patients with acquired immune deficiency syndrome. JAMA 1984;252(7):913–7.
103. Wong B, Gold JW, Brown AE, et al. Central-nervous-system toxoplasmosis in homosexual men and parenteral drug abusers. Ann Intern Med 1984;100(1):36–42.
104. Gray F, Gherardi R, Wingate E, et al. Diffuse "encephalitic" cerebral toxoplasmosis in AIDS. Report of four cases. J Neurol 1989;236(5):273–7.
105. Kupfer MC, Zee CS, Colletti PM, et al. MRI evaluation of AIDS-related encephalopathy: toxoplasmosis vs. lymphoma. Magn Reson Imaging 1990;8(1):51–7.
106. Novati R, Castagna A, Morsica G, et al. Polymerase chain reaction for Toxoplasma gondii DNA in the cerebrospinal fluid of AIDS patients with focal brain lesions. AIDS 1994;8(12):1691–4.
107. Mesquita RT, Ziegler AP, Hiramoto RM, et al. Real-time quantitative PCR in cerebral toxoplasmosis diagnosis of Brazilian human immunodeficiency virus-infected patients. J Med Microbiol 2010;59(Pt 6):641–7.
108. Cinque P, Scarpellini P, Vago L, et al. Diagnosis of central nervous system complications in HIV-infected patients: cerebrospinal fluid analysis by the polymerase chain reaction. AIDS 1997;11(1):1–17.
109. Keiser PB, Nutman TB. Strongyloides stercoralis in the immunocompromised population. Clin Microbiol Rev 2004;17(1):208–17.
110. Walker MD, Zunt JR. Neuroparasitic infections: nematodes. Semin Neurol 2005; 25(3):252–61.
111. Kennedy DH, Fallon RJ. Tuberculous meningitis. JAMA 1979;241(3):264–8.
112. Pormohammad A, Nasiri MJ, McHugh TD, et al. A systematic review and meta-analysis of the diagnostic accuracy of nucleic acid amplification tests for tuberculous meningitis. J Clin Microbiol 2019;57(6):e01113–8.

Functional Seizures

Evie Marcolini, MD[a],*, Benjamin Tolchin, MD, MS[b,c]

KEYWORDS

- PNEA • Psychogenic nonepileptic seizures • PNES • Functional seizures
- Dissociative seizures • Functional neurologic disorders

KEY POINTS

- Functional seizures can look and feel like epileptic seizures, but are distinct in that they are a form of functional neurologic disorder or conversion disorder, with contributing biological, psychological, and social factors. Patients do not consciously produce or "fake" functional seizures.
- The gold standard for distinguishing functional seizures from epileptic seizures is evaluation with long-term video-electroencephalogram (video-EEG) in an epilepsy monitoring unit, showing no epileptiform changes on the EEG immediately before, during, or following typical seizure events. Characteristics of the clinical history and the seizure events themselves are also important in diagnosing functional seizures.
- Untreated functional seizures are associated with significantly elevated mortality and impaired function and quality of life.
- Multiple randomized trials support the efficacy of cognitive behavioral therapy in treating functional seizures, and other forms of psychotherapy, such as mindfulness-based psychotherapy and psychodynamic psychotherapy, may be effective.
- There is no evidence that antiseizure medications provide any benefit in the treatment of functional seizures.

INTRODUCTION

Functional seizures are paroxysmal episodes of altered awareness that may resemble an epileptic seizure, but have no physiologic basis in epilepsy. These attacks are transient, usually involving significant stress, and have been associated with comorbid psychiatric and psychological difficulties, poor quality of life, elevated mortality rates, and frequent use of the health care system.

Multiple names have been used for this disorder, with the goals of accurately describing the pathophysiology, allowing for supportive and productive interaction

[a] Emergency Medicine and Neurology, Geisel School of Medicine, Department of Emergency Medicine, 1 Medical Center Drive, Lebanon, NH 03756, USA; [b] Department of Neurology, Yale School of Medicine, 15 York Street, New Haven, CT 06510, USA; [c] Epilepsy Center of Excellence, VA Connecticut Healthcare System, 950 Campbell Avenue, West Haven, CT 06516, USA
* Corresponding author. Department of Emergency Medicine, 1 Medical Center Drive, Lebanon, NH 03756, USA
E-mail address: emarcolini@gmail.com

Emerg Med Clin N Am 39 (2021) 123–132
https://doi.org/10.1016/j.emc.2020.09.007
0733-8627/21/© 2020 Elsevier Inc. All rights reserved.
emed.theclinics.com

with patients, and dispelling the perception that the patient is "faking" a seizure for alternate gain. The historical term "pseudoseizure" inadvertently created an environment of mistrust between patients and emergency clinicians, and perhaps given the inaccurate impression that the diagnosis itself is fraudulent. This has contributed to patients distrusting clinicians who recommend that psychotherapy is the generally accepted treatment of choice, which only serves to keep patients from successful treatment and improved quality of life.[1] Other terms in use include psychogenic nonepileptic seizure, dissociative seizure, nonepileptic attack disorder, and conversion disorder with attacks or seizures. There is growing recognition that patients and families also find the term "psychogenic" pejorative, leading to a shift away from this terminology and efforts to identify a single unified terminology.[2–5] For the purposes of this review, we use the term "functional seizures," which is acceptable in surveys of patients and clinicians, and accords with the Diagnostic and Statistical Manual of Mental Disorders, 5th Edition (DSM-5), and the broader category of functional neurologic disorders (FND) or conversion disorders.[6] This broader category includes functional seizures, functional movement disorders, functional paralysis, functional cognitive disorders, and other functional disorders The International Classification of Diseases (ICD)-11 uses the term "dissociative" to connote a compartmentalization or detachment of neurologic functioning from normal awareness. For the first time in the history of the ICD, FNDs were placed in the neurology section instead of the psychiatry section.[7] This is groundbreaking in that it will allow neurologists to make functional seizures a positive diagnosis instead of a diagnosis of exclusion. It will also provide a stimulus for research, endorse a nomenclature that will allow for constructive patient-physician encounters, and give patients access to innovative treatments, such as specialist neurologic physiotherapy.

Functional seizures are a common and especially disabling type of FND, and in keeping with the biopsychosocial model of mental illness, are thought to have contributing biological, psychological, and social factors. Contributing psychological factors include severe adverse life events (such as neglect, abuse, and other psychological traumas), which are identified in 91% of people with FNDs.[8] Functional MRI (fMRI) studies are beginning to demonstrate potentially predisposing biological factors, including decreased activity in the amygdala during distress conditions and increased resting state functional connectivity between areas of the brain involved in emotion (amygdala) and areas involved in motor planning (precentral gyrus).[9]

FNDs have challenged clinicians and patients alike, due to the perception that a diagnosis without an associated structural cause must have an intentional or willful component, thus placing "blame" on the patient for the disorder. This mind-body dualism has persisted throughout history, and it is generally accepted that FNDs are involuntary, with symptoms occurring even when patients believe themselves to be unobserved. Therefore, functional seizures and other FNDs should be distinguished from disorders that involve conscious production of symptoms such as malingering or factitious disorder.

The DSM-5 includes functional seizures in the category of FND or conversion disorder with the following criteria:

- One or more symptoms of altered voluntary motor or sensory function
- Clinical findings provide evidence of incompatibility between the symptom and recognized neurologic or medical conditions
- The symptom or deficit is not better explained by another medical or mental disorder

- The symptom or deficit causes clinically significant distress or impairment in social, occupational, or other important areas of functioning or warrants medical evaluation

Of note, the DSM-5 does not include a requirement that an adverse life event or other psychological stressor be identified to make the diagnosis of functional seizures or other FND.[6] This is important because psychological stressors are often not identified by clinicians or patients until extensive psychotherapy is completed. Historically, the average delay to diagnosis of functional seizures has been 7 to 10 years.[10] In that time, the impact to the patient and family can be devastating, including multiple hospital admissions, failed medication trials with concomitant side effects, social ostracization, lost wages, depression, and increased mortality. Therefore, in cases of suspected functional seizures, it is critical to actively seek supporting evidence through neurologic evaluation and video electroencephalography (vEEG). Diagnosis should not be delayed until a psychological stressor is identified or until all other possible diagnoses are definitively ruled out.

EPIDEMIOLOGY

There are an estimated 2 to 33 patients with functional seizures per 100,000 persons annually.[11] However, this relatively small number of patients has frequent recurrent contact with the health care system: functional seizures are diagnosed in 25% of all patients evaluated in epilepsy monitoring units and FND more generally are diagnosed in 16% of patients evaluated in neurology clinics.[12,13] The diagnosis of functional seizures can be challenging, with significant overlap; 12% of people with epilepsy also have functional seizures and 22% of people with functional seizures also have epilepsy.[14]

Most patients with functional seizures are female, with initial presentation in the late teens to early twenties.[15] They typically have a history of trauma or psychological stressors, such as sexual or physical abuse, neglect, and social or family conflict.[16] Because this is a difficult diagnosis affected by clinical presentation, clinician and patient perceptions and lack of access or willingness to pursue psychotherapeutic treatment, most patients presenting to the emergency department (ED) with functional seizures have had multiple related visits and hospital admissions, and have been unsuccessfully treated with antiseizure medications.[10]

The costs of functional seizures are real and devastating for patients, families, and society. In a study of more than 5000 patients diagnosed with vEEG monitoring, mortality for patients with functional seizures was 2.5 times that of the general population, not significantly different from that of patients with drug-resistant epilepsy, and 8.3 times higher in those younger than 30 years.[17] Notably, 20% of deaths in those younger than 50 years were attributed to suicide. Quality of life associated with functional seizures is worse than quality of life in epilepsy, fraught with avoidance of emotions, poor management of internal anger, depression, and dysfunctional family life.[18] Patients with functional seizures have higher health-related social welfare costs, and lower levels of employment. The diagnosis also has a significant impact on partners and family.[19] In a cohort of 698 adults with functional seizures, 67% of patients were unemployed, 56% were receiving disability payments, and more than half lived in economically deprived areas at the time of diagnosis.[20]

EVALUATION

Because a delay in diagnosis predicts worse outcomes, functional seizures should be part of the differential diagnosis for seizure and considered with respect to history, clinical presentation, and EEG if available and appropriate. The International League Against Epilepsy offers guidelines for diagnosing functional seizures with increasing levels of diagnostic certainty on the basis of clinical history, EEG findings, and semiology (what the seizures look and feel like).[21] The diagnosis of functional seizures can be categorized as *possible* if patient or witness reported the event with typical functional seizure semiology, *probable* if a clinician witnessed the event in person or by video, *clinically established* if an experienced epileptologist witnessed an event that was also captured on EEG, or *documented* if an experienced epileptologist witnessed an event with typical functional seizure semiology while the patient was on vEEG to disprove epileptiform activity.[21]

Any seizure event can be broadly categorized as epileptic seizure, functional seizures, or physiologic nonepileptic events, such as a convulsive syncope, hypoglycemic seizure, transient ischemic attack, stroke, sleep disorders, transient global amnesia, and/or migraine. Accurate diagnosis is important to reduce the risk of delayed diagnosis, and to give the patient an opportunity for improved quality of life. The gold standard diagnostic test is vEEG, which is not always available.[21]

HISTORY

In addition to demographic characteristics of patients with functional seizures, other historic and clinical evidence make functional seizures a more likely diagnosis than epileptic seizure. Seventy percent to 80% of people with functional seizures are female, 80% to 90% have additional psychiatric comorbidities, and most have a history of adverse life events.[22] Patients with functional seizures may report a precipitating event such as trauma including mild traumatic brain injury or concussion (75%) or sexual trauma (40%). Patients with functional seizures tend to have a higher frequency of events and recurrent associated hospital admissions. Functional seizures may be triggered by a stressful situation, or medical situation such as a computed tomography scan or EEG. The disorder in general may be triggered by surgery or physical trauma, and up to 40% of patients may exhibit a partial or transient response to antiseizure medications.[21]

In one study, patients who had at least 2 events per week, were not responsive to 2 antiseizure medications, and had 2 normal EEG studies showed 85% positive predictive value for functional seizures.[23] A history of fibromyalgia or chronic pain in a patient presenting for evaluation of seizures also carries a positive predictive value of 75% for functional seizures.[24] Of note, no single historical feature is 100% sensitive or specific for functional seizures. Rather, clusters of multiple historical features can make functional seizures more or less likely.

SEMIOLOGY

A functional seizure is more likely to be hyperkinetic, similar to an epileptic seizure, but less commonly can be hypokinetic, similar to a vasovagal or cardiac syncope event. In the hyperkinetic event, there is typically eye closure, fluctuating movements, asynchronous movements of different body parts, pelvic thrusting, side to side head or body movement, closed eyes, partially retained awareness, ictal crying, and prolonged duration (≥ 2 minutes). One of the most specific discriminatory signs is ictal crying, which can occur during or after the event, may be complex and affective, differentiated from an epileptic seizure in which and ictal cry occurs at the beginning of the event, and is primitive in nature with no emotional expression.[21] As with historical features, no semiological feature is 100% sensitive or specific for functional seizures. Although rare, frontal lobe epileptic seizures can present with many of the characteristics typical of functional seizures, including pelvic thrusting, opisthotonic posturing, bicycling movements, and asynchronous movements. This reinforces the requirement for vEEG for definitive diagnosis.

During a functional seizure, ictal heart rate is typically appropriate for the level of physical activity noted during the event, as opposed to an epileptic seizure, that can have a rapid as well as a rapid increase in heart rate during the seizure.

It is important to note that patients should not be subjected to aggressive or harmful stimuli such as aggressive sternal rub, exposure to ammonia capsules, or other painful stimuli in order to "differentiate" between an epileptic and functional seizure.[1,25] Patients with functional seizures have a high likelihood of traumatic events including abuse, and the aggressive infliction of pain and/or noxious stimulus is not diagnostically helpful, and only serves to potentially create distrust and fear.[26]

LABORATORY FINDINGS

A rise in serum prolactin level to twice normal, if drawn within 20 minutes of the event and compared with a baseline level can be useful to rule out epileptic generalized tonic-clonic seizure but not focal seizures. The absence of a rise in the prolactin level may suggest functional seizures, but not with great sensitivity or specificity, and in particular cannot rule out a focal epileptic seizure. Some have investigated serum white blood cell count, cortisol levels, creatinine kinase, neuron-specific enolase, and dexamethasone suppression testing to identify functional seizures, but none has proven to be sensitive or specific in the diagnosis.[21]

IMAGING

Although there is a growing body of evidence that research protocol MRI can identify subtle functional and structural differences between groups of people with functional seizures and groups of healthy controls, such techniques are not yet clinically useful in diagnosing individual patients.[9,27] At this time, clinical imaging findings cannot be used in the clinical diagnosis or exclusion of functional seizures.

NEUROPHYSIOLOGY

EEG is the gold standard for the diagnosis of functional seizures. The diagnosis of even *possible* functional seizures requires at minimum a routine EEG, obtained interictally (between seizure events), without epileptiform abnormalities, such as sharp and slow-wave discharges.[21] More extensive EEG data can support a greater level of diagnostic certainty, such as *clinically established* or *documented* functional seizures. In particular, to make the most definitive diagnosis of documented functional seizures, it is necessary capture of all typical seizure events without epileptiform abnormalities immediately before, during, or following seizures. In many cases, normal awake brain electrical activity, including a normal posterior dominant rhythm, can be seen during impaired or lost consciousness in functional seizures. Important caveats to keep in mind include frontal lobe epileptic seizures, and focal seizures without impaired awareness, both of which can appear to have no epileptiform correlate on surface EEG. In such cases, it is necessary for experienced neurologists to make the diagnosis solely on the basis of clinical history and semiology. For example, frontal lobe epileptic seizures can be distinguished from functional seizures because frontal lobe seizures are usually much shorter than functional seizures (<30 seconds rather than ≥ 2 minutes), stereotyped (with similar movements occurring in each seizure), with bicycling movements and dystonic posturing of the arms and legs, and frequently occur during sleep.[28]

Extended vEEG evaluations are often accomplished during an extended elective admission in an epilepsy monitoring unit. For patients whose episodes are so infrequent as to make evaluation in an epilepsy monitoring unit difficult or impossible (usually less than 1 seizure per 2 weeks), other modalities of evaluation are under development. Single-channel electromyography (EMG) obtained at home over weeks or months through a wearable device, has shown some promise in distinguishing functional seizures from focal and generalized epileptic seizures, but is not yet widely clinically available.[29]

THERAPEUTIC OPTIONS

The first step in a successful treatment plan for the patient with functional seizures is to carefully and effectively explain to him or her that this is a neurologic diagnosis, it can be definitively established (with vEEG), and is potentially reversible with treatment.[30] This approach will reassure the patient that he or she is being taken seriously, is not being accused of "faking" symptoms, and that the clinician is invested in helping to improve outcome. Communication of the diagnosis is understandably challenging. Demonstrating sincere compassion and empathy for the patient's experiences, and avoiding an accusing or judgmental demeanor are especially important in delivering a diagnosis of functional seizures. Patients with functional seizures have exceptionally high rates of adverse life events, such as neglect and abuse, contributing to distrust and a feeling that clinicians are not taking them seriously when suggesting that their events are not epileptic seizures.[1] Retrospective studies have shown that a significant number of patients stop having functional seizures when the diagnosis is carefully explained, most notably in those who had recent onset, absence of coexisting anxiety, depression, personality disorder, or abuse history and in those who were employed, and not on state benefits.[31–33]

Most patients diagnosed with or suspected to have functional seizures in the ED will benefit from outpatient neurologic and psychiatric follow-up. Emergency medicine physicians play a vital role in the diagnosis and treatment of patients with functional seizures by avoiding unnecessary and potentially harmful treatments with antiseizure medications, by referring patients for outpatient diagnosis and treatment if the patient does not already have outpatient neurologic and psychiatric care, and by compassionate treatment to support the therapeutic alliance between the patient and their long-term outpatient clinicians.

PSYCHOTHERAPY

The accepted standard of care for a patient with functional seizures includes description of the diagnosis with the patient with family or trusted friends present, weaning the patient from antiseizure medications unless indicated for concomitant epilepsy, and referral to an experienced psychiatrist or psychologist.[34]

In a recent multicenter trial, 313 patients with functional seizures were randomized to functional seizure-specific cognitive behavioral therapy (CBT) plus standardized medical care versus standardized medical care alone. The primary outcome, monthly functional seizure frequency, was not different between the groups (both of which showed significant improvement). However, multiple secondary outcomes did show greater improvement in the CBT group, including less bothersome seizure activity, longer period of functional seizure freedom, better health-related quality of life, less impairment in psychosocial functioning, less overall psychological distress, fewer somatic symptoms, and patient-reported greater clinical improvement and treatment satisfaction.[35] This is the largest randomized study to investigate the effectiveness of any treatment for functional seizures, and its positive findings are supported by 2 smaller prior single center randomized trials.[36,37] The improvement in secondary outcomes gives clinicians impetus to consider outcomes other than seizure frequency as markers of improved outcome. Previous research has shown that quality of life for patients with functional seizures is closely linked to mood, anxiety and illness perceptions.[38] It also encourages researchers to pursue further study in CBT, considering the types of symptoms that patients are having to further stratify the type of psychotherapy that might benefit, as opposed to a "one-size-fits-all" categorization of patients with functional seizures.[39]

If psychotherapy is beneficial to patients with functional seizures, one of the major obstacles has been patient adherence. In a prospective study of 105 patients with functional seizures who were referred to receive psychotherapy, adherence to at least 8 sessions in 16 weeks was associated with a reduction in functional seizure frequency, improved quality of life, and fewer ED visits. Self-identified minority status and a history of child abuse contributed to patient nonadherence.[22] Motivational interviewing, before referral to psychotherapy, has been shown in a randomized trial to improve adherence with psychotherapy, functional seizure frequency, and quality of life.[40]

Psychiatric and psychotherapeutic treatment starts with a formal assessment to exclude other psychiatric disorders. This is best accomplished when the psychiatrist is experienced with functional seizures and part of a team of clinicians.[21]

Although CBT is the most extensively studied psychotherapeutic modality in the treatment of functional seizures, and the only modality supported by evidence from randomized trials, observational studies also support other psychotherapeutic modalities: these include hypnotherapy,[41,42] eye movement desensitization (EMDR),[43] EEG biofeedback,[44] mindfulness-based psychotherapy,[45] and group therapy and/or family therapy.

Randomized trials have not shown consistent benefit of psychopharmaceuticals such as selective serotonin reuptake inhibitors in the treatment of functional seizures, but these and other psychopharmaceuticals may be effective in the treatment of comorbid psychiatric conditions such as mood and anxiety disorders.[36]

It is important to wean patients from antiseizure medications unless they are being administered for concomitant epilepsy, mood or anxiety disorder, or psychiatric diagnosis. A randomized trial has demonstrated that patients benefit more from rapid titration off antiseizure medications at the time of diagnosis than from a prolonged titration over weeks or months.[46]

FUTURE DIRECTIONS

Recent data showing the value of CBT, and the transition of functional seizures as a diagnosis from psychiatry to neurology in the ICD sets the stage for increased involvement of neurology and a collaborative partnership between neurologists, emergency physicians, psychiatrists and psychologists in approaching the patient with functional seizures. Future research may target specific subgroups of patients with functional seizures, using an individualized approach based on their propensity to engage with a particular method. Randomized trials of other psychotherapeutic modalities beyond CBT are needed to guide treatment of functional seizures. The development and testing of effective teletherapy and computerized CBT regimens will be important in providing psychotherapy to patients in areas where specialized expertise in CBT is not widely available.

It has also become apparent that frequency of seizures is only one quality of life indicator, and future research may target other outcomes such as quality of life, psychosocial function, pain, fatigue or other mental health symptoms that accompany this diagnosis.

Other tools such as wearable devices, fMRI for diagnosis, and neurostimulation for treatment are potential avenues that may dramatically expand the diagnosis and treatment of functional seizures in the years to come.

SUMMARY

- The role of the emergency clinician in the diagnosis and treatment of functional seizures includes maintaining a compassionate and nonjudgmental relationship, referring the patient to neurology or psychiatry clinicians and minimizing iatrogenic or psychological harm.

CLINICAL CARE POINTS

- Avoid judgment or minimize the presentation of a patient who presents for seizure, especially if he or she carries a presumed diagnosis of functional seizures
- Do not inflict noxious or painful stimuli to attempt to disprove an event as a seizure
- Understand the potential diagnosis and make an attempt to explain it carefully and nonjudgmentally to the patient, with family present if possible
- Do not attempt to diagnose this in the ED; work in tandem with neurology and psychiatry.
- Working collaboratively with neurology and psychiatry, attempt to wean ineffective medications
- Educate prehospital and emergency medicine learners in this diagnosis, which has a strong history of being misunderstood

DISCLOSURE

No disclosures.

REFERENCES

1. Robson C, Lian OS. Blaming, shaming, humiliation": stigmatizing medical interactions among people with non-epileptic seizures. Wellcome Open Res 2017;2:55.
2. Morgan LA, Dvorchik I, Williams KL, et al. Parental ranking of terms describing nonepileptic events. Pediatr Neurol 2013;48(5):378–82.
3. Sahaya K, Dholakia SA, Lardizabal D, et al. Opinion survey of health care providers towards psychogenic non epileptic seizures. Clin Neurol Neurosurg 2012;114(10):1304–7.
4. Stone J, Campbell K, Sharma N, et al. What should we call pseudoseizures? The patient's perspective. Seizure 2003;12(8):568–72.
5. Wichaidit BT, Østergaard JR, Rask CU. Diagnostic practice of psychogenic nonepileptic seizures (PNES) in the pediatric setting. Epilepsia 2015;56(1):58–65.
6. American Psychiatric Association. Diagnostic and statistical manual of mental disorders. 5th edition. Arlington (VA): American Psychiatric Publishing; 2013.
7. Stone J, Hallett M, Carson A, et al. Functional disorders in the neurology section of ICD-11. Neurology 2014;83:2299–301.
8. Nicholson TR, Aybek S, Craig T, et al. Life events and escape in conversion disorder. Psychol Med 2016;46(12):2617–26.
9. Allendorfer JB, Nenert R, Hernando KA, et al. FMRI response to acute psychological stress differentiates patients with psychogenic non-epileptic seizures from

healthy controls - A biochemical and neuroimaging biomarker study. Neuroimage Clin 2019;24:101967.

10. Kerr WT, Janio EA, Le JM, et al. Diagnostic delay in psychogenic seizures and the association with anti-seizure medication trials. Seizure 2016;40:123–6.

11. Benbadis SR, Allen Hauser W. An estimate of the prevalence of psychogenic non-epileptic seizures. Seizure 2000;9(4):280–1.

12. Salinsky M, Spencer D, Boudreau E, et al. Psychogenic nonepileptic seizures in US veterans. Neurology 2011;77(10):945–50.

13. Stone J, Carson A, Duncan R, et al. Who is referred to neurology clinics?—the diagnoses made in 3781 new patients. Clin Neurol Neurosurg 2010;112(9):747–51.

14. Kutlubaev MA, Xu Y, Hackett ML, et al. Dual diagnosis of epilepsy and psychogenic nonepileptic seizures: Systematic review and meta-analysis of frequency, correlates, and outcomes. Epilepsy Behav 2018;89:70–8.

15. Asadi-Pooya AA, Sperling MR. Epidemiology of psychogenic nonepileptic seizures. Epilepsy Behav 2015;46:60–5.

16. Panagos PD, Merchant RC, Robert L. Alunday Psychogenic Seizures: A Focused Clinical Review for the Emergency Medicine Practitioner. Postgrad Med 2010; 122:34–8.

17. Nightscales R, McCartney L, Auvrez C, et al. Mortality in patients with psychogenic nonepileptic seizures. Neurology 2020;95:e643–52.

18. Jones B, Reuber M, Norman P. Correlates of health-related quality of life in adults with psychogenic nonepileptic seizures: A systematic review. Epilepsia 2016; 57(2):171–81.

19. Jennum P, Ibsen R, Kjellberg J. Welfare consequences for people diagnosed with nonepileptic seizures: A matched nationwide study in Denmark. Epilepsy Behav 2019;98:59–65.

20. Goldstein LH, Robinson EJ, Reuber M, et al. Characteristics of 698 patients with dissociative seizures: A UK multicenter study. Epilepsia 2019;60:2182–93.

21. LaFrance WC Jr, Baker GA, Duncan R, et al. Minimum requirements for the diagnosis of psychogenic nonepileptic seizures: a staged approach: a report from the International League Against Epilepsy Nonepileptic Seizures Task Force. Epilepsia 2013;54(11):2005–18.

22. Tolchin B, Dworetzky BA, Martino S, et al. Adherence with psychotherapy and treatment outcomes for psychogenic nonepileptic seizures. Neurology 2019; 92(7):e675–9.

23. Davis BJ. Predicting nonepileptic seizures utilizing seizure frequency, EEG, and response to medication. Eur Neurol 2004;51:153–6.

24. Benbadis SR. A spell in the epilepsy clinic and a history of "chronic pain" or "fibromyalgia" independently predict a diagnosis of psychogenic seizures. Epilepsy Behav 2005;6(2):264–5.

25. KellerJ. Ammonia capsules are a great tool for assessing pseudoseizures. Jail Medicine. 2014. Available at: http://www.jailmedicine.com/ammonia-capsulesare-a-great-tool-for-assessing-pseudoseizures/#more-2559. Accessed February 12, 2019.

26. Tolchin B, Martino S, Hirsch LJ. Treatment of patients with psychogenic nonepileptic attacks. JAMA 2019;321(20):1967–8.

27. McSweeney M, Reuber M, Levita L. Neuroimaging studies in patients with psychogenic non-epileptic seizures: A systematic meta-review. Neuroimage Clin 2017;16:210–21.

28. Kellinghaus C, Lüders HO. Frontal lobe epilepsy. Epileptic Disord 2004;6(4): 223–39.

29. Husain AM, Towne AR, Chen DK, et al. Differentiation of epileptic and psychogenic nonepileptic seizures using single-channel surface electromyography. J Clin Neurophysiol 2020 [Online ahead of print].
30. Espay AJ, Aybek S, Carson A, et al. Current concepts in diagnosis and treatment of functional neurological disorders. JAMA Neurol 2018;75(9):1132–41.
31. Aboukasm A, Mahr G, Gahry BR, et al. Retrospective analysis of the effects of psychotherapeutic interventions on outcomes of psychogenic nonepileptic seizures. Epilepsia 1998;39:470–3.
32. Kanner AM, Parra J, Frey M, et al. Psychiatric and neurologic predictors of psychogenic pseudoseizure outcome. Neurology 1999;53:933–8.
33. Arain AM, Hamadani AM, Islam S, et al. Predictors of early seizure remission after diagnosis of psychogenic nonepileptic seizures. Epilepsy Behav 2007;11:409–12.
34. Mayor R, Smith PE, Reuber M. Management of patients with nonepileptic attack disorder in the United Kingdom: a survey of health care professionals. Epilepsy Behav 2011;21:402–6.
35. Goldstein LH, Robinson EJ, Mellers JDC, et al. Cognitive behavioural therapy for adults with dissociative seizures (CODES): a pragmatic, multicentre, randomized controlled trial. Lancet Psychiatry 2020;7:491–505.
36. LaFrance WC Jr, Baird GL, Barry JJ, et al. Multicenter pilot treatment trial for psychogenic nonepileptic seizures: a randomized clinical trial. JAMA Psychiatry 2014;71(9):997–1005.
37. Goldstein LH, Chalder T, Chigwedere C, et al. Cognitive-behavioral therapy for psychogenic nonepileptic seizures: a pilot RCT. Neurology 2010;74(24):1986–94.
38. Rawlings GH, Brown I, Reuber M. Predictors of health-related quality of life in patients with epilepsy and psychogenic nonepileptic seizures. Epilepsy Behav 2017;68:153–8.
39. Perez D. The CODES trial for dissociative seizures: a landmark study and inflection point. Lancet Psychiatry 2020;7(6):464–5.
40. Tolchin B, Baslet G, Suzuki J, et al. Randomized controlled trial of motivational interviewing for psychogenic nonepileptic seizures. Epilepsia 2019;60(5):986–95.
41. Khan AY, Baade L, Ablah E, et al. Can hypnosis differentiate epileptic from nonepileptic events in the video/EEG monitoring unit? Data from a pilot study. Epilepsy Behav 2009;15:314–7.
42. Harvey SG, Stanton BR, David AS. Conversion disorder: towards a neurobiological understanding. Neuropsychiatr Dis Treat 2006;2(1):13–20.
43. Kelley SD, Benbadis S. Eye movement desensitization and reprocessing in the psychological treatment of trauma-based psychogenic non-epileptic seizures. Clin Psychol Psychother 2007;14:135–44.
44. Swingle PG. Neurofeedback treatment of pseudoseizure disorder. Biol Psychiatry 1998;44:1196–9.
45. Baslet G, Ehlert A, Oser M, et al. Mindfulness-based therapy for psychogenic nonepileptic seizures. Epilepsy Behav 2020;103(Pt A):106534.
46. Oto M, Espie CA, Duncan R. An exploratory randomized controlled trial of immediate versus delayed withdrawal of antiepileptic drugs in patients with psychogenic nonepileptic attacks (PNEAs). Epilepsia 2010;51(10):1994–9.

Emergency Neuropharmacology

Kyle M. DeWitt, PharmD*, Blake A. Porter, PharmD

KEYWORDS

- Pharmacotherapy • Treatment • Medication • Pharmacokinetics • CNS infection
- Status epilepticus • Traumatic brain injury

KEY POINTS

- Benzodiazepines must be optimally dosed and immediately followed by appropriate anti-epileptic medications for status epilepticus, because drug efficacy diminishes with prolonged seizure duration.
- Prompt initiation of empiric anti-infectives with adequate central nervous system penetration is associated with decreased mortality and adverse outcomes.
- Appropriate selection and timely administration of medications to support airway and hemodynamics is critical to decrease secondary neurologic injury for patients presenting with traumatic neurologic emergencies.
- Evidence-based, patient-specific blood pressure goals should be targeted using rapid-acting antihypertensives to decrease hematoma expansion, morbidity, and mortality.

INTRODUCTION

The management of acute neurologic disorders in the emergency department is often multimodal and may require the use of medications to reduce morbidity and mortality secondary to neurologic injury. To optimize patient care, clinicians should form an individualized treatment approach with regard to patient age, weight, comorbidities, drug–drug interactions, and goals of care. Pharmacokinetic properties (drug absorption, distribution, metabolism, and elimination) must be taken into consideration to achieve optimal efficacy and minimize adverse effects. This article focuses on the pharmacotherapy for common neurologic emergencies that present to the emergency department, including traumatic brain injury (TBI), central nervous system (CNS) infections, status epilepticus (SE), hypertensive emergencies, spinal cord injury, and neurogenic shock.

Emergency Medicine, Department of Pharmacy, The University of Vermont Medical Center, 111 Colchester Avenue, Mailstop 272 BA1, Burlington, VT 05401, USA
* Corresponding author.
E-mail address: Kyle.DeWitt@uvmhealth.org
Twitter: @EmergPharm (K.M.D.); @RxEmergency (B.A.P.)

Emerg Med Clin N Am 39 (2021) 133–154
https://doi.org/10.1016/j.emc.2020.09.008
0733-8627/21/© 2020 Elsevier Inc. All rights reserved.

emed.theclinics.com

STATUS EPILEPTICUS

SE is defined as continuous seizure activity that persists beyond 5 minutes or recurrent seizures without recovery to baseline. Rapid initiation of appropriate pharmacotherapy, in conjunction with supportive care measures, is paramount to prevent neurologic sequelae and reduce mortality.[1,2] Choice of treatment depends on several factors, including the availability of parenteral access, duration of seizure activity, individualized patient characteristics, and institutional formulary and policy. Many antiepileptics are prone to drug interactions among themselves (**Fig. 1**) and other drugs that are metabolized via the hepatic cytochrome system (eg, diltiazem, warfarin, protease inhibitors). Historically, algorithms have categorized treatment into emergent, urgent, and refractory SE. Management of seizures induced by specific toxicologic agents or those that persist beyond 24 hours despite intravenous (IV) anesthetics, defined as super-refractory SE, are beyond the scope of this review.

Emergent Treatment

Benzodiazepines (BZD) are standard of care for initial treatment of SE. BZDs modulate type A gamma-aminobutyric acid receptors to suppress seizure activity and are more likely to be effective when administered soon after seizure onset, as receptors begin to internalize with prolonged seizure duration.[3,4] In adults without IV access, intramuscular midazolam is preferred.[1,5] To date, no significant differences in efficacy or safety between IV lorazepam or diazepam have been established. Phenobarbital may be used as an alternative if BZDs are not readily available.

Inadequate dosing of BZDs is common and associated with higher rates of respiratory complication and progression to refractory SE.[6–9] A full dose of IV lorazepam or diazepam may be repeated once within 5 to 10 minutes if termination of the seizure is not achieved. Dosing and administration considerations are outlined in **Table 1**.

Urgent Treatment

A second-line antiepileptic medication is recommended if seizures do not abate with adequate doses of BZDs. Fosphenytoin, levetiracetam, or valproic acid are all viable

	CBZ	CLOB	LTG	MID	OXC	PHT	PHNBRB	VPA
CBZ			↓ LTG	↓ MID	↓ CBZ	↓ PHT/↓ CBZ	↓ CBZ	↓ VPA/↑ CBZ
CLOB						↑ PHT		
LTG	↓ LTG				↓ LTG	↓ LTG	↓ LTJ	SJS/TENS
MID	↓ MID					↓ MID	↓ MID	
OXC	↓ CBZ		↓ LTG			↓ OXC/↑ PHT	↓ OXC	↓ OXC
PHT	↓ PHT/↓ CAR	↑ PHT	↓ LTG	↓ MID	↓ OXC/↑ PHT		↓ PHT	↓ VPA
PHNBRB	↓ CBZ		↓ LTG	↓ MID	↓ OXC	↓ PHT		↓ VPA
VPA	↓ VPA/↑ CBZ		SJS/TENS		↓ OXC	↓ VPA	↓ VPA	

Fig. 1. Select antiepileptic drug–drug interactions. CBZ, carbamazepine; CLOB, clobazam; LTG, lamotrigine; MID, midazolam; PHNBRB, phenobarbital; PHT, phenytoin and fosphenytoin; SJS, Stevens-Johnson Syndrome; TEN, toxic epidermal necrolysisl; VPA, valproic acid. *Red boxes* indicate a major interaction, which may be life threatening and/or require medical intervention to minimize or prevent serious adverse effects. *Yellow boxes* indicate a moderate interaction which may result in exacerbation of the patient's condition. *Green boxes* indicate minor or clinically insignificant interactions. (*Data from* Micromedex: Drug Interactions Tool. Truven Health Analytics; 2020.)

Table 1
Pharmacologic therapies for SE

	Initial Dose	Administration	Goal Serum Concentration	Serious Adverse Effects/ Considerations
Emergent				
Lorazepam	0.1 mg/kg (max 4 mg/dose) may repeat once	IVP up to 2 mg/min	N/A	Hypotension, respiratory depression, contains propylene glycol
Midazolam	10 mg for >40 kg 5 mg for 13–40 kg	IM	N/A	Hypotension, respiratory depression
Diazepam	0.2 mg/kg (max 10 mg/dose) may repeat once	IVP up to 5 mg/min	N/A	Hypotension, respiratory depression, contains propylene glycol
Urgent				
Phenobarbital	15–20 mg/kg	IV up to 100 mg/min	15–40 μg/mL	Hypotension, respiratory depression, contains propylene glycol
Phenytoin	20 mg/kg (max 1500 mg/dose)	IV up to 50 mg/min	Total: 10–20 mcg/mL Free: 1–2 μg/mL	Arrhythmia, hypotension, hepatotoxicity, purple glove syndrome, contains propylene glycol
Fosphenytoin	20 mg PE/kg (max 1500 mg/dose)	IV up to 150 mg PE/min	Total: 10–20 μg/mL Free: 1–2 μg/mL	Arrhythmia, hypotension, hepatotoxicity
Levetiracetam	60 mg/kg (max 4500 mg/dose)	IV up to 450 mg/min	N/A	Rare
Valproic acid	40 mg/kg (max 3000 mg/dose)	IV up to 6 mg/kg/min	50–150 μg/mL	Hepatotoxicity, hyperammonemia, pancreatitis, thrombocytopenia
Refractory				
Clobazam	10 mg twice daily	Enteral only	N/A	Hypotension, respiratory depression

(continued on next page)

Table 1
(continued)

	Initial Dose	Administration	Goal Serum Concentration	Serious Adverse Effects/ Considerations
Topiramate	200–400 mg every 6–12 h (max 1600 mg/d)	Enteral only	5–20 µg/mL (not routinely monitored)	Metabolic acidosis
Lacosamide	200–400 mg	IV over 15–30 min	N/A	Bradycardia, PR prolongation, dizziness
Ketamine	1–2 mg/kg bolus then 1–10 mg/kg/ h infusion	Slow IV push followed by infusion	N/A	Hypertension, tachycardia, salivation, laryngospasm, transient apnea, psychiatric
Midazolam	0.2 mg/kg then 0.05–2 mg/kg/h infusion	IV bolus followed by continuous infusion	N/A	Tachyphylaxis after prolonged use
Propofol	1–2 mg/kg then 20–200 µg/kg/min infusion	IV bolus followed by continuous infusion, titrated based on EEG	N/A	Requires intubation, hypotension, bradycardia, respiratory depression, metabolic acidosis, rhabdomyolysis, renal failure, hypertriglyceridemia
Pentobarbital	5–15 mg/kg then 0.5–5 mg/kg/h infusion	IV bolus followed by continuous infusion, titrated based on EEG	N/A	Requires intubation, hypotension, bradycardia, respiratory depression, paralytic ileus, contains propylene glycol

Abbreviations: EEG, electroencephalography; IM, intramuscular; IVP, intravenous push; N/A, not applicable.
Data from Refs.[1,10–12]

options. The Established Status Epilepticus Treatment Trial (ESETT) randomized children and adults with BZD-refractory SE to receive fosphenytoin 20 mg/kg, levetiracetam 60 mg/kg, or valproic acid 40 mg/kg.[10] The primary outcome, clinical cessation of SE with improvement in mental status at 60 minutes after the start of the drug infusion, was similar between all groups (45%, 47%, and 46%, respectively). Of note, approximately 70% of initial BZD doses in ESETT were inadequate and may have contributed to overall response rates.[8] Greater rates of intubation and hypotension occurred in the fosphenytoin arm (26.4% and 3.2%, respectively) and more deaths occurred in the levetiracetam arm compared with others; however, these differences were not statistically significant. Two similar trials conducted in pediatric patients found no difference in the cessation of seizures between phenytoin and levetiracetam.[13,14]

Fosphenytoin can be infused at a higher rate compared with phenytoin, and is associated with less hypotension, cardiac arrhythmias, and infusion site pain; however, there are insufficient data regarding the comparative efficacy.[15] Thus, fosphenytoin is preferred owing to patient tolerability; however, phenytoin is considered an effective alternative.[1]

Given the relatively low success rates of all antiepileptic agents, clinicians must initiate these agents early (preferably with or immediately subsequent to the second dose of BZD) and be prepared for endotracheal intubation with ketamine or propofol if termination of seizure is not achieved. IV phenobarbital is a reasonable alternative to the aforementioned agents, but is associated with higher rates of adverse events.

Refractory Status Epilepticus

Seizures that do not respond to a BZD plus 1 antiepileptic drug are considered refractory SE. There is no robust evidence to guide therapy in this stage and clinical response rate to a third medication may be as low as 2%.[4] Continuous infusion sedatives (midazolam, propofol, ketamine, and pentobarbital) have been used in conjunction with electroencephalography monitoring in those with general tonic–clonic refractory SE. Data are insufficient to suggest any superiority of specific treatments and combinations of medications with unique mechanisms of action may be required.

CENTRAL NERVOUS SYSTEM INFECTIONS

Infections of the CNS are neurologic emergencies that require prompt recognition and treatment. Clinicians in the emergency department should be cognizant of common pathogens, empiric treatments, CNS penetration of anti-infectives, and the role of adjunctive agents such as glucocorticoids. The key goals of treatment include eradication of infection, mitigation of symptoms, and prevention of complications, such as deafness and coma.[16] We review treatment considerations for bacterial meningitis, encephalitis, brain and spinal abscesses, and ventriculitis.

Timing of Antibiotic Administration

Delayed initiation of antibiotics for the treatment of acute meningitis is strongly associated with adverse outcomes and increased mortality.[17,18] Current guidelines strongly recommend administration of empiric antibiotics within 1 hour of suspected diagnosis.[19] When possible, cerebral spinal fluid (CSF) and blood cultures should be obtained before antibiotic administration in an effort to identify a causative pathogen. Data regarding the impact of antibiotics on time to CSF sterilization are conflicting and range from as early as 15 minutes to 4 hours.[20–23]

Central Nervous System Penetration

For antibiotics to reach the site of infection within the CNS at therapeutic concentrations, they must penetrate the blood–brain and/or blood–CSF barrier(s). Several factors govern a drug's ability to do so, including the extent of meningeal inflammation, affinity to drug efflux pumps, molecular weight, lipophilicity, ionization, and protein binding. **Table 2** provides a comparison of CNS penetration between anti-infectives.

In general, medications that are ideal for treatment of CNS infections have smaller molecular weights, moderate lipophilicity, low protein binding, and exist in a nonionized form.[24] The pH of CSF can be significantly lower than blood pH in cases of severe bacterial meningitis; therefore, weak acids such as cephalosporins and penicillins diffuse more readily out of the CNS compartments and into the blood.[25] Larger cephalosporins such as ceftriaxone, have minimal affinity to drug efflux pumps and thus can still achieve adequate CNS concentration.[26] Vancomycin is hydrophilic with a high molecular weight and must be dosed aggressively to achieve optimal bactericidal CSF concentration. A loading dose of 20 to 35 mg/kg actual body weight (not to exceed 3000 mg) should be administered for critically ill patients.[27]

Bacterial Meningitis

Empiric antibiotics should target the most likely bacterial pathogens known to cause meningitis. Common pathogens of bacterial meningitis include *S pneumoniae,* group B *Streptococcus, Neisseria meningitidis, Haemophilus influenzae,* and *Listeria monocytogenes*; however, the etiology depends on age, vaccination status, past medical history, and the presence of additional risk factors (**Table 3**).[28] Therapy should be

Table 2
Comparative CNS penetration

Agents that Achieve Therapeutic CSF Concentration with or Without Inflammation	Agents that Achieve Therapeutic CSF Concentration with Inflammation	Agents with Poor CSF Concentration
Acyclovir	Ampicillin ± sulbactam aztreonam	Aminoglycosides
Ciprofloxacin	Cefepime	Amphotericin B
Fluconazole	Ceftazidime	Cephalosporins (first and second generation)[a]
Foscarnet	Ceftriaxone	Clavulanic acid
Ganciclovir	Cefuroxime	Doxycycline
Isoniazid	Colistin	Itraconazole[b]
Linezolid	Daptomycin	Sulbactam
Metronidazole	Ethambutol	Tazobactam
Moxifloxacin	Imipenem	
Pyrazinamide	Meropenem	
Rifampin	Nafcillin	
Sulfonamides	Ofloxacin	
Trimethoprim	Penicillin G	
Voriconazole	Piperacillin/tazobactam	
	Ticarcillin ± clavulanic acid	
	Vancomycin	

[a] Cefuroxime is an exception.
[b] Effective against *Cryptococcus neoformans.*
Data from Nau R, Sorgel F and Eiffert H. Penetration of drugs through the blood-cerebrospinal fluid/blood-brain barrier for treatment of central nervous system infections. Clin Microbiol Rev. 2010; 23(4): 858-83.

Table 3
Common pathogens and empiric therapy based on risk factor

Risk Factor	Common Pathogens	Empiric Therapy
Age		
<1 mo	Group B streptococcus, *E coli, K pneumoniae, L monocytogenes*	Ampicillin + ceftazidime or aminoglycoside
1 mo to <2 y	*S pneumoniae,* group B Streptococcus, *N meningitidis, H influenzae, E coli*	Vancomycin + ceftriaxone or ceftazidime
≥2 y to <50 y	*S pneumoniae, N meningitidis*	Vancomycin + ceftriaxone or ceftazidime
≥50 y	*S pneumoniae, N meningitidis, L monocytogenes,* aerobic Gram-negative bacilli	Vancomycin + ceftriaxone or ceftazidime + ampicillin
Basilar skull fracture	*S pneumoniae, H influenzae,* group A beta-hemolytic *streptococci*	Vancomycin + ceftriaxone or ceftazidime
Immunocompromised	*S pneumoniae, N meningitidis,* aerobic gram-negative bacilli, *L monocytogenes*	Ceftriaxone or ceftazidime + ampicillin
Penetrating head trauma, CSF shunt, postneurosurgery	*S aureus* (methicillin-resistant *S aureus*), coagulase-negative staphylococci (methicillin-resistant *S epidermidis*), aerobic gram-negative bacilli (*P aeruginosa*)	Vancomycin + ceftazidime or cefepime or meropenem
Pregnancy	*S pneumoniae, L monocytogenes, N meningitidis*	Vancomycin + ceftriaxone or ceftazidime + ampicillin

Data from Tunkel AR, Hartman BJ, Kaplan SL et al. Practice guidelines for the management of bacterial meningitis. Clin Infect Dis. 2004; 39(9): 1267-84.

continued for at least 48 to 72 hours or until an infectious process has been excluded. Historically, cefotaxime was the cephalosporin of choice in neonates; however, in 2019 it was discontinued by the last remaining manufacturer in the United States. Ceftazidime may be used as an alternative third-generation cephalosporin in this population or in those with risk factors for *Pseudomonas*.

Role of Dexamethasone

Inflammation of the subarachnoid space is thought to be a contributing factor to morbidity and mortality. Thus, adjunctive corticosteroids have been used to attenuate this inflammatory response. A meta-analysis of 25 randomized controlled trials (including 4121 adults and children) determined that corticosteroids significantly decreased hearing loss (13.8% vs 19.0%) and neurologic sequelae (17.9% vs 21.6%) in patients with bacterial meningitis in high-income countries. Corticosteroids did not reduce mortality in the overall population; however, death was significantly lower in a subgroup analysis of adults with *S pneumoniae*.[29]

Dexamethasone has been most commonly studied, with a recommended dose of 0.15 mg/kg (maximum, 10 mg) every 6 hours for 2 to 4 days.[19,28] To prevent additional inflammation caused by antibiotic-induced bacteriolysis, the Infectious Disease Society of America guidelines recommend that steroids be administered with, or 10 to 20 minutes before, antibiotics.[28,30] European guidelines allow for administration up to 4 hours after the initiation of antibiotics; however, this recommendation is based on expert opinion; randomized controlled trials evaluating the timing of corticosteroids have not yet been conducted.[19] Dexamethasone should be discontinued if bacterial meningitis is ruled out or if the pathogen causing meningitis is a bacterium other than *H influenzae* type b or *S pneumoniae*. Data to support the routine use of dexamethasone in neonates are insufficient.[31]

Encephalitis

Herpes simplex virus, West Nile virus, and enteroviruses are the most commonly diagnosed etiologies of encephalitis in the United States.[32] In addition to supportive care measures, IV acyclovir is considered the standard of care for herpes simplex virus encephalitis. Acyclovir requires dose adjustment in patients with renal insufficiency and adequate hydration is recommended to decrease the risk of acyclovir-induced nephrotoxicity. Transplant patients on immunosuppressive therapy and those with human immunodeficiency virus are at higher risk for cytomegalovirus and may require treatment with a combination of antivirals, including ganciclovir and foscarnet.[33] There is not a routine role for corticosteroids in the treatment of encephalitis, unless severe edema is present.

Brain Abscess

Bacteria account for more than 95% of brain abscesses in immunocompetent patients.[16] Abscesses are most frequently polymicrobial and empiric therapy must provide coverage against gram-negative, gram-positive, and anaerobic bacteria.[34,35] IV ceftriaxone combined with metronidazole is acceptable for most patients. Vancomycin should be added if the patient has risk factors for methicillin-resistant *S aureus* and ceftazidime or cefepime may be used in place of ceftriaxone if *Pseudomonas* is suspected. Patients with immunosuppression are at a higher risk of infection caused by fungi, yeast, and toxoplasmosis; therefore, voriconazole and trimethoprim-sulfamethoxazole should be added for empiric treatment until a definitive pathogen is identified. Duration of therapy is variable, but prolonged courses of antibiotics for 6 to 8 weeks are often required.

Adjunctive dexamethasone may reduce antibiotic penetration through the blood-brain barrier and subsequently prolong treatment. Corticosteroids are only recommended for patients with profound perifocal edema with midline shift or those at risk of herniation.[36] Although seizures are a frequent complication of brain abscesses, prophylactic antiepileptic medication is not routinely recommended.[34,37]

Ventriculitis and Cerebrospinal Fluid Shunt Infections

Broad-spectrum antibiotics that provide coverage against methicillin-resistant *Staphylococcus aureus* and *Pseudomonas* bacteria are paramount for empiric treatment of these infections until a causative pathogen is identified. Regimens should include a β-lactam with activity against *Pseudomonas* (eg, ceftazidime, cefepime, meropenem) plus vancomycin. Piperacillin–tazobactam does not achieve adequate CNS penetration and should be avoided. Intraventricular instillation of antibiotics may be required in patients who do not respond to systemic antibiotics.[38]

TRAUMATIC BRAIN INJURY

TBI is defined as an alteration in brain function or other evidence of brain injury caused by an external force.[39] Emergency care involves airway, breathing, and circulatory management to prevent hypoxemia and hypotension, prevention of post-traumatic seizures, intracranial pressure (ICP) management, correction of coagulopathy, and analgesic and sedative administration as required. Timely pharmacotherapeutic interventions in this population can help to decrease secondary injury, morbidity, and mortality.[39,40]

Airway and Hemodynamic Management

Hypoxemia and hypotension lead to worsened cerebral ischemia and have been associated with increases in morbidity and mortality.[41–44] The cerebral perfusion pressure (CPP) must be adequate to decrease cerebral ischemia. This is done by maintaining or increasing the mean arterial pressure (MAP) and decreasing the ICP. See **Table 4** for specific blood pressure targets in patients with TBI.[40,41,45] The MAP can be increased via multiple mechanisms to achieve adequate CPP. IV isotonic crystalloid fluids are the mainstay of initial resuscitation for trauma patients with hypotension, especially in resource-limited settings.[46] However, hypotonic fluids (eg, dextrose 5%, sodium chloride 0.45%, lactated Ringers solution) should be avoided because they may worsen cerebral edema.[47] If the blood pressure target has not been achieved after adequate resuscitation with crystalloids and/or blood products, vasopressors (eg, phenylephrine, norepinephrine) may be used to maintain MAP (ie, CPP).[48–50]

Care should be taken in the selection of induction and paralytic agents for patients with TBI requiring intubation. Premedication with fentanyl and its analogues have been shown to blunt the sympathetic response that occurs during intubation, which may help to minimize the secondary effects of rapid sequence intubation on ICP.[51–54] Historically, lidocaine has been used for this indication; however, its benefits in blunting the sympathetic response and effects on ICP have recently been called into question.[54–57] The medications listed in **Table 5** are common sedatives and paralytics used for rapid sequence intubation with differing kinetic and adverse event profiles. Propofol can significantly decrease blood pressure after a single bolus and therefore should typically be avoided in this population.[61] Ketamine has historically been avoided owing to the thought that it may increase ICP; however, more recent data support the use of ketamine in this population because it may have a neutral or lowering effect on ICP.[62–65]

Although rocuronium is not thought to increase ICP, its extended duration over succinylcholine may limit management-changing neurologic examinations.[66–68] Sugammadex may play a role in this setting.[69,70] Succinylcholine has been demonstrated to increase ICP and 1 retrospective review demonstrated increased mortality in patients with severe TBI receiving succinylcholine compared with rocuronium.[71,72] However, this single-center retrospective study has limitations that prevent practice-changing conclusions from being made.[71]

Post-Traumatic Seizure Prevention

Post-traumatic seizures can be classified as early or late defined as occurring within 7 days or beyond 7 days from the event, respectively.[40] Post-traumatic seizures

Table 4 Blood pressure targets in TBI	
Age (y)	**Systolic Blood Pressure (mm Hg)**
15–49	>110
50–69	>100
≥70	>110

Data from Carney N, Totten AM, O'Reilly C et al. Guidelines for the management of severe traumatic brain injury, fourth edition. Neurosurgery. 2017; 80(1): 6-15.

Table 5
Rapid sequence intubation medications

Drug (Mechanism)	Dosing	Kinetics	ADE and Considerations
Induction			
Ketamine (NMDA antagonist)	1.5–2 mg/kg IV	Onset: <1–2 min Duration: 5–15 min	ADE: emergence reaction, catecholamine surge, hypersalivation MAP: Increase ICP: Neutral
Etomidate (GABA)	0.3 mg/kg IV	Onset: <60 s Duration: 5–10 min	ADE: Inhibits cortisol production, decrease seizure threshold MAP: Neutral ICP: Decrease
Propofol (GABA)	1–2 mg/kg IV	Onset: <30 s Duration: 5–10 min	ADE: Hypotension, myocardial depression MAP: Decrease ICP: Decrease
Paralysis			
Succinylcholine (DP NMB)	1–1.5 mg/kg IV	Onset: 30 s Duration: 5–15 min	ADE: May increase ICP Avoid: Hyperkalemia, myopathy, neuropathy, denervation, history of malignant hyperthermia
Rocuronium (NDP NMB)	1–1.2 mg/kg IV	Onset: <1 min Duration: 45 min	Prolonged duration
Vecuronium (NDP NMB)	0.1 mg/kg IV	Onset: 2–3 min Duration: 30–45 min	Slow onset, prolonged duration

Abbreviations: ADE, adverse effects; DP NMB, depolarizing neuromuscular blocker; GABA, gamma-aminobutyric acid; NDP NMB, nondepolarizing neuromuscular blocker.
Data from Refs.[58–60]

may occur clinically in up to 12% of patients and subclinically on electroencephalography in up to 25% of patients with severe TBI.[40] Risk factors for developing early post-traumatic seizures have been identified and may be helpful in determining which patients to initiate prophylactic therapy[40,73]:

- Risk factors for early post-traumatic seizures
  - Glasgow Coma Scale of 10 or less
  - Immediate seizures
  - Linear or depressed skull fracture(s)
  - Post-traumatic amnesia for more than 30 minutes
  - Penetrating head injury
  - Subdural, epidural, or intracerebral hematoma
  - Cortical contusion
  - Age 65 years or younger
  - Chronic alcoholism

The administration of antiepileptics for primary prophylaxis of early post-traumatic seizures is warranted in patients with TBI, particularly if it is severe (Glasgow Coma Scale of ≤8). Common antiepileptics used for post-traumatic seizures prophylaxis include phenytoin or fosphenytoin and levetiracetam (**Table 6**). Temkin and

Table 6
Antiepileptic recommendations for early post-traumatic seizures

Drug	Dosing	Duration	2016 BTF Recommendations
Phenytoin/fosphenytoin[a]	See **Table 1**	7 d	Recommended for early post-traumatic seizures (level IIA[b])
Levetiracetam[a]	Load: 20 mg/kg IV Maintenance: 500–1000 mg IV q12h	7 d	Not recommended over phenytoin (insufficient evidence)

Abbreviation: BTF, brain trauma foundation.
[a] See **Table 1** for further guidance on dosing, administration, target serum concentrations, and adverse effects.
[b] Level IIA defined as a "moderate-quality body of evidence."
Data from Carney N, Totten AM, O'Reilly C et al. Guidelines for the management of severe traumatic brain injury, fourth edition. Neurosurgery. 2017; 80(1): 6-15; and Szaflarski JP, Sangha KS, Lindsell CJ et al. Prospective, randomized, single-blinded comparative trial of intravenous levetiracetam versus phenytoin for seizure prophylaxis. Neurocrit Care. 2010; 12(2): 165-72.

colleagues[74] demonstrated an absolute decrease in early post-traumatic seizures of 10.6% in patients with moderate to severe TBI receiving phenytoin versus placebo (3.6% vs 14.2% respectively; $P<.001$). The incidence of late post-traumatic seizures was not different between groups. **Table 6** includes antiepileptics commonly administered for early post-traumatic seizures. Of note, prophylaxis for late post-traumatic seizures is not recommended, because the current literature does not support this practice.[40,74]

Intracranial pressure management
ICP is the pressure inside the cranial vault and is normally less than 10 to 15 mm Hg in healthy adults.[75] An ICP of greater than 22 mm Hg is associated with increased mortality and treatments should be initiated to decrease and maintain ICP below this threshold.[40,76] Hyperosmolar therapies can be given acutely to decrease cerebral edema and elevated ICP. IV hypertonic sodium solutions and mannitol are the most extensively studied agents for this indication (**Table 7**). Although both agents have a

Table 7
Hyperosmolar therapy

Drug	Dosing	Considerations	Adverse Effects
Mannitol	Bolus: 0.25–1 g/kg IV Redose every 4–6 h	Duration: 1.5–6 h In-line filter required Goal osmolar gap <20 mOsm/kg	Rebound ICP, AKI, hypotension, hypovolemia, electrolyte losses
Hypertonic sodium chloride solutions	Bolus dosing: 3%: 3–5 mL/kg IV 5%: 2.5–5 mL/kg IV 7.5%: 2 mL/kg IV 23.4%: 30 mL IV Continuous infusion may be considered, however controversial[79]	Duration: 1.5–4.0 h Central access required for continuous infusion or concentrations >3% Avoid hypernatremia (>160 mEq/L)	Heart failure, pulmonary edema, AKI, hypernatremia, metabolic acidosis, phlebitis, osmotic demyelination

Abbreviation: AKI, acute kidney injury.
Data from Refs.[12,40,77,78]

role, it is yet to be determined which agent, if any, is more effective in improving patient-oriented neurologic outcomes.[40,80,81] However, The Neurocritical Care Society's 2020 Guideline for the Acute Treatment of Cerebral Edema conditionally recommends hypertonic sodium solutions over mannitol based on low-quality evidence demonstrating it to be as effective and safe with possible advantages (quicker onset, volume expansion, a more profound and sustained reduction, and ICP decrease after mannitol failure).[80,82,83] Mannitol may be preferred in select patients with volume overload (eg, decompensated heart failure) or severe hypernatremia.[80]

Pain and sedation

Pain, anxiety, and agitation should be treated judiciously in a patient with TBI, especially after intubation. Analgesia and sedation should be used to provide patient comfort, decrease ICP and cerebral oxygen consumption, facilitate mechanical ventilation, and decrease sympathetic hyperactivity.[58] This concern must be balanced against the risk of hypotension, decreased CPP, and impaired neurologic examinations. Analgosedation (analgesics first, sedation second) should be used with short-acting, hemodynamically neutral medications when able. No specific analgosedation strategy has demonstrated clear advantages; however, opioids such as fentanyl or remifentanil and sedatives such as propofol or short-acting BZD are reasonable initial choices. Deep sedation (ie, barbiturate coma) should be reserved for patients with an elevated ICP refractory to standard measures.

Coagulopathy

The incidence of coagulopathy in TBI is directly proportional to the severity of TBI.[84,85] It has been associated with intracranial hematoma expansion and worse outcomes.[86–88] There are multiple mechanisms of coagulopathy of TBI and the management of preexisting coagulopathy (ie, antithrombotics) is discussed elsewhere.[89] An acquired coagulopathy can develop soon after TBI owing to intrinsic mechanisms (eg, tissue factor release) and rapid assessment and management is required.[88] One such therapy, tranexamic acid (TXA), has been studied extensively in patients with TBI.[90,91] The effect of TXA for TBI in 9202 patients was recently published and found no difference in the primary outcome of head injury–related death within 28 days of injury.[91] However, a subgroup analysis of patients with mild to moderate head injury (Glasgow Coma Scale of 9–15) demonstrated a decrease in mortality when given TXA (relative risk, 0.78; 95% confidence interval, 0.64–0.95).[91] Although TXA cannot be recommended for all patients presenting with a TBI, administration within this select population may be reasonable and should be considered.

TRAUMATIC SPINAL CORD INJURY

Key concepts in emergency care include airway, breathing, and circulatory assessment; spinal motion restriction; spinal and motor/sensory examination; imaging; and surgical decompression. Although decompression is the mainstay in management of severe traumatic spinal cord injury (TSI), consideration of pharmacotherapy should be made surrounding airway and hemodynamic management. The risks and benefits of corticosteroids for this indication are also discussed.

Airway and Hemodynamic Considerations

Many of the same pharmacotherapeutic interventions for TBI should be considered when managing the airway and hemodynamics of a patient experiencing TSI; however, some differences do exist. Patients with TSI occurring above the T4 level are more likely to result in a loss of sympathetic tone leading to neurogenic shock.[92]

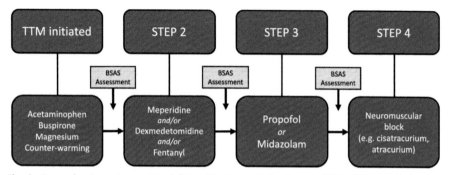

Fig. 2. Example step-wise protocol for anti-shiver medications in TTM. BSAS, bedside shivering assessment scale. (*Data from* Choi HA, Ko SB, Presciutti M et al. Prevention of shivering during therapeutic temperature modulation: The Columbia anti-shivering protocol. Neurocrit Care. 2011; 14(3): 389-94.)

Norepinephrine, dopamine, or epinephrine are preferred and should be titrated to maintain a MAP greater than 85 to 90 mm Hg for 7 days after injury to improve spinal cord perfusion.[93] Phenylephrine should be avoided as monotherapy for TSI above T4 because it lacks beta activity and may worsen bradycardia via reflexive mechanisms.[94]

Clinicians should avoid medications for rapid sequence intubation that may exacerbate this issue (see **Table 5**). Atropine and/or vasopressors should be considered around the time of rapid sequence intubation to mitigate further bradycardia and hypotension. Push-dose pressors have been used for decades in the operating theater and may be considered here. However, their benefits in an emergency setting are yet to be determined and the risks of dosing and administration errors have previously been described.[95,96] Succinylcholine may be used within 48 hours of injury because the upregulation of acetylcholine receptors is unlikely to have occurred early on in the injury-process based on expert consensus.[97]

Corticosteroids

Corticosteroids were historically considered beneficial for patients experiencing TSI owing to a decrease in the inflammatory process leading to improved neurologic function from the original injury. The NASCIS II trial demonstrated improved neurologic benefit when high-dose methylprednisolone was given to patients within 8 hours of TSI.[98] A significant debate over the validity of this trial's results with the inability of

Table 8	
Blood pressure targets in select neurologic emergencies	
Condition	**Target Blood Pressure (mm Hg)**
Spontaneous ICH	SBP <140–180
Aneurysmal SAH	SBP <140–160
Ischemic Stroke (no thrombolytic) Before a thrombolytic Post-thrombolytic administration	SBP <220 SBP <185 *and* DBP <110 SBP <180 *and* DBP <105

Abbreviations: DBP, diastolic blood pressure; ICH, intracranial hemorrhage; SAH, subarachnoid hemorrhage; SBP, systolic blood pressure.
   Data from Refs.[106–108,114,115]

Table 9
Antihypertensives for neurologic emergencies

Drug (Mechanism)	Dosing	Kinetics	ADE and Considerations
Nicardipine (CCB)	Initial: 2.5 mg/h Titrate: 2.5 mg/h every 15 min to goal BP Max: 15 mg/h	Onset: 15 min Duration: 0.5–2.0 h	ADE: Reflex tachycardia, phlebitis, headache, flushing Dose stacking may occur with rapid titration, reduce rate once at goal Avoid: Severe aortic stenosis
Clevidipine (CCB)	Initial: 1–2 mg/h Titrate: Every 90 s Max: 21 mg/h	Onset: 2 min Duration: 90 s	ADE: Reflex tachycardia 2 Kcal/mL of lipid Avoid: egg/soy allergy, severe aortic stenosis
Sodium nitroprusside (VD)	Initial: 0.3–0.5 µg/kg/min Titrate: 0.5 µg/kg/min every 3 min Max: 3 µg/kg/min	Onset: <2 min Duration: 1–2 min	ADE: cyanide toxicity (>3 µg/kg/min, AKI), methemoglobinemia Avoid: AKI, elevated ICP, CAD (coronary steal)
Hydralazine (VD)	10–20 mg IV push every 4–6 h	Onset: 5–20 min Duration: 2–12 h	ADE: Reflex tachycardia, flushing, headache Profound hypotension may occur in slow acetylators
Esmolol (BB)	Initial: 500–1000 µg/kg optional bolus, 50 µg/kg/min infusion Titrate: 50 µg/kg/min every 3–5 min Max: 300 µg/kg/min	Onset: 1–2 min Duration: 10–30 min	ADE: Bradycardia, heart block, headache, flushing Avoid: Bradycardia, heart block, cardiogenic shock, decompensated heart failure Bolus may be administered at each increase in infusion rate
Labetalol (BB)	Initial: 10–20 mg IV push Titrate: Double IV dose every 10 min to target BP Max single dose: 80 mg IV Max cumulative dose: 300 mg IV	Onset: 2–5 min Duration: 2–4 h	ADE: Bronchospasm, heart failure exacerbation, bradycardia, heart block Dose stacking may occur with rapid titration Continuous infusion difficult to titrate

Abbreviations: AKI, acute kidney injury; ADE, adverse effects; BB, beta-blocker; BP, blood pressure; CAD, coronary artery disease; CCB, calcium channel blocker; VD, vasodilator.
Data from Refs.[12,106,107,114]

more recent evidence to confirm this finding led to major organizations recommending against this therapy.[99,100] Further supporting this updated recommendation was evidence demonstrating harms associated with high-dose steroids (eg, infection).[101,102] At this time, corticosteroids should not be routinely administered to patients presenting with TSI.

PHARMACOTHERAPY ADJUNCTS FOR TARGETED TEMPERATURE MANAGEMENT
Antishivering Medications

Targeted temperature management (TTM) includes targeted hypothermia, maintaining normothermia, and preventing fever. Fever contributes to secondary neurologic injury and worsens morbidity and mortality in patients with a primary neurologic insult.[103] For adult patients, it is most commonly performed and supported by evidence in comatose patients achieving return of spontaneous circulation after cardiac arrest.[104] TTM has been explored in patients presenting with ischemic stroke, TBI, and intracranial hemorrhage with conflicting results.[105] Major organizational guidelines currently recommend maintaining normothermia for these indications and saving therapeutic hypothermia for salvage therapy or patients in clinical studies.[106–108] Although TTM may not be used routinely in these populations, it is critical to understand management of shivering when TTM is implemented. Shivering increases the rate of metabolism, oxygen consumption, and carbon dioxide production, which may counteract the benefits of TTM.[109] Common medications used to counteract shivering include analgesics, sedatives, and neuromuscular blockers. The reader is referred elsewhere for a comprehensive review of these medications.[12] An example protocol for implementation of these medications in a stepwise fashion is shown in **Fig. 2**. Nonpharmacologic measures may also be instituted to decrease the shiver response (eg, skin and extremity counterwarming).

ANTIHYPERTENSIVES FOR NEUROLOGIC EMERGENCIES

Certain neurologic emergencies require increases in blood pressure to maintain CPP (ie, TBI) whereas others (eg, intracranial hemorrhage, thrombolytic administration for ischemic stroke) necessitate antihypertensive therapy to decrease the risk of bleeding, hematoma expansion, and mortality.[110–113] Blood pressure targets are indication specific and many times should be tailored for each patient (**Table 8**). A variety of antihypertensives are available, but the choice depends on the condition being managed. **Table 9** lists common antihypertensives used for neurologic emergencies.

DISCLOSURE

The authors have nothing to disclose.

REFERENCES

1. Glauser T, Shinnar S, Gloss D, et al. Evidence-based guideline: treatment of convulsive status epilepticus in children and adults: Report of the guideline committee of the American Epilepsy Society. Epilepsy Curr 2016;16(1):48–61.

2. Jagoda A, Riggio S. Refractory status epilepticus in adults. Ann Emerg Med 1993;22(8):1337–48.

3. Goodkin HP, Yeh JL, Kapur J. Status epilepticus increases the intracellular accumulation of GABA-A receptors. J Neurosci 2005;25(23):5511–20.

4. Treiman DM, Meyers PD, Walton NY, et al. A comparison of four treatments for generalized convulsive status epilepticus. Veterans affairs status epilepticus cooperative study group. N Engl J Med 1998;339(12):792–8.
5. Silbergleit R, Lowenstein D, Durkalski V, et al. Neurological Emergency Treatment Trials (NETT) Investigators. Rampart (rapid anticonvulsant medication prior to arrival trial): a double-blind randomized clinical trial of the efficacy of intramuscular midazolam versus intravenous lorazepam in the prehospital treatment of status epilepticus by paramedics. Epilepsia 2011;52(Suppl 8):45–7.
6. Rao SK, Mahulikar A, Ibrahim M, et al. Inadequate benzodiazepine dosing may result in progression to refractory and non-convulsive status epilepticus. Epileptic Disord 2018;20(4):265–9.
7. Kellinghaus C, Rossetti AO, Trinka E, et al. Factors predicting cessation of status epilepticus in clinical practice: data from a prospective observational registry (sense). Ann Neurol 2019;85(3):421–32.
8. Sathe AG, Tillman H, Coles LD, et al. Underdosing of benzodiazepines in patients with status epilepticus enrolled in established status epilepticus treatment trial. Acad Emerg Med 2019;26(8):940–3.
9. Alldredge BK, Gelb AM, Isaacs SM, et al. A comparison of lorazepam, diazepam, and placebo for the treatment of out-of-hospital status epilepticus. N Engl J Med 2001;345(9):631–7.
10. Kapur J, Elm J, Chamberlain JM, et al. Randomized trial of three anticonvulsant medications for status epilepticus. N Engl J Med 2019;381(22):2103–13.
11. Brophy GM, Bell R, Claassen J, et al. Guidelines for the evaluation and management of status epilepticus. Neurocrit Care 2012;17(1):3–23.
12. Brophy GM, Human T. Pharmacotherapy pearls for emergency neurological life support. Neurocrit Care 2017;27(Suppl 1):51–73.
13. Lyttle MD, Rainford NEA, Gamble C, et al. Levetiracetam versus phenytoin for second-line treatment of paediatric convulsive status epilepticus (eclipse): a multicentre, open-label, randomised trial. Lancet 2019;393(10186):2125–34.
14. Dalziel SR, Borland ML, Furyk J, et al. Levetiracetam versus phenytoin for second-line treatment of convulsive status epilepticus in children (CONSEPT): an open-label, multicentre, randomised controlled trial. Lancet 2019; 393(10186):2135–45.
15. DeToledo JC, Ramsay RE. Fosphenytoin and phenytoin in patients with status epilepticus: improved tolerability versus increased costs. Drug Saf 2000; 22(6):459–66.
16. Koutsari C, Dilworth TJ, Holt J, et al. Central Nervous System Infections. In: DiPiro JT, Yee GC, Posey L, et al. eds Pharmacotherapy: a pathophysiologic approach, 11e. McGraw-Hill; Available at: https://accesspharmacy.mhmedical.com/content.aspx?bookid=2577&sectionid=219306888. Accessed June 24, 2020.
17. Aronin SI, Peduzzi P, Quagliarello VJ. Community-acquired bacterial meningitis: risk stratification for adverse clinical outcome and effect of antibiotic timing. Ann Intern Med 1998;129(11):862–9.
18. Proulx N, Frechette D, Toye B, et al. Delays in the administration of antibiotics are associated with mortality from adult acute bacterial meningitis. QJM 2005; 98(4):291–8.
19. van de Beek D, Cabellos C, Dzupova O, et al. ESCMID guideline: diagnosis and treatment of acute bacterial meningitis. Clin Microbiol Infect 2016;22(Suppl 3): S37–62.

20. Geiseler PJ, Nelson KE, Levin S, et al. Community-acquired purulent meningitis: a review of 1,316 cases during the antibiotic era, 1954-1976. Rev Infect Dis 1980;2(5):725–45.
21. Kanegaye JT, Soliemanzadeh P, Bradley JS. Lumbar puncture in pediatric bacterial meningitis: defining the time interval for recovery of cerebrospinal fluid pathogens after parenteral antibiotic pretreatment. Pediatrics 2001;108(5): 1169–74.
22. Michael B, Menezes BF, Cunniffe J, et al. Effect of delayed lumbar punctures on the diagnosis of acute bacterial meningitis in adults. Emerg Med J 2010;27(6): 433–8.
23. Rogers T, Sok K, Erickson T, et al. Impact of antibiotic therapy in the microbiological yield of healthcare-associated ventriculitis and meningitis. Open Forum Infect Dis 2019;6(3):ofz050.
24. Nau R, Sorgel F, Eiffert H. Penetration of drugs through the blood-cerebrospinal fluid/blood-brain barrier for treatment of central nervous system infections. Clin Microbiol Rev 2010;23(4):858–83.
25. Thea D, Barza M. Use of antibacterial agents in infections of the central nervous system. Infect Dis Clin North Am 1989;3(3):553–70.
26. Spector R. Ceftriaxone pharmacokinetics in the central nervous system. J Pharmacol Exp Ther 1986;236(2):380–3.
27. Rybak MJ, Le J, Lodise TP, et al. Therapeutic monitoring of vancomycin for serious methicillin-resistant staphylococcus aureus infections: a revised consensus guideline and review by the American Society of Health-System Pharmacists, the Infectious Diseases Society of America, the Pediatric Infectious Diseases Society, and the Society of Infectious Diseases Pharmacists. Am J Health Syst Pharm 2020;77(11):835–64.
28. Tunkel AR, Hartman BJ, Kaplan SL, et al. Practice guidelines for the management of bacterial meningitis. Clin Infect Dis 2004;39(9):1267–84.
29. Brouwer MC, McIntyre P, Prasad K, et al. Corticosteroids for acute bacterial meningitis. Cochrane Database Syst Rev 2015;9:CD004405.
30. de Gans J, van de Beek D, European Dexamethasone in Adulthood Bacterial Meningitis Study Investigators. Dexamethasone in adults with bacterial meningitis. N Engl J Med 2002;347(20):1549–56.
31. Mathur NB, Garg A, Mishra TK. Role of dexamethasone in neonatal meningitis: a randomized controlled trial. Indian J Pediatr 2013;80(2):102–7.
32. Bloch KG, Glaset CA. Encephalitis surveillance through the emerging infections program, 1997-2010. Emerg Infect Dis 2015;21:1562–7.
33. Tunkel AR, Glaser CA, Bloch KC, et al. The management of encephalitis: clinical practice guidelines by the Infectious Diseases Society of America. Clin Infect Dis 2008;47:303–27.
34. Brouwer MC, van de Beek D. Epidemiology, diagnosis, and treatment of brain abscesses. Curr Opin Infect Dis 2017;30(1):129–34.
35. Sonneville R, Ruimy R, Benzonana N, et al. An update on bacterial brain abscess in immunocompetent patients. Clin Microbiol Infect 2017;23(9):614–20.
36. Brouwer MC, Tunkel AR, McKhannGM 2nd, et al. Brain abscess. N Engl J Med 2014;371:447–56.
37. Tremont-Lukats IW, Ratilal BO, Armstrong T, et al. Antiepileptic drugs for preventing seizures in people with brain tumors. Cochrane Database Syst Rev 2008;(2):CD004424.

38. Tunkel AR, Hasbun R, Bhimraj A, et al. 2017 Infectious Diseases Society of America's Clinical Practice Guidelines for Healthcare-Associated Ventriculitis and Meningitis. Clin Infect Dis 2017;64:e34–65.
39. Garvin R, Mangat HS. Emergency neurological life support: severe traumatic brain injury. Neurocrit Care 2017;27(Suppl 1):159–69.
40. Carney N, Totten AM, O'Reilly C, et al. Guidelines for the management of severe traumatic brain injury, fourth edition. Neurosurgery 2017;80(1):6–15.
41. Berry C, Ley EJ, Bukur M, et al. Redefining hypotension in traumatic brain injury. Injury 2012;43(11):1833–7.
42. Brenner M, Stein DM, Hu PF, et al. Traditional systolic blood pressure targets underestimate hypotension-induced secondary brain injury. J Trauma Acute Care Surg 2012;72(5):1135–9.
43. Butcher I, Murray GD, McHugh GS, et al. Multivariable prognostic analysis in traumatic brain injury: results from the impact study. J Neurotrauma 2007; 24(2):329–37.
44. Spaite DW, Hu C, Bobrow BJ, et al. The effect of combined out-of-hospital hypotension and hypoxia on mortality in major traumatic brain injury. Ann Emerg Med 2017;69(1):62–72.
45. Carney NA, Chesnut R, Kochanek PM, et al. Guidelines for the acute medical management of severe traumatic brain injury in infants, children, and adolescents. Pediatr Crit Care Med 2003;4(3 Suppl):S1.
46. Tan PG, Cincotta M, Clavisi O, et al. Review article: prehospital fluid management in traumatic brain injury. Emerg Med Australas 2011;23(6):665–76.
47. Shackford SR, Zhuang J, Schmoker J. Intravenous fluid tonicity: effect on intracranial pressure, cerebral blood flow, and cerebral oxygen delivery in focal brain injury. J Neurosurg 1992;76(1):91–8.
48. Ract C, Vigue B. Comparison of the cerebral effects of dopamine and norepinephrine in severely head-injured patients. Intensive Care Med 2001;27(1):101–6.
49. Steiner LA, Johnston AJ, Czosnyka M, et al. Direct comparison of cerebrovascular effects of norepinephrine and dopamine in head-injured patients. Crit Care Med 2004;32(4):1049–54.
50. Sookplung P, Siriussawakul A, Malakouti A, et al. Vasopressor use and effect on blood pressure after severe adult traumatic brain injury. Neurocrit Care 2011; 15(1):46–54.
51. Chung KS, Sinatra RS, Halevy JD, et al. A comparison of fentanyl, esmolol, and their combination for blunting the haemodynamic responses during rapid-sequence induction. Can J Anaesth 1992;39(8):774–9.
52. Cork RC, Weiss JL, Hameroff SR, et al. Fentanyl preloading for rapid-sequence induction of anesthesia. Anesth Analg 1984;63(1):60–4.
53. Dahlgren N, Messeter K. Treatment of stress response to laryngoscopy and intubation with fentanyl. Anaesthesia 1981;36(11):1022–6.
54. Kim JT, Shim JK, Kim SH, et al. Remifentanil vs. Lignocaine for attenuating the haemodynamic response during rapid sequence induction using propofol: double-blind randomised clinical trial. Anaesth Intensive Care 2007;35(1):20–3.
55. Bachofen M. [suppression of blood pressure increases during intubation: lidocaine or fentanyl?]. Anaesthesist 1988;37(3):156–61.
56. Samaha T, Ravussin P, Claquin C, et al. [prevention of increase of blood pressure and intracranial pressure during endotracheal intubation in neurosurgery: esmolol versus lidocaine]. Ann Fr Anesth Reanim 1996;15(1):36–40.
57. Yano M, Nishiyama H, Yokota H, et al. Effect of lidocaine on ICP response to endotracheal suctioning. Anesthesiology 1986;64(5):651–3.

58. Moheet A, Lovett M, Qualls S, et al. Emergency neurological life support: airway, ventilation, and sedation. Neurocrit Care 2017;(Suppl 1):4–28.

59. Hampton JP. Rapid-sequence intubation and the role of the emergency department pharmacist. Am J Health Syst Pharm 2011;68(14):1320–30.

60. Kramer N, Lebowitz D, Walsh M, et al. Rapid sequence intubation in traumatic brain-injured adults. Cureus 2018;10(4):e2530.

61. Dietrich SK, Mixon MA, Rogoszewski RJ, et al. Hemodynamic effects of propofol for induction of rapid sequence intubation in traumatically injured patients. Am Surg 2018;84(9):1504–8.

62. Bourgoin A, Albanese J, Leone M, et al. Effects of sufentanil or ketamine administered in target-controlled infusion on the cerebral hemodynamics of severely brain-injured patients. Crit Care Med 2005;33(5):1109–13.

63. Bourgoin A, Albanese J, Wereszczynski N, et al. Safety of sedation with ketamine in severe head injury patients: comparison with sufentanil. Crit Care Med 2003;31(3):711–7.

64. Kolenda H, Gremmelt A, Rading S, et al. Ketamine for analgosedative therapy in intensive care treatment of head-injured patients. Acta Neurochir (Wien) 1996;138(10):1193–9.

65. Mayberg TS, Lam AM, Matta BF, et al. Ketamine does not increase cerebral blood flow velocity or intracranial pressure during isoflurane/nitrous oxide anesthesia in patients undergoing craniotomy. Anesth Analg 1995;81(1):84–9.

66. Schramm WM, Strasser K, Bartunek A, et al. Effects of rocuronium and vecuronium on intracranial pressure, mean arterial pressure and heart rate in neurosurgical patients. Br J Anaesth 1996;77(5):607–11.

67. TEVA. Rocuronium injection, for intravenous use: US prescribing information. Available at: https://www.accessdata.fda.gov/drugsatfda_docs/label/2008/078717s000lbl.pdf. Accessed May 25, 2020.

68. HOSPIRA Inc. Succinylcholine chloride injection, USP [package insert]. Lake forest, il: 2004. Available at: https://www.accessdata.fda.gov/drugsatfda_docs/label/2010/008845s065lbl.pdf. Accessed May 25, 2020.

69. Curley JM, Ciceri DP, Culp WC Jr. Sugammadex administration to facilitate timely neurologic examination in the traumatic brain injury patient. Neurocrit Care 2020;32(3):880–2.

70. Smack MA, Moore M, Hong C, et al. Ultra-rapid reversal of rocuronium-induced paralysis with sugammadex in the emergency department. J Emerg Nurs 2018;44(5):529–31.

71. Patanwala AE, Erstad BL, Roe DJ, et al. Succinylcholine is associated with increased mortality when used for rapid sequence intubation of severely brain injured patients in the emergency department. Pharmacotherapy 2016;36(1):57–63.

72. Minton MD, Grosslight K, Stirt JA, et al. Increases in intracranial pressure from succinylcholine: prevention by prior nondepolarizing blockade. Anesthesiology 1986;65(2):165–9.

73. Temkin NR. Risk factors for posttraumatic seizures in adults. Epilepsia 2003;44(s10):18–20.

74. Temkin NR, Dikmen SS, Wilensky AJ, et al. A randomized, double-blind study of phenytoin for the prevention of post-traumatic seizures. N Engl J Med 1990;323(8):497–502.

75. Rangel-Castilla L, Gopinath S, Robertson CS. Management of intracranial hypertension. Neurol Clin 2008;26(2):521–41, x.

76. Sorrentino E, Diedler J, Kasprowicz M, et al. Critical thresholds for cerebrovascular reactivity after traumatic brain injury. Neurocrit Care 2012;16(2):258–66.

77. Forsyth LL, Liu-DeRyke X, Parker D Jr, et al. Role of hypertonic saline for the management of intracranial hypertension after stroke and traumatic brain injury. Pharmacotherapy 2008;28(4):469–84.

78. Papangelou A, Lewin JJ 3rd, Mirski MA, et al. Pharmacologic management of brain edema. Curr Treat Options Neurol 2009;11(1):64–73.

79. Asehnoune K, Lasocki S, Seguin P, et al. Association between continuous hyperosmolar therapy and survival in patients with traumatic brain injury - a multicentre prospective cohort study and systematic review. Crit Care 2017; 21(1):328.

80. Cook AM, Morgan Jones G, Hawryluk GWJ, et al. Guidelines for the acute treatment of cerebral edema in neurocritical care patients. Neurocrit Care 2020; 32(3):647–66.

81. Chen H, Song Z, Dennis JA. Hypertonic saline versus other intracranial pressure-lowering agents for people with acute traumatic brain injury. Cochrane Database Syst Rev 2020;(1):CD010904.

82. Harutjunyan L, Holz C, Rieger A, et al. Efficiency of 7.2% hypertonic saline hydroxyethyl starch 200/0.5 versus mannitol 15% in the treatment of increased intracranial pressure in neurosurgical patients - a randomized clinical trial [isrctn62699180]. Crit Care 2005;9(5):R530–40.

83. Li M, Chen T, Chen S, et al. Comparison of equimolar doses of mannitol and hypertonic saline for the treatment of elevated intracranial pressure after traumatic brain injury: a systematic review and meta-analysis. Medicine (Baltimore) 2015; 94(17):e668.

84. Lustenberger T, Talving P, Kobayashi L, et al. Early coagulopathy after isolated severe traumatic brain injury: relationship with hypoperfusion challenged. J Trauma 2010;69(6):1410–4.

85. Cap AP, Spinella PC. Severity of head injury is associated with increased risk of coagulopathy in combat casualties. J Trauma 2011;71(1 Suppl):S78–81.

86. Stein SC, Young GS, Talucci RC, et al. Delayed brain injury after head trauma: significance of coagulopathy. Neurosurgery 1992;30(2):160–5.

87. Engstrom M, Romner B, Schalen W, et al. Thrombocytopenia predicts progressive hemorrhage after head trauma. J Neurotrauma 2005;22(2):291–6.

88. Stein SC, Smith DH. Coagulopathy in traumatic brain injury. Neurocrit Care 2004;1(4):479–88.

89. Marcolini E, Stretz C, DeWitt KM. Intracranial hemorrhage and intracranial hypertension. Emerg Med Clin North Am 2019;37(3):529–44.

90. Zehtabchi S, Abdel Baki SG, Falzon L, et al. Tranexamic acid for traumatic brain injury: a systematic review and meta-analysis. Am J Emerg Med 2014;32(12): 1503–9.

91. CRASH-3 Trial Collaborators. Effects of tranexamic acid on death, disability, vascular occlusive events and other morbidities in patients with acute traumatic brain injury (CRASH-3): a randomised, placebo-controlled trial. Lancet 2019; 394(10210):1713–23.

92. Velmahos GC, Toutouzas K, Chan L, et al. Intubation after cervical spinal cord injury: to be done selectively or routinely? Am Surg 2003;69(10):891–4.

93. Ryken TC, Hurlbert RJ, Hadley MN, et al. The acute cardiopulmonary management of patients with cervical spinal cord injuries. Neurosurgery 2013;72(Suppl 2):84–92.

94. Stein DM, Knight WAt. Emergency neurological life support: traumatic spine injury. Neurocrit Care 2017;27(Suppl 1):170–80.
95. Acquisto NM, Bodkin RP, Johnstone C. Medication errors with push dose pressors in the emergency department and intensive care units. Am J Emerg Med 2017;35(12):1964–5.
96. Cole JB, Knack SK, Karl ER, et al. Human errors and adverse hemodynamic events related to "push dose pressors" in the emergency department. J Med Toxicol 2019;15(4):276–86.
97. Consortium for Spinal Cord Medicine. Early acute management in adults with spinal cord injury: a clinical practice guideline for health-care professionals. J Spinal Cord Med 2008;31(4):403–79.
98. Bracken MB, Shepard MJ, Collins WF Jr, et al. Methylprednisolone or naloxone treatment after acute spinal cord injury: 1-year follow-up data. Results of the second national acute spinal cord injury study. J Neurosurg 1992;76(1):23–31.
99. Coleman WP, Benzel D, Cahill DW, et al. A critical appraisal of the reporting of the national acute spinal cord injury studies (ii and iii) of methylprednisolone in acute spinal cord injury. J Spinal Disord 2000;13(3):185–99.
100. Hurlbert RJ, Hadley MN, Walters BC, et al. Pharmacological therapy for acute spinal cord injury. Neurosurgery 2013;72(Suppl 2):93–105.
101. Gerndt SJ, Rodriguez JL, Pawlik JW, et al. Consequences of high-dose steroid therapy for acute spinal cord injury. J Trauma 1997;42(2):279–84.
102. Galandiuk S, Raque G, Appel S, et al. The two-edged sword of large-dose steroids for spinal cord trauma. Ann Surg 1993;218(4):419–25 [discussion: 25–7].
103. Greer DM, Funk SE, Reaven NL, et al. Impact of fever on outcome in patients with stroke and neurologic injury: a comprehensive meta-analysis. Stroke 2008;39(11):3029–35.
104. Arrich J, Holzer M, Havel C, et al. Hypothermia for neuroprotection in adults after cardiopulmonary resuscitation. Cochrane Database Syst Rev 2016;(2):CD004128.
105. Madden LK, Hill M, May TL, et al. The implementation of targeted temperature management: an evidence-based guideline from the neurocritical care society. Neurocrit Care 2017;27(3):468–87.
106. Powers WJ, Rabinstein AA, Ackerson T, et al. 2018 guidelines for the early management of patients with acute ischemic stroke: a guideline for healthcare professionals from the American Heart Association/American Stroke Association. Stroke 2018;49(3):e46–110.
107. Hemphill JC 3rd, Greenberg SM, Anderson CS, et al. Guidelines for the management of spontaneous intracerebral hemorrhage: a guideline for healthcare professionals from the American Heart Association/American Stroke Association. Stroke 2015;46(7):2032–60.
108. Connolly ES Jr, Rabinstein AA, Carhuapoma JR, et al. Guidelines for the management of aneurysmal subarachnoid hemorrhage: a guideline for healthcare professionals from the American Heart Association/American Stroke Association. Stroke 2012;43(6):1711–37.
109. Badjatia N, Strongilis E, Gordon E, et al. Metabolic impact of shivering during therapeutic temperature modulation: the bedside shivering assessment scale. Stroke 2008;39(12):3242–7.
110. Qureshi AI. The importance of acute hypertensive response in ICH. Stroke 2013; 44(6 Suppl 1):S67–9.
111. Dandapani BK, Suzuki S, Kelley RE, et al. Relation between blood pressure and outcome in intracerebral hemorrhage. Stroke 1995;26(1):21–4.

112. Anderson CS, Huang Y, Arima H, et al. Effects of early intensive blood pressure-lowering treatment on the growth of hematoma and perihematomal edema in acute intracerebral hemorrhage: the intensive blood pressure reduction in acute cerebral haemorrhage trial (INTERACT). Stroke 2010;41(2):307–12.
113. Butcher K, Christensen S, Parsons M, et al. Postthrombolysis blood pressure elevation is associated with hemorrhagic transformation. Stroke 2010; 41(1):72–7.
114. Qureshi AI, Palesch YY, Barsan WG, et al. Intensive blood-pressure lowering in patients with acute cerebral hemorrhage. N Engl J Med 2016;375(11):1033–43.
115. Rose JC, Mayer SA. Optimizing blood pressure in neurological emergencies. Neurocrit Care 2006;4(1):98.

Diagnosis of Coma

Anna Karpenko, MD*, Joshua Keegan, MD

KEYWORDS

- Coma • Neurocritical care • Disorders of consciousness

KEY POINTS

- The differential diagnosis for the comatose patient is broad and includes structural abnormality, seizure, encephalitis, metabolic derangements, and toxicologic etiologies.
- Obtaining a good collateral history and physical examination are imperative for identifying the correct diagnosis.
- We discuss the diagnostic testing and treatment considerations for each cause of coma.

INTRODUCTION

Coma may be defined as a state of prolonged unresponsive unconsciousness. As such, it is not a disease process, but rather a symptom that may be caused by a variety of disease processes. Causes include structural, metabolic, toxicologic, and infectious etiologies; prognosis varies substantially with the underlying cause. The common pathway resulting in coma is thought to include disruption of neuronal function or pathways from the ascending reticular activating system through the thalami to the cortex.[1] It is important to note that only lesions affecting the ascending reticular activating system or bilateral hemispheres result in coma and coma should never be attributed to unilateral cortical lesions.

Coma is by definition a medical emergency, because it impairs the patient's ability to protect the airway; many underlying causes of coma are also independently emergent. In a study of *International Classification of Diseases,* 9th edition, codes, coma was responsible for 29 emergency department visits per 100,000 population,[2] a decreasing number that likely represents under-reporting as emergency department workup to identify an underlying cause is improving.

Treatment of coma is targeted toward immediate stabilization, identification in particular of reversible underlying etiologies, and correcting alterations in normal physiologic processes. This article contains a differential diagnosis for coma etiologies, prioritized by acuity and reversibility, along with suggested diagnostic and stabilization strategies. In all cases, information obtainable from the patient will be limited,

Dartmouth Hitchcock Medical Center, 1 Medical Center Drive, Lebanon, NH 03756, USA
* Corresponding author.
E-mail address: Anna.Karpenko@hitchcock.org

Emerg Med Clin N Am 39 (2021) 155–172
https://doi.org/10.1016/j.emc.2020.09.009   emed.theclinics.com
0733-8627/21/© 2020 Elsevier Inc. All rights reserved.

and consequently the initial differential must be formed on the basis of historical information from surrogates and physical examination.

HISTORY AND PHYSICAL EXAMINATION PEARLS
History

The patient's history should provide the majority of information needed to narrow the diagnosis. In addition to knowing the right questions to ask, knowing the order in which to ask them will help to triage the patient and to formulate a plan at the same time. In some cases collateral information will be unavailable resulting in reliance solely on physical examination and ancillary testing.

- Acuity and onset
  - Was the change sudden?
  - Was the patient showing earlier signs such as excessive sleepiness, confusion, or memory problems before coma onset?
  - Was the patient experiencing other symptoms such as fevers, unusual movements, weakness, numbness or tingling, headaches, light sensitivity, or neck or back pain?
  - What was the patient doing when this occurred?
  - When was the last time seen in their usual state of health?
- History of brain surgery?
- Vascular risk factors
  - Hypertension, hyperlipidemia, diabetes mellitus, coronary artery disease, smoking history, obstructive sleep apnea, atrial fibrillation, history of stroke or intracerebral hemorrhage, family history of aneurysms, or history of thrombosis or thromboembolism?
- Seizure risk factors
  - Personal or family history of seizures or status epilepticus?
  - Febrile seizures as a child?
  - History of head trauma with loss of consciousness?
  - History of central nervous system infection?
- History of psychiatric disease?
  - History of depression or suicidal ideations?
  - Prescribed psychiatric medications?
  - Compliant with medications?
  - When was the last refill and how much is left?
- History of substance abuse?
  - Which substances?
  - How much?
  - Use of injectable drugs?

Physical Examination

Vital signs

Tachycardia is nonspecific and may reflect hemodynamic compromise. The patient may have an elevated heart rate owing to pain, seizure, or intoxication with an adrenergic or anticholinergic substance. Rapid atrial fibrillation may be reactive but should raise concern for ischemic stroke as the cause of altered sensorium.

Bradycardia may result in cerebral hypoperfusion when associated with relative hypotension. Additionally, particularly when seen in conjunction with hypertension and decreased or irregular breathing, known as Cushing's triad, it may signify elevated intracranial pressure.

Hypertension, similarly, may directly cause encephalopathy and thus leads to a diagnosis of hypertensive emergency. However, hypertensive encephalopathy is usually relatively mild and the diagnosis should be reached only after excluding other acute processes. In acute brain injury blood pressure is augmented by the brain's intrinsic autoregulatory mechanism to maintain cerebral blood flow. Hypertension can also be seen in patients with seizures or those with ingestion of adrenergic or anticholinergic substances.

Hypotension may result in cerebral hypoperfusion and coma. It is otherwise a nonspecific finding with a broad differential diagnosis, including various forms of end-organ dysfunction such as shock, end-stage kidney disease, or end-stage liver disease. It may also be seen in the setting of opiate, barbiturate or benzodiazepine intoxication, overdose of antihypertensive medication, or loss of sympathetic tone from a spinal cord injury.

Tachypnea may be a central phenomenon known as central neurogenic hyperventilation, occurring in response to a lesion in the midbrain or diencephalon. However, tachypnea is more frequently a result of a primary pulmonary process, a pain response, or as compensation for a metabolic acidosis as seen in sepsis and drug intoxication (Kussmaul's breathing).

Apnea or irregular breathing patterns, when central in origin, have multiple variants including:

- Cheyne–Stokes respirations: Periods of "crescendo–decrescendo" tachypnea with periods of apnea, which can be seen in metabolic encephalopathy, supratentorial lesions, and lesions of the midbrain or diencephalon.
- Apneustic: Prolonged inspiration and expiration separated by periods of apnea, which can be seen in pontine lesions.
- Ataxic (Biot's): Periods of tachypnea and apnea lacking the crescendo–decrescendo quality of Cheyne–Stokes respirations and is associated with lesions in the medulla. This breathing pattern usually carries a poor prognosis.

Additional examination findings

Hiccups may be seen with medullary lesions. Additionally, outside of gastrointestinal disease, vomiting may be indicative of hydrocephalus with increased pressure to the area postrema located on the floor of the fourth ventricle.

Head, Eyes, Ears, Nose, and Throat

Fundoscopic examination may show papilledema suggestive of elevated intracranial pressure. Presence of retinal hemorrhage or detachment is suggestive of head trauma. Periorbital ecchymosis ("raccoon eyes"), mastoid ecchymoses ("Battle's sign"), and hemotympanum are concerning for basal skull fracture. Dry mucosal membranes may be a result of dehydration or intoxication with antidepressants, anticholinergics, neuroleptics, antihistamines, muscle relaxants, seizure medications, or antihypertensives. Conversely, excessive salivation, lacrimation, and diaphoresis can point to cholinergic intoxication. Finally, scleral icterus may be a sign of end-stage liver disease or hepatic encephalopathy with or without cerebral edema.

Neurologic Examination

Pupils

Anisocoria is present in the general population and may be a benign finding, especially if reactivity is intact. A unilateral dilated and nonreactive pupil may suggest uncal herniation with compression of cranial nerve III, or a midbrain lesion affecting the third nerve nucleus. Abnormal pupillary constriction or dilation can be caused by medications with adrenergic or cholinergic effects. When accompanying coma, miotic ("pinpoint") pupils most commonly indicate intoxication with opiates or benzodiazepines, cholinergic substances such as organophosphates, or a structural lesion in the pons. Bilateral dilated pupils with decreased or absent pupillary constriction may be indicative of a severe diffuse cerebral process; however, this finding can also be found in profound intoxication, sedation, or hypothermia (**Table 1**).

Extraocular motion
Vestibulo-ocular reflex Loss of this reflex suggests an abnormality in the brain stem or higher cortical function, but is nonspecific in etiology. This condition can be assessed with oculocephalic maneuver or cold caloric testing. Forced gaze deviation or gaze preference involves functional disruption for the frontal eye fields. The patient will gaze toward the side of stroke or away from the seizure focus. Dysconjugate gaze is generally nonspecific for diagnostic purposes, although skew deviation is a vertical misalignment of the eyes and is a sign of a brain stem or cerebellar lesion. Although unilateral nystagmus may be seen in peripheral vestibular disease, when it is bidirectional, vertical or rotatory, and nonfatiguing, it is indicative of a cerebellar or brain stem lesion or substance intoxication such as phencyclidine. A downward fixed gaze, also known as "setting sun sign," is caused by a midbrain lesion (Parinaud syndrome). Ocular bobbing is associated with pontine lesions.

Other cranial nerve findings
Absence of the corneal, cough, or gag reflexes is another sign of severe diffuse cerebral dysfunction, but the etiology is nonspecific. Central facial asymmetry, in which eyebrow raise is preserved, is seen with cortical or subcortical injury. Head version may be indicative of a focal seizure originating from the contralateral hemisphere.

Motor and sensory findings
In comatose patients, the sensory portion of the neurologic examination is limited to their response to stimulation, which is performed during the motor examination. Increased tone or rigidity can indicate serotonin syndrome, neuroleptic malignant syndrome, malignant hyperthermia, subacute or chronic brain injury, seizure, or chronic spinal cord injury. Spontaneous and purposeful movement is often times a reassuring finding. Response to noxious stimulation in the upper extremities can be categorized as either localization, withdrawal, decorticate, or decerebrate posturing. Response to noxious stimulation in the lower extremities can be categorized as either spontaneous, withdrawal, or triple flexion. Triple flexion is a nonsustained, stereotyped flexion at the hip, knee, and ankle and is a brain stem–mediated response reflecting a loss of cortical involvement. Absence of motor responses is nonspecific and could indicate organic disease or other severe metabolic disease or intoxication.

Reflex testing
Hyperreflexia or clonus may be seen as part of serotonin syndrome, neuroleptic malignant syndrome, malignant hyperthermia or tetanus. Hyporeflexia may be seen in acute brain or spinal cord injury or a neuromuscular process such as botulism.

DIFFERENTIAL DIAGNOSIS
Structural Causes

It is critical in patients with undifferentiated coma to exclude structural causes, because they form some of the most acute and in many cases very treatable causes of coma. Broadly speaking, structural causes of coma can be grouped into vascular

Table 1
Abnormal eye findings and causes

Bilateral miosis "pinpoint pupils"	Opiates
	Benzodiazepines
	Barbiturates
	Cholinomimetic substances (pilocarpine, carbachol, etc.)
	Cholinesterase inhibiters (neostigmine, organophosphates, etc)
	Clonidine
	Phenothiazine
	Ergot derivatives
	Pontine lesion
Bilateral mydriasis	Anticholinergics (atropine, diphenhydramine, scopolamine)
	Sympathomimetics (cocaine, methamphetamines, MDMA, dopamine, phenylephrine, norepinephrine)
	Serotonergics (selective serotonin reuptake inhibitors, psilocybin, d-lysergic acid diethylamide, dextromethorphan)
	Opioid or benzodiazepine withdrawal
	Oxytocin
	Increased intracranial pressure with bilateral cranial nerve III compression (nonreactive)
	Botulinum toxin
	Post-traumatic iridoplegia
	Diabetic neuropathy
Anisocoria	May be a normal finding, especially if minimal difference in size and both reactive
	Unilateral cranial nerve III compression (herniation)
	Midbrain lesion affecting the cranial nerve III nucleus
	Posterior communicating artery aneurysm
	Horner's syndrome
	Adie's tonic pupil
	Post-traumatic irido plegia
	Diabetic neuropathy
Conjugate gaze deviation	Structural lesion involving the frontal lobe ipsilateral to direction of gaze
	Rarely, can be caused by pontine lesion
	Seizure involving the frontal lobe contralateral to direction of gaze
Skew	Brain stem or cerebellar lesion
Nystagmus	Bidirectional and sustained, vertical or rotatory - brain stem or cerebellar lesion
Sunset Sign	Loss of vertical gaze - dorsal midbrain lesion or hydrocephalus
Ocular bobbing	Extensive pontine lesion, associated with poor prognosis

lesions, space-occupying lesions, and lesions causing diffusely elevated intracranial pressure through cerebrospinal fluid outflow obstruction. Some lesions may span multiple categories, such as a space-occupying intracranial hemorrhage owing to a ruptured arteriovenous malformation.

All patients presenting with coma should undergo an emergent head computed tomography (CT) scan to exclude space-occupying structural lesions and hydrocephalus; this is especially true for those with focal neurologic deficits, such as cranial nerve findings. The decision to perform neuroimaging must be made on clinical grounds and not delayed for results of laboratory testing, because many identifiable structural causes require time-critical treatment.

Comatose patients will have a decreased intrinsic ability to maintain their airway, and most will require intubation to ensure safety for neuroimaging. Any with overt evidence of elevated intracranial pressure such as a herniation syndrome warrant empiric osmotic therapy before neuroimaging, especially since this imaging requires prolonged supine positioning.

The identification of a discrete space-occupying lesion will usually require specialist consultation, because classification into operative versus nonoperative lesions is beyond the scope of most emergency medicine practitioners. Any lesion causing substantial mass effect, herniation, or suspicion for globally elevated intracranial pressure should be treated with osmotic therapy such as mannitol or hypertonic saline while awaiting neurosurgical consultation. If this situation requires central line placement, the subclavian site is preferred to limit potential obstructions of cerebral venous outflow. Steroid administration should be reserved for vasogenic edema owing to underlying tumor and is not recommended for edema surrounding hemorrhages.[3,4] Hydrocephalus severe enough to result in coma, particularly if caused by intraventricular hemorrhage or cerebrospinal fluid outflow obstruction, will likely require emergent endoventricular drain placement by neurosurgery. It should be mentioned that procedural management of infratentorial lesions is controversial and may include either endoventricular drain or suboccipital decompression at the discretion of the neurosurgical team.

If an intracranial hemorrhage is diagnosed, reversal of anticoagulation is recommended. Reversal of antiplatelet agents for intraparenchymal hemorrhages has been shown to double the risk of death or dependency[5] and has therefore been removed as a routine practice recommendation.[5] This development does not mean to imply that specific individual patients (such as those with active arterial bleeding or undergoing neurosurgical procedures) may not derive some benefit. A cornerstone of management of intracranial hemorrhage is careful management of blood pressure. A goal of systolic blood pressure is controversial, although targeting to less than 160 has been shown to decrease hematoma expansion without significant repercussions to renal function.[6,7] There is no evidence for the use of prophylactic antiepileptic drugs. Last, in patients with intracranial hemorrhage identified on noncontrast CT scan, CT angiography may identify a responsible neurovascular lesion warranting intervention.

Neurovascular etiologies of coma warrant specific discussion owing to their time-sensitive and treatable nature. Basilar system thrombosis carries an extremely poor untreated prognosis, and in the neurointerventional era has time-critical and potentially effective treatments. The sensitivity of a noncontrast head CT scan for basilar thrombosis has been reported to be as high as 50% to 70%[8,9] with high clinical pretest probability and when reviewed by expert neuroradiologists. In many clinical scenarios even this moderate sensitivity will not be achievable, and consequently CT angiography is increasingly becoming a standard diagnostic evaluation for comatose patients and especially those with cranial nerve findings. Identifying acute basilar clot has significant impact on outcomes, with 45% to 46%[10,11] of those treated via endovascular therapy having good outcomes (modified Rankin Scale of 0–2, functional independence) versus an untreated historical norm of approximately 10%.

In some cases, pontine injury may cause locked-in syndrome, which can be difficult to differentiate from coma. In this syndrome, motor function is impaired but sensory function and consciousness are preserved; patients may be able to use their eyes to communicate and have variably preserved cranial nerve function depending on the exact level of the lesion. Careful attention to cranial nerve and particularly the oculomotor components of the examination will ensure that locked-in syndrome is not mistaken for coma. Although most strokes causing acute coma are basilar in nature, there are uncommon supratentorial causes as well. These by necessity must be bilateral, and may include strokes affecting multiple territories. Possible etiologies include cardioembolic strokes as well as strokes arising from the artery of Percheron, which is an anatomic variant in which the arterial supply of the bilateral paramedian thalami arises unilaterally.

Depending on local institutional practices and resources, MRI may be considered in the evaluation of structural causes of coma. This modality may be particularly helpful in identifying brain stem pathology, including early infarction in the absence of overt large vessel occlusion, as well as diffuse axonal injury from traumatic brain injury. In most cases, this determination will not result in an immediate treatment change and so may be deferred in many institutions; however, early identification of brain stem infarct may obviate a comprehensive search for other etiologies, inform code status discussions, and change disposition (ie, medical intensive care unit for undifferentiated coma vs neurologic intensive care unit for infarct vs trauma or neurotrauma intensive care unit for diffuse axonal injury or traumatic brain injury) (**Table 2**).

Nonconvulsive Status Epilepticus Versus Postictal State

Status epilepticus is defined as at least 5 minutes of clinical or electrographic seizure activity, or multiple seizures without a return to neurologic baseline. Status epilepticus is further divided into convulsive or nonconvulsive. Generalized convulsive status epilepticus is characterized by tonic or tonic–clonic movements accompanied by an altered mental status. In contrast, nonconvulsive status epilepticus does not have obvious signs suggesting prolonged seizures, but rather is defined electrographically. Patients with nonconvulsive status epilepticus may have subtle signs of seizures such as facial or extremity twitching, eye deviation or nystagmus, or it may manifest only as an abnormal mental status. Alternatively, the patient may present with agitation, aphasia, staring, confusion or coma.

Uncontrolled generalized convulsive status epilepticus may transition into nonconvulsive status epilepticus; therefore, timely recognition and treatment are essential.

Table 2 Structural causes of Coma		
Ischemic	**Hemorrhagic**	**Other**
Bilateral anterior cerebral artery strokes	Subarachnoid hemorrhage	Traumatic brain injury
Basilar occlusion	Thalamic hemorrhage	Hydrocephalus
Vasculitis	Pontine hemorrhage	Midbrain tumor
		Central pontine myelinolysis
		Supratentorial mass causing herniation
		Multiple sclerosis

Patients who present with nonconvulsive status epilepticus usually have underlying comorbidities and are acutely ill. The differential of the inciting disease is broad and includes toxic or metabolic derangements, infection, or structural brain lesions. Nonconvulsive status epilepticus is also generally more refractory to treatment.[12]

Diagnostic testing

A noncontrast CT scan of the head is standard of care to rule out acute structural etiologies. MRI of the brain with and without contrast can be considered once the patient has been stabilized.

An electroencephalogram (EEG) is the only definitive method of making the diagnosis of nonconvulsive status epilepticus, and to differentiate nonconvulsive status epilepticus from postictal state. Continuous EEG monitoring is preferred over routine EEG. The duration of EEG monitoring is uncertain; however, for patients who have risk factors for developing status epilepticus, 24 hours of monitoring should be considered.[13]

Laboratory testing should include glucose, basic metabolic panel, complete blood count, lactate, and creatine kinase levels, which may be elevated in prolonged seizure. Serum prolactin level is nonspecific for the diagnosis of status epilepticus; however, it may be useful in differentiating patients with epileptic seizures from those with psychogenic nonepileptic seizures if drawn at most 20 minutes from the time of seizure.[14] Antiepileptic drug levels should be obtained when appropriate.

A lumbar puncture may be of value to acutely exclude central nervous system infection. It may also allow for testing of infrequent causes, such as autoimmune encephalitis or occult malignancy when the etiology is uncertain. If a lumbar puncture is performed in the setting of suspected or confirmed status epilepticus additional cerebrospinal fluid should be banked to facilitate possible specialized testing.

Treatment

After initial stabilization and airway attainment, targeted therapy includes the following. Benzodiazepines are the first-line treatment for status epilepticus. Intravenous (IV) or intramuscular lorazepam or midazolam are preferred for their favorable pharmacodynamics. Lorazepam should be dosed at 0.1 mg/kg, divided into multiple doses to attenuate subsequent hypotension and respiratory depression. Similarly, midazolam should be dosed at 0.2 mg/kg.

Concurrently, the patient should receive an antiepileptic drug, including:

- Levetiracetam 1000 to 3000 mg
  - Minimal side effects
- Lacosamide 200 to 400 mg
  - Minimal side effects
- Phenytoin 20 mg/kg load, may repeat 5 to 10 mg/kg dose in 10 minutes
  - Phenytoin load may result in arrhythmias or hypotension; for this reason fosphenytoin is preferred
- Valproate 20 to 40 mg/kg
  - Side effects include hepatotoxicity, thrombocytopenia, and pancreatitis
- Phenobarbital 15 to 20 mg/kg
  - Side effects include hypotension and respiratory depression

If the patient continues to seize despite appropriate benzodiazepine dosing and at least one antiepileptic drug, they are defined as having refractory status epilepticus. A continuous infusion should be initiated and titrated to seizure suppression on EEG.

- Propofol: Load with a 1 to 2 mg/kg bolus followed by infusion starting at 20 μg/kg/min.

- ○ Side effects include hypotension, respiratory depression, and propofol infusion syndrome including metabolic acidosis, rhabdomyolysis, cardiac and renal failure.
- Midazolam: 0.2 mg/kg dose followed by infusion starting at 0.05 to 2 mg/kg/h.
  - ○ Side effects include hypotension and respiratory depression.
- Pentobarbital: 5 to 15 mg/kg loading dose followed by continuous infusion at 0.5 to 5 mg/kg/h, at a maximum rate of 50 mg/min.
  - ○ Side effects include hypotension, cardiac depression, respiratory depression, and ileus.

The choice for preferred antiepileptic drug administration is a topic of debate, although IV administration is vital for urgent seizure control. Traditionally phenytoin, valproate, and phenobarbital were considered the agents of choice[15] and were selected based on their side effect profile and ease of administration. Newer agents including levetiracetam, brivaracetam and lacosamide have since gained popularity owing to their relatively lower incidence of side effects. A recent randomized clinical trial[16] was stopped early for futility and showed that levetiracetam was as efficacious as phenytoin and valproate in aborting status epilepticus. Despite the excellent tolerability of brivaracetam and lacosamide, there is currently a paucity of strong evidence to support their use in standard of care.

Encephalitis

Meningoencephalitis must be considered when a patient presents in a comatose state. Both infectious and noninfectious etiologies should be reviewed and additional history obtained to narrow the scope of treatment. Meningitis on its own does not manifest with an altered mental status and presents instead with meningismus: headache, neck stiffness, and photosensitivity. Encephalitis, in contrast, affects the brain focally or diffusely and may present with a myriad of signs, including confusion, lethargy, personality changes, motor or sensory deficits, or seizures. Cerebritis describes regionalized inflammation of the brain and is associated with infectious etiologies. Immunosuppressed patients may have primary or coinfections with rare or atypical diseases. Aseptic meningitis may include drug-induced, postinfectious or paraneoplastic etiologies (**Table 3**).

Diagnostic testing

A CT scan of the head may not be abnormal in meningitis or encephalitis, but may have a localized area of hypodensity reflecting vasogenic edema surrounding an abscess. It is also necessary to exclude a mass lesion to ensure safe lumbar puncture. An MRI of the brain with and without contrast may be considered once the patient has been treated empirically for potential reversible causes.

Routine serum laboratory tests may reveal a leukocytosis and lactic acidosis.

Lumbar puncture must be performed in a timely manner to isolate the offending agent. Cerebrospinal fluid findings and their significance are listed in **Table 4**. Basic cerebrospinal fluid studies include glucose, protein, cell count with differential, herpes simplex virus polymerase chain reaction, varicella zoster virus polymerase chain reaction and antibodies, cytomegalovirus polymerase chain reaction, Epstein–Barr virus polymerase chain reaction, and bacterial culture. Opening pressure is important because it can be suggestive of a specific underlying process. Additional studies may be sent if atypical or rare infections are considered, or if there is concern for autoimmune encephalitis.

An EEG should be performed to exclude nonconvulsive status epilepticus in comatose patients with evidence of central nervous system infection (see **Table 4**).

Table 3
Causes of Meningoencephalitis

Bacterial	Viral	Fungal	Parasitic	Autoimmune	Drug Induced	Other
Borrelia species	Herpes simplex	*Aspergillus species*	*Acanthamoeba species*	Anti-AMPA	Allopurinol	Acute Disseminated Encephalomyelitis
Escherichia coli	Varicella zoster	*Blastomyces dermatitidis*	*Balamuthia mandrillaris*	Anti-Ampithysin	Azathioprine	Carcinomatous meningitis
Group B Streptococcus	Cytomegalovirus	*Candida species*	*Naegleria fowleri*	Anti-ANGA	Carbamezepine	Central nervous system vasculitis
Haemophilus influenzae	Epstein-Barr virus	*Cocciodes immitis*	*Taenia solium*	Anti-ANNA	Cephalosporins	Creutzfeldt–Jakob disease
Klebsiella species	Human herpes virus-6	*Cryptococcus species*	*Toxoplasma gondii*	Anti-CASPR2	Ciprofloxacin	Fabry disease
Leptospira species	Coxackie	*Histoplasma capsulatum*	*Trypanosoma brucei*	Anti-CRMP	Intrathecal chemotherapy agents	Incomplete treatment of previous infection
Listeria monocytogenes	Echovirus			Anti-DPPX	Isoniazid	Lymphoma
Mycobacterium tuberculosis	Human enteroviruses			Anti-GABA	Intravenous immunoglobulin	Neurosarcoidosis
Mycoplasma pneumoniae	Rotavirus			Anti-GAD65	Lamotrigine	Progressive multifocal Leukoencephalopathy
Neisseria meningitidis	Adenovirus			Anti-GFAP	Metronidazole	
Rickettsia species	Respiratory syncytial virus			Anti-LGi1	Nnonsteroidal anti-inflammatory drugs	
Staphylococcus aureus	Rhinovirus			Anti-mGluR1	Penicillins	
Streptococcus pneumoniae	Influenza A and B			Anti-NMDA	Pyrazinamide	
Treponemia pallidum	Parainfluenza viruses			Anti-PCA	Pyridium	
	Human immunodeficiency virus			Striated muscle antibody	Sulfasalazine	
	Powassan virus				Trimethoprim–sulfamethoxazole	
	Colorado tick fever virus					

Western equine encephalitis
Venezuelan equine encephalitis
St. Louis encephalitis
Eastern equine encephalitis
California encephalitis virus
La Crosse encephalitis
West Nile virus
Human T-cell lymphotropic virus 1 and 2
Parvovirus
Hepatitis A and B virus
Lymphocytic choriomeningitis
Rabies virus
Measles
Mumps
Rubella

Table 4
Toxicologic causes of Coma

Environmental	Drugs	Metabolic
Carbon monoxide poisoning	Alcohol	Hypoglycemia
Hypothermia	Benzodiazepines	Hyperglycemia/diabetic ketoacidosis
Organophosphate poisoning	Barbiturates	Uremia
	Opiates	Hepatic encephaopathy
	Anticholinergics	Hypercalcemia
	Toxic alcohols	Hypocalcemia
		Myxedema coma
		Hypercapneic respiratory failure
		Wernicke's encephalopathy

Treatment

If there is suspicion for infectious cause, steroids and empiric antimicrobial medication should be started without delay. For streptococcal meningitis, steroids have been shown to reduce mortality if given before or with the initial dose of antibiotics.[17]

The recommended empiric regimen includes:

- Dexamethasone 0.15 mg/kg every 6 hours for 2 to 4 days
- Vancomycin: 15 to 20 mg/kg every 8 to 12 hours
- Third generation cephalosporin:– for example, ceftriaxone 2 g every 12 hours
- Acyclovir 10 mg/kg every 8 hours
- If the patient is more than 50 years old or immunosuppressed, ampicillin should be added for coverage of atypical organisms
- If the patient has had a recent neurosurgical procedure, a fourth-generation cephalosporin such as cefepime should replace the third-generation cephalosporin

Fever should be treated to avoid secondary brain injury. Prophylaxis with antiseizure medication is not recommended unless the patient has clinical or electrographic seizures. Autoimmune encephalitides are treated acutely with high dose steroids (methylprednisolone 1 g/d for 5 days), intravenous immunoglobulin (2 g/kg divided over 5 days) or plasma exchange. Steroid-sparing agents may be considered if there is a good clinical response to acute treatment.

Toxicologic Causes

Because coma may be caused by numerous toxins and laboratory identification of them is time consuming and at times misleading (eg, having limited ability to differentiate acute drug toxicity from recent ingestion), an initial differential diagnosis must be formed and empiric therapy begun based solely on history and physical examination, with urine toxicologic screens and other laboratory testing serving primarily purposes of confirmation and assisting in longitudinal care. The more common, time-sensitive, and treatable toxicologic causes of coma are discussed in detail elsewhere in this article. A wide range of uncommon toxins exist and require supportive care while seeking expert consultation (**Table 5**).

One of the most common and most immediately reversible etiologies is opiate toxicity, in which case coma is usually accompanied by miosis and decreased respiratory drive. Although most frequent in recreational drug users, iatrogenic opiate toxicity, for example, among elderly patients with fluctuating renal function, should also be considered. Clinicians should have a low threshold for administration of

Table 5
Cerebrospinal fluid findings

	Opening Pressure (cmH$_2$O)	Glucose (mg/dL)	Protein (mg/dL)	White Blood Cell Count	Differential
Normal	5–20	>50 or 2/3 serum glucose	<50	<5	No differential
Bacterial	Elevated	<50	elevated	>500	Neutrophilic predominance
Viral	Normal	Normal	Normal or slightly elevated	<1000	Lymphocytic predominance
Fungal or tuberculosis	Elevated	Normal or low	Elevated	<1000	Lymphocytic predominance
Autoimmune	Normal	Normal	Elevated	<500	Lymphocytic predominance

naloxone, a competitive opiate antagonist, because it has a benign side effect profile and may help to avoid intubation. It should be noted that meperidine and propoxyphene result in mydriasis; naloxone administration should not be withheld solely on the basis of this physical examination finding. Last, naloxone has a short half-life, often shorter than that of the opiate itself, and especially in the context of an unknown opiate ingestion patients must be monitored for recurrence of toxicity as the naloxone is metabolized.

Benzodiazepines are another medication class with substantial potential to cause coma, particularly in intentional/suicidal ingestions. Benzodiazepines taken in isolation are rarely fatal and there are no pathognomonic physical examination findings[18]; suspicion must be based on historical clues. The main physical examination finding consistent with benzodiazepine toxicity is depressed mental status, which may be as severe as complete electroencephalographic silence on EEG. Compromised respirations are possible but much less common than with opiate or barbiturate ingestions. Flumazenil is a competitive antagonist that can be used to reverse cases of known acute-only benzodiazepine toxicity, but should be avoided in cases of unknown or chronic benzodiazepine administration to avoid precipitating potentially life-threatening withdrawal and intractable seizures. Care in such cases is primarily supportive while awaiting toxin metabolism.

Barbiturate ingestion presents similarly to benzodiazepine toxicity but with more pronounced respiratory and cardiovascular suppression; no specific reversal agent is available and care is supportive including mechanical ventilation and vasopressor support.

Acute alcohol intoxication may result in coma when blood levels exceed 0.3%; approximately 1% of all alcohol intoxication visits require critical care,[19] which is generally supportive and may include management of accompanying bradycardia and hypotension. Rapid testing of exhaled breath levels or blood levels is commonly available and may assist with risk stratification and disposition decisions. Rapid testing for toxic alcohols such as methanol, ethylene glycol, and isopropyl alcohol is largely unavailable; elevated osmolar gap and anion gap metabolic acidosis (in the cases of methanol and ethylene glycol) should raise clinical suspicion. When clinical suspicion exists, empiric administration of fomepizole, an alcohol dehydrogenase inhibitor preventing breakdown to toxic metabolites, should be initiated while awaiting confirmatory testing. Last, Wernicke encephalopathy has been reported to cause reversible coma[20,21] and thiamine should be administered empirically to comatose patients with suspicion of alcohol use disorders.

Severe carbon monoxide poisoning may also result in coma; again there are no pathognomonic findings and high clinical suspicion must be maintained. Although more common in the winter owing to higher home heating needs, 30% carbon monoxide poisoning is intentional[22] and may therefore occur at all times of the year. Diagnosis is supported by pulse co-oximetry or laboratory spectrophotometry, but owing to poisoning of the oxidative phosphorylation pathway symptoms may persist after blood carbon monoxide levels have returned to baseline. As a result, normal level should not be used to exclude toxicity in an appropriate clinical context. When available and performed from the emergency department, MRI showing restricted diffusion specifically in the region of the globus pallidus is strongly supportive of carbon monoxide poisoning. Aside from supportive care, specific treatment includes oxygen supplementation and consideration of hyperbaric oxygen therapy.

Metabolic Causes

Hypoglycemia is one of the most common and most immediately reversible causes of coma. Any patient presenting with coma should either have a fingerstick glucose checked or empiric administration of dextrose (preceded by thiamine if the clinical context suggests concurrent alcohol abuse). Patients who are chronically hyperglycemic may become symptomatic even with low-normal glucose levels. An underlying explanation for hypoglycemia such as insulin overdose should always be sought; in the case of accidental overdose of short-acting insulin, emergency department observation and discharge may be all that is indicated, whereas patients with intentional overdoses, overdoses of long-acting insulin, and unexplained hypoglycemia should be admitted for more prolonged monitoring and further workup.

Hypercarbic respiratory insufficiency also frequently leads to depressed mental status and coma. At times patients may present with clinically evidence hypoventilation as a cause; pulmonary disease such as chronic obstructive pulmonary disease may also play a less overt role. Given that venous carbon dioxide cannot be lower than arterial carbon dioxide, a normal venous blood gas is sufficient to exclude clinically significant hypercarbia. If the venous carbon dioxide is elevated an arterial blood gas should generally be performed to confirm this finding. Although depressed mental status is a contraindication to unsupervised biphasic positive airway pressure, cases of hypercarbia attributed to neuromuscular disease or respiratory muscle fatigue may benefit from a short-term (20–30 minutes) trial of biphasic positive airway pressure under direct observation to determine if improved carbon dioxide clearance will result in a mental status suitable for longer term biphasic positive airway pressure. Worsening hypercarbia or failure of mental status changes to resolve should prompt intubation. As opposed to neuromuscular causes, cases of central hypoventilation will generally not respond to biphasic positive airway pressure and mechanical ventilation will be required. Once hypercarbia has been resolved, patients should be reevaluated to exclude additional contributors to coma (eg, opiate administration leading to hypercarbia).

When severe, numerous electrolyte abnormalities may result in coma. Routine laboratory evaluation should include serum electrolytes, including calcium and magnesium levels. Correction of identified abnormalities should be initiated in the emergency department before admission; most patients will likely require inpatient management. Evaluation for underlying causes of electrolyte abnormalities can generally be deferred to the inpatient setting. Last, although usually obvious from historical or environmental clues, hypothermia may also result in coma and it should be ensured that all comatose patients have a core temperature documented as part of their initial evaluation.

Hepatic Encephalopathy

Any patient with history or clinical examination stigmata (such as jaundice or spider telangiectasias) of liver disease presenting with coma should have an ammonia level checked to determine if hepatic encephalopathy may be responsible. The pathogenesis of hepatic encephalopathy is incompletely understood and the degree of hyperammonemia does not directly correlate with degree of encephalopathy. Consequently, for those with any ammonia elevation, treatment with lactulose should be initiated and continued until clinical resolution of symptoms; rifaximin may be a useful adjunct and is thought to decrease intestinal bacterial ammonia production. Contributing conditions such as upper gastrointestinal tract bleeding should be identified and corrected. Administration of flumazenil may be considered because it has been shown to improve symptoms of hepatic encephalopathy, even in the absence of benzodiazepine use; however, this effect may often be transient and no statistically significant effect on mortality has been demonstrated.[23]

Endocrine

Thyroid dysfunction in the form of severe decompensated hypothyroidism can result in an entity termed "myxedema coma." This syndrome includes hypoactive delirium or coma, hypoventilation, bradycardia, hypotension, hypothermia, thick coarse skin, and thinning hair. Seizures may occur as well, especially in the setting of severe metabolic derangements. It is important to also investigate precipitating factors such as infection, cold exposure, and recent trauma. An association exists between decompensated hypothyroidism and intoxication with opioids or other classes of sedating medications, as well as with amiodarone use.

Diagnostic testing

The mainstay of diagnosis is confirmatory thyroid function tests: serum thyroid-stimulating hormone (elevated in primary hypothyroidism but reduced in secondary hypothyroidism), free thyroxine (reduced). Cortisol is often decreased as a result of either primary or secondary adrenal insufficiency and in this case cosyntropin stimulation test may be helpful. Hypoglycemia may result from decreased gluconeogenesis and adrenal insufficiency. Hyponatremia is usually a result of coexisting syndrome of inappropriate diuretic hormone. Elevated creatine kinase and a reduced glomerular filtration rate may be present. Furthermore, hypoxemia and hypercapnia may be seen on blood gas. The electrocardiogram may show sinus arrhythmias and QT prolongation. Therefore, continuous monitoring is recommended. Additionally, EEG monitoring should be performed to exclude nonconvulsive status epilepticus. Lumbar puncture, if performed incidentally, may have an elevated protein but is otherwise diagnostically nonspecific. There are usually no specific abnormalities seen on neuroimaging.

Treatment

Because incidence of myxedema coma is relatively low, there is clinical equipoise as to the exact treatment regimen. Though traditionally a large dose of levothyroxine was the preferred approach, there exist alternative regimens combining tri-iodothyronine and thyroxine replacement. One such regimen is listed here.[24]

After appropriate laboratory testing has been drawn:

- Levothyroxine 200 to 300 µg IV, followed by daily doses of 1.6 µg/kg
- Tri-iodothyronine 10 to 25 µg IV, followed by 2.5 to 10 µg every 8 hours
- Hydrocortisone 100 mg every 8 hours until exclusion of adrenal insufficiency
- Supportive care including ventilator and circulatory support, passive rewarming or IV dextrose as needed
- Treatment of underlying infection
- Treatment of arrhythmias

Psychogenic Causes

Psychiatric or psychological causes of coma may be considered once all medically treatable conditions have been considered and addressed. Such causes include catatonia, psychogenic nonepileptic seizures, conversion disorder, factitious disorder or malingering. The patient's physical examination is the most telling diagnostic test for these entities and consultation with an experienced neurologist may be helpful.

THE FUTURE OF COMA

The Curing Coma Campaign was launched in 2019 and consists of a multidisciplinary scientific advisory committee dedicated to furthering our understanding and treatment of coma. The campaign is organized into 3 pillars. The first pillar includes classification, or endotyping, of different types of coma based on pathophysiology. The second pillar focuses on continuing investigation of neuroprognostic biomarkers, the refinement of which would inform the treating clinician of the expected clinical recovery for each endotype of coma. Finally, the third pillar centers on the efforts to implement proof-of-concept trials targeted at pharmacologic and electrophysiologic interventions to improve outcomes for patients with disorders of consciousness.[25] This concerted international mission holds the potential to advance our current prognostication practice patterns and to improve the long-term outcomes of comatose patients.

DISCLOSURE

The authors have nothing to disclose.

REFERENCES

1. Edlow BL, Takahashi E, Wu O, et al. Neuroanatomic connectivity of the human ascending arousal system critical to consciousness and its disorders. J Neuropathol Exp Neurol 2012;71(6):531–46.
2. Skinner HG, Blanchard J, Elixhauser A. Trends in emergency department visits, 2006–2011: statistical brief #179. In: Healthcare cost and utilization project (HCUP) statistical briefs. Rockville (MD): Agency for Healthcare Research and Quality (US); 2014.
3. Poungvarin N, Bhoopat W, Viriyavejakul A, et al. Effects of dexamethasone in primary supratentorial intracerebral hemorrhage. N Engl J Med 1987;316(20): 1229–33.
4. Hemphill JC 3rd, Greenberg SM, Anderson CS, et al. Guidelines for the management of spontaneous intracerebral hemorrhage: a guideline for healthcare professionals from the American Heart Association/American Stroke Association. Stroke 2015;46(7):2032–60.

5. Baharoglu MI, Cordonnier C, Al-Shahi Salman R, et al. Platelet transfusion versus standard care after acute stroke due to spontaneous cerebral haemorrhage associated with antiplatelet therapy (PATCH): a randomised, open-label, phase 3 trial. Lancet 2016;387(10038):2605–13.

6. Qureshi AI, Palesch YY, Barsan WG, et al. Intensive Blood-Pressure Lowering in Patients with Acute Cerebral Hemorrhage. N Engl J Med 2016;375(11):1033–43.

7. Anderson CS, Huang Y, Arima H, et al. Effects of early intensive blood pressure-lowering treatment on the growth of hematoma and perihematomal edema in acute intracerebral hemorrhage: the Intensive Blood Pressure Reduction in Acute Cerebral Haemorrhage Trial (INTERACT). Stroke 2010; 41(2):307–12.

8. Goldmakher GV, Camargo EC, Furie KL, et al. Hyperdense basilar artery sign on unenhanced CT predicts thrombus and outcome in acute posterior circulation stroke. Stroke 2009;40(1):134–9.

9. Mortimer AM, Saunders T, Cook JL. Cross-sectional imaging for diagnosis and clinical outcome prediction of acute basilar artery thrombosis. Clin Radiol 2011; 66(6):551–8.

10. Kang DH, Jung C, Yoon W, et al. Endovascular thrombectomy for acute basilar artery occlusion: a multicenter retrospective observational study. J Am Heart Assoc 2018;7(14):e009419.

11. Gory B, Eldesouky I, Sivan-Hoffmann R, et al. Outcomes of stent retriever thrombectomy in basilar artery occlusion: an observational study and systematic review. J Neurol Neurosurg Psychiatry 2016;87(5):520–5.

12. Brophy GM, Bell R, Claassen J, et al. Guidelines for the evaluation and management of status epilepticus. Neurocrit Care 2012;17(1):3–23.

13. Herman ST, Abend NS, Bleck TP, et al. Consensus statement on continuous EEG in critically ill adults and children, part I: indications. J Clin Neurophysiol 2015; 32(2):87–95.

14. Chen DK, So YT, Fisher RS. Therapeutics and Technology Assessment Subcommittee of the American Academy of Neurology. Use of serum prolactin in diagnosing epileptic seizures: report of the Therapeutics and Technology Assessment Subcommittee of the American Academy of Neurology. Neurology 2005;65(5):668–75.

15. Treiman DM, Meyers PD, Walton NY, et al. A comparison of four treatments for generalized convulsive status epilepticus. Veterans Affairs Status Epilepticus Cooperative Study Group. N Engl J Med 1998;339(12):792–8.

16. Kapur J, Elm J, Chamberlain JM, et al. Randomized Trial of Three Anticonvulsant Medications for Status Epilepticus. N Engl J Med 2019;381(22):2103–13.

17. Brouwer MC, McIntyre P, Prasad K, et al. Corticosteroids for acute bacterial meningitis. Cochrane Database Syst Rev 2015;(9):CD004405.

18. Kang M, Galuska MA, Ghassemzadeh S. Benzodiazepine toxicity. In: StatPearls. Treasure Island (FL): StatPearls Publishing; 2020.

19. Klein LR, Cole JB, Driver BE, et al. Unsuspected Critical Illness Among Emergency Department Patients Presenting for Acute Alcohol Intoxication. Ann Emerg Med 2018;71(3):279–88.

20. Wallis WE, Willoughby E, Baker P. Coma in the Wernicke-Korsakoff syndrome. Lancet 1978;2(8086):400–1.

21. Gibb WR, Gorsuch AN, Lees AJ, et al. Reversible coma in Wernicke's encephalopathy. Postgrad Med J 1985;61(717):607–10.

22. Rose JJ, Wang L, Xu Q, et al. Carbon monoxide poisoning: pathogenesis, management, and future directions of therapy. Am J Respir Crit Care Med 2017;

195(5):596–606 [published correction appears in Am J Respir Crit Care Med. 2017;196(3):398-399].

23. Goh ET, Andersen ML, Morgan MY, et al. Flumazenil versus placebo or no intervention for people with cirrhosis and hepatic encephalopathy. Cochrane Database Syst Rev 2017;(7):CD002798.

24. Wiersinga WM. Myxedema and coma (severe hypothyroidism). In: Feingold KR, Anawalt B, Boyce A, et al, editors. Endotext [Internet]. South Dartmouth (MA): MDText.com, Inc; 2000. Available at: https://www.ncbi.nlm.nih.gov/books/NBK279007/.

25. Provencio JJ, Hemphill JC, Claassen J, et al. The Curing Coma Campaign: framing initial scientific challenges—proceedings of the First Curing Coma Campaign Scientific Advisory Council Meeting. Neurocrit Care 2020;33:1–12.

Approach to Acute Weakness

Deena Khamees, MD, William Meurer, MD*

KEYWORDS

• Weakness • Neurologic emergency • Stroke • Neuromuscular • CNS • Motor
• Malaise

INTRODUCTION, HISTORY, DEFINITIONS, AND BACKGROUND
Background

Weakness can represent the initial stage of many emergency conditions. The differential diagnosis is broad and includes many etiologies that are decidedly non-neurologic. In this review, we discuss a general emergency medicine approach to neurologic causes of weakness. Our focus is on both common neurologic conditions and uncommon conditions with a high likelihood of morbidity or mortality if the diagnosis is delayed.

Definitions

We consider a variety of external and internal causes of neurologic weakness. We define weakness as decreased or lost muscular strength resulting in an inability to act with normal or desired force.[1] Neurologic weakness, specifically, is due to specific dysfunction in any of the following locations: the neuromuscular junction, peripheral nerves (including brachial plexus), spinal cord, or brain. We do not discuss generalized malaise, often referred to as "weakness" by patients, because this entity is most frequently attributable to or associated with a primary medical cause such as anemia or hypoglycemia. We define external causes to represent infectious diseases, trauma, and toxins (including drug effects). Internal causes broadly include autoimmune, vascular (including stroke), neoplastic, metabolic, and genetic. Idiopathic causes might represent as yet undefined internal or external causes. Localization is the process by which we use the signs and symptoms to determine what part or parts of the nervous system are likely to be the source of the new problem.

History

The now-known causes of weakness were, at some point in history, newly discovered or described. This continues today, because new diseases may present with

Emergency Medicine, University of Michigan Medical School, 1500 East Medical Center Drive, Ann Arbor, MI 48109-5303, USA
* Corresponding author.
E-mail address: wmeurer@med.umich.edu

Emerg Med Clin N Am 39 (2021) 173–180
https://doi.org/10.1016/j.emc.2020.09.010
0733-8627/21/© 2020 Elsevier Inc. All rights reserved.

weakness of unclear etiology. Acute flaccid myelitis, particularly in children, is an example.[2] Evolving technologies, such as methods to isolate viruses and other pathogens or molecular techniques to detect pathologic antibodies that lead to autoimmunity, continue to uncover such previously unknown or unclear etiologies. This historical context importantly highlights that the inability to identify a cause in the emergency department does not mean there is no medical or organic etiology.

DISCUSSION
History Features

As with all neurologic conditions, a careful, focused history can assist in organizing areas to query further with physical examination and diagnostic testing. Ask the patient or accompanying history-provider about the location of the weakness, duration and pattern of symptoms, and association with other symptoms such as blurry vision or pain. Ask about particular tasks or movements that are most impaired or that highlight the weakness. For example, difficulty with standing from a seated position or ascending stairs points to an etiology resulting in a proximal muscle weakness. Inquire about any medications, such as diuretics, that may cause pertinent electrolyte disturbances, with particular emphasis on newly started, changed, or discontinued medications.

Ask:
1. Where is the weakness (note unilateral vs bilateral involvement)?
2. When did this start?
3. Is the weakness persistent or intermittent or is there some consistent pattern?
4. What activities make the weakness more noticeable?
5. What other symptoms accompany the weakness?

Physical Features

The clinician's first duty is to assess for emergent or urgent conditions necessitating timely action. For patients with a suspected neurologic cause, respiratory status is particularly at risk given the propensity for altered mental status or diaphragmatic or accessory respiratory muscle weakness. Note that tachypnea often presents sooner than, and may herald other signs of, impending respiratory failure.[3]

Look for:
1. Abnormal or poor mentation
2. Difficulty with speech or weak voice
3. Drooling or other indication of difficulty handling secretions
4. Inability to lift head off the bed
5. Weak, rapid, or shallow breaths or use of accessory muscles

If rapid sequence intubation is deemed necessary, consider avoiding depolarizing neuromuscular blocking agents such as succinylcholine. These agents carry the risk of potentially fatal hyperkalemia in those with neurologic disease by amplifying the succinylcholine-related cellular potassium release.[4,5] For most relevant conditions, this response occurs in those with symptoms or illness for 3 or more days. Succinylcholine is considered safe in myasthenia gravis, although it should be noted that the emergency physician may not always be certain of the etiology at the time rapid sequence intubation is performed. Nondepolarizing agents such as rocuronium and vecuronium may be preferable in such suspected or unknown cases. On a related note, there may also be some degree of autonomic dysfunction or instability secondary to the suspected or known neurologic process that requires some support or resuscitation until the underlying issue can be identified and managed.

In the absence of emergent or critical findings, a more thorough neurologic examination can be illuminating. This process includes an assessment of the cranial nerves, reflex testing, sensory and motor examinations, coordination, and gait. Any one or combination of these components may be key in narrowing the differential and guiding testing, as well as determining any necessary emergent interventions.

The localization of the culprit lesion as an upper versus lower motor neuron (UMN and LMN, respectively) can be made partly or even completely on the basis of the physical examination. Hyperreflexia, increased muscle tone (spasticity), and a positive or present Babinski sign (the extensor plantar response resulting in a fanning of the toes) indicate UMN involvement. Decreased or absent reflexes and/or muscle tone and an absent Babinski reflex indicate LMN involvement. Note that, in early UMN disease, there may initially be hyporeflexia and decreased muscle tone before the more characteristic spasticity and hyperreflexia develop. These distinctions, coupled with pertinent anatomy, can be helpful in the emergency department. For example, recall that in the adult the spinal cord terminates at L1. Below this point is the cauda equina, at which point an insult would result in an LMN-patterned examination. A patient presenting with bilateral leg weakness, hyperreflexia, and a positive Babinski sign (consistent with a UMN-level lesion) would thus be extremely unlikely to have a lesion at L1 or lower. Consequently, limiting this patient's imaging to an MRI lumbar spine, presumably to identify cauda equina syndrome, would not reveal the etiology. We provide an overview of a localization paradigm as **Fig. 1**.

Strength testing may seem an obvious cornerstone of the physical examination in the acutely weak patient, but its yield is greater when looking for patterns that can narrow the differential diagnosis. The first indication of a pattern may be found in the patient's history, as alluded to elsewhere in this article, look to corroborate this on examination if possible. If the complaints or examination reveal some hemiparesis, consider a central lesion in the brain. Paraplegia is more likely secondary to a spinal cord lesion. Proximal muscle weakness suggests a myopathy. Oculomotor and/or bulbar dysfunction or weakness point to a neuromuscular junction problem such as myasthenia gravis. Fatigability—diminishing strength with repeated normal use or testing of the muscle—is also highly suspicious for neuromuscular junction disease.

Laboratory Tests, Imaging, and Adjuncts

For patients who are ill appearing, presenting with generalized weakness (as opposed to discrete and localized complaints), or are suspected or known to have a potentially dangerous diagnosis, we expect initial diagnostics to be broad screening examinations. These include:

Complete blood count: anemia or signs of infection
Serum electrolyte panel: hypoglycemia, electrolyte derangements including potassium, sodium, and calcium
Electrocardiogram: acute coronary syndrome or abnormalities secondary to electrolyte disturbances
Urinalysis
Blood and urine cultures
Arterial or Venous blood gas

For patients in whom a more narrowed differential may be considered, intentional use of some less common testing may be helpful. A lumbar puncture with cerebral spinal fluid collection is emergently indicated in cases of suspected bacterial meningitis,

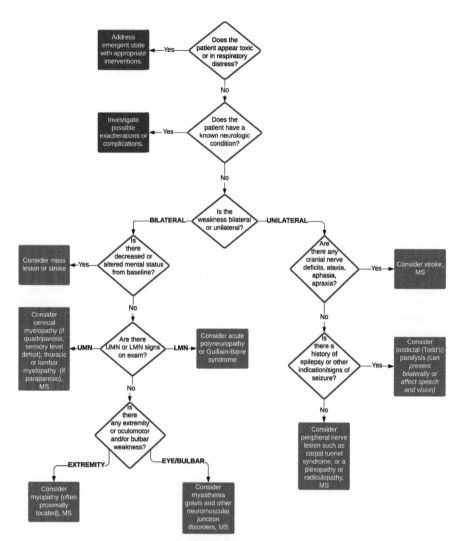

Fig. 1. Approach to undifferentiated weakness in the emergency department. MS, multiple sclerosis. (*Modified from* Asimos, Andrew, Birnbaumer, Diane, et al. Weakness: A Systematic Approach to Acute, Non-traumatic, Neurologic And Neuromuscular Causes. Emerg. med. pract.. 2002;4(12):1-26; with permission.)

particularly because treatment diminishes returns on microbial cultures. Cerebral spinal fluid analysis can be revealing in cases of Guillain–Barre syndrome, myelitis, and demyelinating peripheral neuropathy, although conditions these may not necessarily require an emergent lumbar puncture in the emergency department. In case of suspected myopathy and subsequent muscle damage, serum creatinine phosphokinase may be elevated.

The most frequently utilized neuroradiography in the emergency department is a computed tomography. Computed tomography imaging of the head without contrast can reveal intracranial hemorrhage, mass lesions, cerebral edema, and midline shift. Head computed tomography scans with contrast are often more illustrative of mass lesions and other malignancy-related processes, cerebral enhancing lesions which may be due to infectious causes such as abscess, neurocysticercosis, toxoplasma, or noninfectious etiologies such as demyelination or subacute infarct.[6]

MRI of the brain may be used to assess for acute ischemic stroke, because small and early infarcts may not be identified on computed tomography imaging for several days.[7] MRI of the spinal cord should be obtained in the emergency department for emergent cord and nerve root problems, such as compression, abscess, or transverse myelitis; less time-critical diagnoses such as multiple sclerosis may also be identified via MRI.

Tests of respiratory muscle strength, particularly vital capacity and maximal inspiratory pressure, can be performed in the emergency department to identify those with impending respiratory failure. The vital capacity is the maximal amount of air expired after maximal inhalation. The maximal inspiratory pressure (MIP), also known as the negative inspiratory force, indicates diaphragmatic strength, or lack thereof. Normal ranges for the MIP vary widely based on patient sex and age and is generally lower in women and the elderly.[7,8] The data from such tests are best used in conjunction with the clinical appearance and other information and singular measurements may be less helpful than trending these over time. Certainly these are not necessary before intubation if clear respiratory distress or failure exists on clinical examination. In less apparent cases, these may help with decisions regarding elective intubation; a common example of this occurs in myasthenic crisis.[9,10] In such an instance, acceptable cutoff values have been proposed as follows: a vital capacity of less than 15 to 20 mL/kg and MIP between 0 and -30 cmH$_2$O.[11] Reliance on the MIP should be weighed carefully as it relates to elective intubation; there is good negative predictive value (a normal MIP reliably excludes significant respiratory muscle weakness) but poor positive predictive value (a low MIP cannot confirm respiratory muscle weakness).[12]

Differential Diagnosis

Although outside the scope of this article, recall that a generalized malaise, compared with a true neuromuscular weakness, can and often results from such non-neurologic causes such as sepsis, dehydration, or anemia. Assuming a true neurologic disorder exists, begin by determining if the patient requires any immediate interventions such as intubation, or has any known chronic neurologic condition; if so, consider if this may be the most likely culprit compared with a new, additional condition (see *Considerations for Those with Known Chronic Conditions* elsewhere in this article).

If the patient is well-appearing and without any previously diagnosed relevant condition, a more methodical approach may be used. Assuming an objective weakness exists on examination, determine if the weakness is unilateral or bilateral. If bilateral with decreased or altered mental status, consider a significant cerebral event such as mass lesions or stroke. If bilateral with normal or baseline mental status, next determine if UMN or LMN signs are present on examination. Signs of UMN disease with weakness in all 4 extremities (quadriparesis), usually with some sensory level deficit, is concerning for cervical myelopathy. If the weakness is found to be in the bilateral lower extremities (paraparesis) instead of all 4, consider a thoracic or lumbar myelopathy. Signs of LMN disease with bilateral weakness should prompt suspicion of acute polyneuropathy or Guillain–Barre syndrome.

For patients who present with bilateral weakness but without obvious UMN or LMN signs, differentiate between extremity weakness and oculomotor and bulbar weakness on examination. The former, when more proximally localized, is consistent with a myopathy. The latter is most commonly associated with neuromuscular junction disorders such as myasthenia gravis.

For patients with unilateral weakness, the approach may be comparatively simpler. Central lesions may result in a variety of examination signs such as cranial nerve deficits (brainstem), motor and ataxic hemiparesis (lacunae), or aphasia, apraxia, hemineglect, or other visual deficits (cortex). For patients with a history of epilepsy, postictal paralysis (Todd's paralysis) is a consideration, particularly if the onset of unilateral weakness was sudden and unwitnessed. Note that postictal paralysis can present bilaterally and/or with speech or vision deficits.

If none of these are present on examination, look for a peripheral lesion in form of a peripheral nerve entrapment such as carpal tunnel syndrome, a plexopathy such as a brachial plexus injury, or a radiculopathy which would be expected to follow a clear myotomal distribution.

Remember that multiple sclerosis can present variably across patients and so may not fit an algorithmic approach well. Generally, there is variable presentation of motor, sensory, visual, and cerebellar deficits, but the duration of symptoms, pattern (relapsing–remitting, progressive, and a variations of these), location of the deficit, and other factors may all differ greatly. Frequently, patients report a subacute period of other or similar deficits, relative to the acute presentation, that have self-resolved.

Certain toxins may induce generalized weakness. Botulism toxin in adults can distinctively manifest as bilateral cranial neuropathies, with progression to flaccid paralysis. Carbon monoxide poisoning may present with weakness and other vague symptoms when early, and is another potential consideration. Other neurotoxins such as sarin or VX typically have a more dramatic presentation with seizures and altered mental status.

Considerations for Those with Known Chronic Conditions

Patients with known neurologic conditions may present with an acute exacerbation of the condition, or a complication of such. In these cases, assess for some triggering event such as infection, recently started or discontinued medications, new dosages of current medications, pregnancy, recent childbirth, trauma, or uncontrolled comorbid diseases that may impact a neuromuscular condition. The redemonstration of once-resolved or worsening of persistent deficits from a prior stroke secondary to a new pneumonia is a common example.

Flares of myasthenia gravis may be characterized by increasing weakness, dysphagia, dyspnea, and other signs and symptoms of ocular and bulbar weakness. Exacerbations range from the very mild to the severe myasthenic crisis, with potential for neuromuscular respiratory failure. Consider additional workup if there is evidence of sensory, reflex, pupillary, or cerebellar deficits; these symptoms are not expected in myasthenia gravis.

Patients with multiple sclerosis often present with an exacerbation similar to those experienced in the past, and although these symptoms may be relatively consistent for any given patient, flares are likely to vary markedly between patients. Carefully consider additional workup for patients whose symptoms do not match prior flares, or are accompanied by a change in mental status.

A history of Guillain–Barre syndrome is important to note in patients presenting with new or continuing weakness. The Guillain–Barre syndrome variant chronic inflammatory demyelinating polyneuropathy may persist or progress from an initial diagnosis of Guillain–Barre syndrome (specifically acute inflammatory demyelinating polyneuropathy, the most common form of Guillain–Barre syndrome), or present as a series of relapses.

SUMMARY

The chief complaint of weakness can be difficult to address in the emergency department, but may be the only clue to one of many life-threatening diagnoses. Always start with the identification of those in critical condition who may require intubation or other immediate interventions upon assessment. Carefully gather a history and detailed neurologic examination where possible, with an emphasis on differentiating factors discussed in this article, such as the distribution and quality of the weakness. These findings may be more revealing than imaging and laboratory testing, but certainly they may contribute significantly. Remember there exists a spectrum of patient presentations such that you will encounter those with known neurologic disorders in an acute exacerbation, as well as those whose weakness is both significant and unidentifiable in origin in the emergency department.

CLINICAL CARE POINTS

- Carefully differentiate between true neuromuscular weakness and the more common generalized malaise in the patient presenting with weakness because this markedly impacts the differential.
- Assess for critically ill or emergent conditions, with special attention to the respiratory status.
- For those critically ill or with consistent clinical presentations, consider the potentially life-threatening diagnoses of ischemic or hemorrhagic stroke, myasthenia gravis, Guillain–Barré syndrome, cord compression, and infection such as bacterial meningitis or epidural abscess.
- If pursuing rapid sequence intubation, consider a nondepolarizing agent such as rocuronium or vecuronium instead of the depolarizing neuromuscular blocking agent succinylcholine, which may cause respiratory arrest owing to severe hyperkalemia in the neurologically ill or injured.
- A targeted but detail-oriented history and physical are key in shaping and narrowing the differential; pay attention to that which differentiates unilateral versus bilateral weakness and UMN from LMN, and note signs of central versus peripheral nervous system involvement.
- Exercise caution when using the vital capacity and/or MIP to determine the need for intubation in patients with potential or known respiratory muscle weakness.

DISCLOSURE

The authors of this article have no conflicts of interest to disclose.

REFERENCES

1. Goetz CG. Textbook of clinical neurology. Elsevier Health Sciences; 2007. Available at: https://books.google.com/books/about/Textbook_of_Clinical_Neurology.html?hl=&id=LrxCs3G_wHEC.
2. Greninger AL, Naccache SN, Messacar K, et al. A novel outbreak enterovirus D68 strain associated with acute flaccid myelitis cases in the USA (2012–14): a retrospective cohort study. Lancet Infect Dis 2015;15:671–82.
3. Juel VC, Bleck TP. Neuromuscular disorders in the ICU. In: Textbook of critical care. 2011. p. 212–9. https://doi.org/10.1016/b978-1-4377-1367-1.00037-9.
4. Orebaugh SL. Succinylcholine: adverse effects and alternatives in emergency medicine. Am J Emerg Med 1999;17:715–21.

5. Tobey RE, Jacobsen PM, Kahle CT, et al. The Serum Potassium Response to Muscle Relaxants in Neural Injury. Anesthesiology 1972;332–7. https://doi.org/10.1097/00000542-197209000-00009.

6. Lin EC, Escott E. Practical differential diagnosis for CT and MRI. Thieme; 2011. Available at: https://play.google.com/store/books/details?id=fVK3XJDuNGMC.

7. Stewart M, Bhuta S. Diffusion weighted MRI in acute stroke. 2020. Available at: https://radiopaedia.org/articles/diffusion-weighted-mri-in-acute-stroke-1?lang=us. Accessed August 20, 2020.

8. Harik-Khan RI, Wise RA, Fozard JL. Determinants of maximal inspiratory pressure. The Baltimore Longitudinal Study of Aging. Am J Respir Crit Care Med 1998;158:1459–64.

9. Rabinstein AA, Wijdicks EFM. Warning signs of imminent respiratory failure in neurological patients. Semin Neurol 2003;23:97–104.

10. Juel VC. Myasthenia gravis: management of myasthenic crisis and perioperative care. Semin Neurol 2004;24:75–81.

11. American Thoracic Society/European Respiratory Society. ATS/ERS Statement on respiratory muscle testing. Am J Respir Crit Care Med 2002;166:518–624.

12. Hughes JMB. Lung Function Tests. Physiological Principles and Clinical Applications. 1999. Available at: https://ci.nii.ac.jp/naid/10024821778/. Accessed August 31, 2020.

Diagnosis of Patients with Acute Dizziness

Kiersten L. Gurley, MD[a,b,c,*], Jonathan A. Edlow, MD[a,b]

KEYWORDS

- Posterior circulation stroke • Dizziness • Vertigo • Misdiagnoses • Diagnostic error
- Nystagmus • Vestibular neuritis • HINTS

KEY POINTS

- Summarize the current diagnostic paradigm and its origins.
- Promote a new evidence-based algorithmic approach that better serves clinicians.
- Discuss the extent of and reasons for misdiagnosis.
- Describe physical examination techniques that aid bedside diagnosis.
- Clarify limitations of diagnostic imaging.

INTRODUCTION

Dizziness, the chief complaint in approximately 3% of emergency department (ED) patients,[1] has a broad differential diagnosis. Although most of the causes are benign, serious cerebrovascular conditions account for a small but significant proportion. Emergency physicians are tasked with accurately distinguishing benign from serious causes while being parsimonious with resource utilization.

The traditional diagnostic paradigm is faulty and may actually contribute to misdiagnosis. Brain computed tomography (CT) is often used but has extremely limited utility. Recent studies show that physical examination can be extremely useful in distinguishing benign from serious causes of dizziness. Because treatment follows a correct diagnosis, this article's focus includes the following:

- Summarize the current diagnostic paradigm and its origins
- Promote a new evidence-based algorithmic approach that better serves clinicians
- Discuss the extent of and reasons for misdiagnosis
- Describe physical examination techniques that aid bedside diagnosis

Grant funding: None to report. There are no conflicts of interest to report.
a Harvard Medical School, Boston, MA, USA; b Department of Emergency Medicine, Beth Israel Deaconess Medical Center, Boston, MA, USA; c Anna Jaques Hospital, Newburyport, MA, USA
* Corresponding author. Harvard Medical School, Boston, MA.
E-mail address: kgurley@bidmc.harvard.edu

Emerg Med Clin N Am 39 (2021) 181–201
https://doi.org/10.1016/j.emc.2020.09.011
0733-8627/21/© 2020 Elsevier Inc. All rights reserved.
emed.theclinics.com

- Clarify limitations of diagnostic imaging

HISTORY, DEFINITIONS, AND BACKGROUND

The traditional "symptom quality" approach to diagnose patients with dizziness starts by asking the patient, "What do you mean by 'dizzy'?" Their response (true vertigo vs lightheadedness vs imbalance/disequilibrium vs "other") drives the differential diagnosis and the evaluation. This diagnostic paradigm stems from a study published in 1972.[2]

The investigators established a "dizziness clinic" to which patients were referred and underwent several days of clinical evaluation. Based on these results, the lead author assigned a diagnosis. Despite serious flaws and no prospective validatation,[3,4] the "symptom quality" approach became the prevailing paradigm. Newer evidence shows that its underlying logic is faulty[5] and that a newer paradigm based on "timing and triggers" is more consistent with current evidence.

RELEVANT ANATOMY, PHYSIOLOGY, AND PATHOPHYSIOLOGY

Dizziness from general medical causes may be mediated by neural dysfunction due to factors such as fever, hypotension, anemia, medication side effects, electrolyte abnormalities, and others. Dizziness due to vestibular and neurologic causes have more clear-cut mechanisms that require some familiarity of basic anatomy and physiology.

The end organs in the labyrinth, the peripheral vestibular apparatus including semicircular canals, utricle, and saccule (organ of balance), and the cochlea (organ of hearing) lie in the temporal bone (**Fig. 1**). The vestibular apparatus includes 3 paired semicircular canals that sense rotational motion and the utricle and saccule that sense linear motion (**Fig. 2**). These interconnected structures are filled with endolymph. Hair

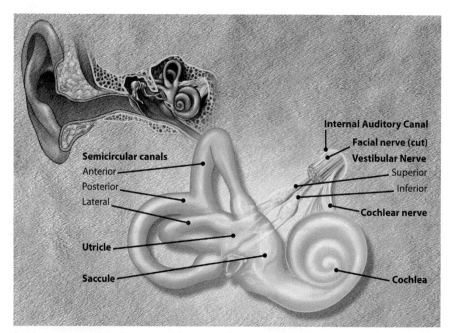

Fig. 1. Anatomy of the inner ear. (*Courtesy of* Marie Rossettie.)

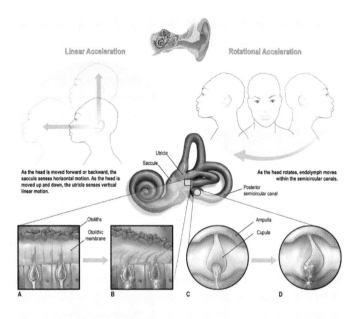

Fig. 2. Physiology of perception of motion. Displacement of the cupula. (*Courtesy of* Marie Rossettie.)

cells in the utricle and saccule are covered by a gelatinous otolithic membrane in which calcium carbonate particles (otoliths) are embedded. As fluid moves in a semi-circular canal, it displaces the cupula (see **Fig. 2**), which generates the sense of motion.

The vestibular nerves supply the end organs in the labyrinth.

With linear head movement (see **Fig. 2**), gravity causes the heavier otoliths to move, displacing the hair cells in the utricle (vertical movement) and saccule (horizontal movement). With angular motion, fluid motion displaces the cupula that lies within the dilated end portion of the semicircular canals (ampulla). This displacement of the cupula is transduced into electrical energy, which is transmitted to the brainstem via the vestibular nerve.

Benign paroxysmal positional vertigo (BPPV) is caused by dislodged otoliths from the utricle that migrate into one of the semicircular canals, most commonly 1 of the 2 posterior canals because they are the most gravity dependent, therefore simulating motion that is nonexistent[6] (**Fig. 3**).

The eighth cranial nerve comprises the vestibular and the cochlear nerves. Signals from the vestibular labyrinth travel through the vestibular nerve to the vestibular nuclei in the brainstem, then connects with the cerebellum, oculomotor system, cortex, and spinal cord.

The connections with the oculomotor system contain a reflex arc, the vestibulo-ocular reflex (VOR), that helps to fix one's gaze on a visual target when the head is moving, an important survival trait. The horizontal head impulse test (HIT), which was first described in 1988, tests the VOR.[7] This arc does not loop through the cerebellum, which is why the HIT is "negative" in cerebellar stroke. However, the cerebellum does modulate the VOR due to connections between the vestibular nuclei and the cerebellum.

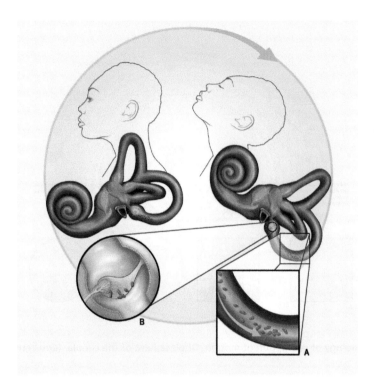

Fig. 3. Pathophysiology of BPPV. Displaced otoliths that have fallen into the posterior canal causing BPPV. (*Courtesy of* Marie Rossettie.)

The posterior circulation is fed by paired vertebral arteries that ascend in the neck and fuse to form the basilar artery. Just before fusing, they give off the posterior inferior cerebellar artery (PICA), the anterior inferior cerebellar artery (AICA), and the superior cerebellar artery. These are the major branches of the basilar artery before it splits into terminal branches—the paired posterior cerebral arteries. The PICA nourishes the lateral medulla and inferior cerebellum. The AICA nourishes the lateral pons including the vestibular nerve root entry zone. A branch of the AICA, the labyrinthine artery, supplies the peripheral labyrinth (**Fig. 4**). This explains why strokes of the lateral pons and the labyrinth are associated with a "positive" or falsely "reassuring" HIT.

CURRENT EVIDENCE

The evidence base for diagnosis of dizzy patients is weak[8] and because it specifically relates to routine emergency medicine practice, even weaker. In some of the most important articles about the diagnosis of dizzy patients, the interventions were done by neuro-otologists. That said, the evidence base for the diagnosis of dizziness is growing.[9]

DIFFERENTIAL DIAGNOSIS AND MISDIAGNOSIS

The individual causes of dizziness are too numerous to be clinically useful. Instead, one must use an organized diagnostic method. In an analysis of 9472 patients from

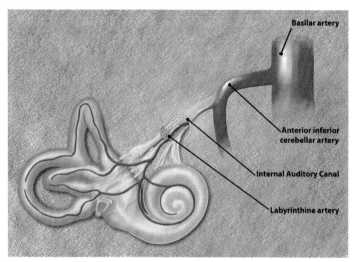

Fig. 4. Posterior circulation cerebrovascular anatomy. (*Courtesy of* Marie Rossettie.)

a large National Hospital Ambulatory Medical Care Survey database[1] of ED patients, the causes of dizziness listed in the charts by the attending emergency physicians were as follows:

- General medical (toxic, metabolic, and infectious) conditions: 49%
- Otologic or vestibular conditions: 33%
- Cardiovascular causes: 21%
- Respiratory conditions: 12%
- Neurologic diseases: 7%
- Cerebrovascular causes: 4%

Predefined "dangerous" diagnoses (mostly serious cardiovascular, cerebrovascular, and general medical conditions) accounted for 15% of cases and were twice as likely in patients older than 50 years of age.[1]

Misdiagnosis of patients with acute dizziness, especially misdiagnosis of cerebellar and brainstem stroke, is a common problem not restricted to emergency physicians.[9] In a German study of 475 ED patients with dizziness assessed by a neurologist, nearly 50% of diagnoses were changed by a second neurologist (blinded to the initial diagnosis) on follow-up.[10] Importantly, evolution of the clinical course over time after the initial evaluation (obviously not available to physicians who are first diagnosing the patients) was a factor in 70% of the misdiagnosed patients.[10]

Patients with anterior circulation strokes often present with lateralizing weakness, which scores more points on the National Institute of Health Stroke Scale and receives more attention in the medical literature[11] than posterior circulation strokes. The latter are misdiagnosed more than twice as often as anterior circulation events.[12] Our use of stroke heuristics emphasizes lateralizing deficits, which are often subtle or absent in patients with posterior circulation strokes.[9]

Another reason for misdiagnosis is the "needle in the haystack" phenomenon. Very few ED patients with dizziness are having strokes. In one study of 1666 adult ED patients with dizziness, fewer than 1% of those with isolated dizziness had a cerebrovascular cause.[13] Other studies found that of ED patients with dizziness who are discharged with a peripheral vestibular diagnosis, less than a half of 1% (range = 0.14–0.5%) are subsequently hospitalized with a stroke.[14–17] Although low, given the high number of dizzy patients, the absolute number is significant.

Other studies that "look backwards," analyzing patients who are ultimately diagnosed with strokes (only focusing on the needles), show that between 28% to 59% of patients with cerebellar strokes are missed in the ED.[18–20] In one study of 240 patients with cerebellar strokes, 10% (25 patients) presented with isolated dizziness that mimicked peripheral lesions.[21] Misdiagnosis rates look very different depending on whether or not the study looks "forward" or "backward."[22] Factors associated with misdiagnoses of patients with dizziness include use of the traditional symptom quality approach, lack of familiarity with eye movement examinations, overweighting of age and other traditional vascular risk factors, and overreliance on CT scanning,[23] as well as younger age, vertebral dissection as a cause and a presentation of dizziness.[12,24,25]

Lack of familiarity with some of the eye findings is an important knowledge gap. Nystagmus in particular, is often underutilized or incorrectly utilized by emergency clinicians. The presence or absence of nystagmus is important, but the details of the nystagmus are far more important diagnostically. In a study of 1091 dizzy patients in US EDs, physicians used templates to document the presence or absence of nystagmus in 887 (80%).[26] Nystagmus was documented as present in 185 (21%), of which, diagnostically meaningful information was recorded in only 10 (5.4%). Of patients given a peripheral vestibular diagnosis, the nystagmus description often conflicted with that diagnosis in 81%.[26]

Finally, it should be emphasized that CT scanning, the typical ED "go to" brain imaging test, is of extremely limited utility in these patients, often giving false reassurance. In a study of ED patients with dizziness who were discharged with a benign ICD-9 "dizzy" diagnosis and followed-up for 30 days, patients who returned with a stroke were 2.3 times more likely to have had a CT on the first visit, suggesting that physicians were correctly determining worrisome patents but then applying the wrong diagnostic test.[27]

DIAGNOSTIC APPROACH

According to traditional "symptom quality" paradigm, patients will select either vertigo, lightheadedness, disequilibrium, or other.[2] The first group has vestibular problems; the second group, cardiovascular or general medical problems; the third group, neurologic problems; and the last group, psychiatric disease.

For traditional approach to work, patients must be able to consistently select a single "type" of dizziness, and each dizziness type is tightly associated with specific diagnoses. Neither proposition is true. In a study of ED patients with dizziness, researchers asked questions about the type of dizziness and the timing and triggers of the dizziness.[28] When they reasked the same questions but in a different sequence an average of 6 minutes later, 50% of patients changed the "type" of dizziness that they had selected just minutes before. Frequently, they selected 2 or 3 different dizziness types. However, they were far more consistent about the timing of the dizziness and the factors that triggered it.

In addition, the use of one term versus another (eg, vertigo vs lightheadedness) is not diagnostically meaningful. In the ED study of 1666 acutely dizzy patients, use of the word "vertigo" was not associated with a cerebrovascular diagnosis.[13] In another study of patients with BPPV, 27% endorsed "dizziness" and *not* "vertigo," far more commonly in elderly patients.[29] In another review of patients with cardiovascular conditions with dizziness, nearly 40% endorsed vertigo (not lightheadedness, which the traditional paradigm would predict).[30]

Timing and Triggers Approach

Not only is a timing and triggers paradigm more consistent with current evidence but it is the way we take histories from every other patient. One would never base the differential diagnosis of a chest pain patient solely on the descriptor that the patient uses. One elicits the onset, the evolution, the constant or intermittent nature, and factors that trigger or alleviate the pain. For example, it is less important that a patient endorses sharp or dull or even tearing chest pain but rather if it has been intermittent, only occurring with exertion and is relieved by rest.

Rather than basing a differential diagnosis on the descriptive word a patient uses (vertigo or lightheadedness or imbalance), a more logical strategy is based on the timing and the triggers of the dizziness.[6,23,31–33]

The "ATTEST" algorithm uses an evidence-based systematic approach to diagnose acutely dizzy patients. The first three letters in the ATTEST pneumonic (Associated symptoms, Timing, and Triggers) refer to historical information: "What happened?" "When?" "Is the dizziness continuous or intermittent?" "Are there associated symptoms?" "What is the broader context?" (**Fig. 5**).

Patients without an obvious general medical cause usually fall into 1 of 3 categories: the acute vestibular syndrome (AVS) (acute onset persistent, continuously present dizziness), the triggered episodic vestibular syndrome (t-EVS) (brief episodes of dizziness caused by some obligate trigger), and the spontaneous episodic vestibular syndrome (s-EVS) (spontaneous episodes of variable duration dizziness not triggered by anything).

A = associated symptoms
TT = timing and triggers
ES = examination signs
T = (confirmatory) testing

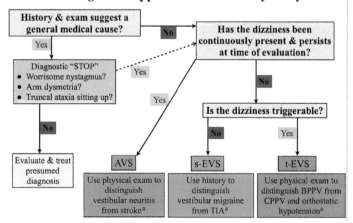

Fig. 5. ATTEST diagnostic algorithm. [a] For each vestibular syndrome, only the most common benign and dangerous diagnosis is listed. (*From* Edlow JA, Gurley KL, Newman-Toker DE. A New Diagnostic Approach to the Adult Patient with Acute Dizziness. *J Emerg Med.* 2018;54(4):469-483. https://doi.org/10.1016/j.jemermed.2017.12.024; with permission.)

Although this approach has not been validated in routine ED practice, it is consistent with the way other chief complaints are approached, is rooted in vestibular and neurologic physiology and pathophysiology, and is consistent with current evidence.[5]

Asking about timing and triggers yields 3 acute vestibular categories that are tightly associated with a specific differential diagnosis (**Table 1**).[3,6,31,34] Patients may have an AVS, an s-EVS, or a t-EVS (see **Table 1**).

For practical purposes in patients with an AVS, the major distinction to be made is neuritis versus stroke because approximately 95% of patients with AVS have 1 of those 2 diagnoses.[35] Two to three percent have an initial presentation of multiple sclerosis.[35,36] The remainder may have a long list of very uncommon diagnoses.[35] One important uncommon cause is Wernicke encephalopathy (thiamine deficiency).[37]

For patients with an s-EVS, the most common diagnosis by far is vestibular migraine but the important serious diagnosis is TIA. Although posterior circulation TIA presenting as isolated dizziness was long thought to not exist, mounting evidence demonstrates that it does.[38–42] In one study of 1141 stroke patients, brief episodes of symptoms occurring within the 2 days before the stroke that could be ascribed to posterior circulation ischemia were 36 times more likely in patients who had vertebrobasilar strokes compared with those with anterior circulation strokes.[39]

For patients with a t-EVS, BPPV and non–life-threatening causes of orthostatic hypotension are the common benign causes, and central paroxysmal positional vertigo (CPPV) and serious causes of orthostasis are the life-threatening causes. CPPV is caused by small lesions (mass, multiple sclerosis, or tumor) in the region of the fourth ventricle that can mimic BPPV.[43,44]

General Medical Causes

History and vital signs usually suggest the roughly 50% of patients whose dizziness is caused by general medical causes. The particular descriptive word used by the patient (eg, lightheadedness or vertigo or imbalance) to describe their dizziness is not diagnostically useful.

Consider the following histories in patients who endorse dizziness plus:

- Heavy ibuprofen use and black stools
- New antihypertensive or anticonvulsant medication use
- Moderate mechanism motor vehicle crash
- Abdominal pain, vaginal bleeding, and positive pregnancy test
- Chest pain and dyspnea in a patient with Factor V Leiden

Each situation suggests a diagnosis or group of diagnoses that would require confirmatory testing. Similarly, the vital signs inform this diagnostic process. If a general medical diagnosis is likely, the authors recommend a brief diagnostic "STOP" that takes less than 1 minute to perform (see **Fig. 5**).[6,31] In order to identify disorders that might mimic a general medical condition, the 3 components of the "STOP" are testing for worrisome nystagmus (described in detail later), arm dysmetria, and truncal ataxia. To test for truncal ataxia, simply have the patient sit up in the stretcher without holding onto the side rails. If the "STOP" is reassuring, proceed with management for the presumed condition. If it is worrisome, consider various vestibular or central conditions.

Acute Vestibular Syndrome

If the history does not suggest a general medical condition (or if the "STOP" is worrisome), then the next question to pose is, "is the dizziness persistently present and still present at the time of ED evaluation?" A "yes" answer identifies patients with the AVS,

Table 1
Timing-and-trigger–based "vestibular[a] syndromes" in acute dizziness and their corresponding differential diagnosis[b]

Syndrome	Description	Common Benign Causes	Common Serious Causes	Important Rare Causes
AVS	Acute, continuous dizziness lasting days, accompanied by nausea, vomiting, nystagmus, head motion intolerance, and gait unsteadiness	Vestibular neuritis Labyrinthitis	Posterior circulation ischemic stroke	Multiple sclerosis Wernicke encephalopathy Drug/medication side effects or toxicity
s-EVS	Episodic dizziness that occurs spontaneously, is not triggered, and usually last minutes to hours	Vestibular migraine Menière disease	Posterior circulation TIA	Cardiac dysrhythmia Pulmonary embolism Panic attacks
t-EVS	Episodic dizziness triggered by a specific, obligate trigger (typically a change in head position or standing up), and usually lasting <1 min	BPPV Orthostatic hypotension caused by benign problems	CPPV Orthostatic hypotension due to serious medical illness	Superior canal dehiscence Postural tachycardia syndrome Panic attacks Vertebral artery rotation (Bow Hunters syndrome)

Abbreviation: TIA, transient ischemic attack.

[a] The word "vestibular" here connotes vestibular symptoms (dizziness or vertigo or imbalance), rather than underlying vestibular diseases (eg, BPPV or vestibular neuritis).

[b] This table lists the more common and most important conditions and is not intended to be exhaustive.

From Gurley, K.L. and J.A. Edlow, *Acute Dizziness.* Semin Neurol, 2019. **39**(1): p. 27–40; with permission.

who have the abrupt or rapid onset of dizziness that has lasted hours to days and is still present at the time of examination even when the patient is lying still. The dizziness may decrease when lying still and worsen with head movement, a common occurrence that does *not* mean that the dizziness has a peripheral cause.

Although the strict definition of the AVS includes the presence of nystagmus, some patients who otherwise fulfill the AVS definition (such as many with cerebellar stroke) do not have nystagmus. Its presence or absence is a key distinction because it affects how one interprets the HIT.[3,31,32,34] Bedside eye findings in these symptomatic patients to distinguish central (stroke) from peripheral (neuritis) causes, referred to as Head Impulse–Nystagmus–Test of Skew (HINTS) testing in patients with AVS. An important caveat is that most of the studies that examine the utility of HINTS have been done with neuro-otologists performing the examinations.[45,46] A potential source of confusion, the HINTS acronym, is similar to but different from the abbreviation for the HIT, a component of HINTS.

Although one study found that vascular neurologists can be trained to effectively use the HINTS examination[47] and other European studies of emergency physicians (who received 12 hours of special training using Frenzel lenses to interpret the eye findings) showed the same,[48,49] HINTS accuracy in routine practice has not been fully validated. The authors therefore recommend 2 additional components to the examination of patients with the AVS[3,31]—a targeted posterior circulation examination and gait testing.

Five questions are posed when doing the physical examination (intentionally in the following sequence) (**Fig. 6**):

- Is there a central pattern of nystagmus?
- Is skew deviation present?
- Is the HIT worrisome for a central process (ie, absent corrective saccade)?

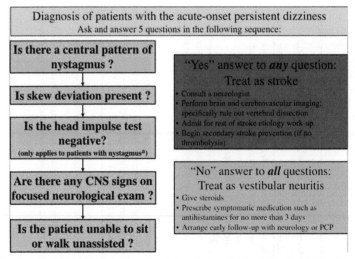

Fig. 6. Physical examination testing algorithm for patients with the AVS. [a] In patients *without* nystagmus, the head impulse test may give misleading results; the focused neurological exam and gait assessment become more important in this group (see text). (*From* Edlow JA. Diagnosing Patients With Acute-Onset Persistent Dizziness. Ann Emerg Med. 2018;71(5):625-631. https://doi.org/10.1016/j.annemergmed.2017.10.012; with permission.)

- Are there central nervous system (CNS) findings on the targeted posterior circulation examination?
- Can the patient sit up or walk without assistance?

Because none of these tests is 100% sensitive, patients with a "yes" answer to *any one* of the questions means the cause is central (likely stroke) and should be admitted to the hospital for further management.[3,31,32,34] If the answer to *all five* questions is "no," then the patient likely has neuritis and can be safely discharged on oral prednisone with outpatient follow-up.

The HINTS acronym notwithstanding do not start with the HIT but rather with nystagmus. First, nystagmus testing is easy for the patient. Secondly, if nystagmus is absent, interpretation of the HIT is problematic because it has only been validated in patients WITH nystagmus and also, vestibular neuritis and labyrinthitis are very unlikely (early presenting patients almost always display nystagmus).

To test for nystagmus, ask the patient to open their eyes and look forward. Observe if there is any jerk nystagmus, in which the eyes drift in one direction, then snap quickly back. By convention, nystagmus is named for its rapid phase. If a patient looks forward and their eyes drift to the left then snap back to the right, they have "right-beating horizontal nystagmus." This is usually easy to see, especially in the first few days from symptom onset. Next ask the patient to follow the examiner's finger, going 30° to the right, then the left—this is called "gaze-evoked nystagmus." Also observe for vertical or pure torsional nystagmus. In patients with the AVS, nystagmus, which is vertical, torsional, or that changes direction with the direction of gaze, is central (**Table 2**).[6,32]

Next, check for skew deviation using the alternate cover test, also easy for the patient. One stands in front of the patient, instructing them to focus on the tip of your nose, and then alternately covers one eye then the other multiple times, covering one eye then the next every second or so. The presence of skew deviation—a small vertical correction in the eye when it is uncovered—indicates a brainstem localization. It is easiest if one focuses on only one eye (both eyes will display the vertical correction, one going down, whereas the other going up).

The third component of the examination is the HIT (**Fig. 7**). The patient is instructed to relax their head and neck and to focus on the examiner's nose. The examiner holds the patient's head on both sides and very rapidly snaps it in one direction or the other over a very small arc of only ~15°.[3,7,31,32] Ideally, hold the head 15° from the midline and then move it very quickly to the midline. The "normal" or "negative" HIT (eyes remain focused on the examiner's nose) is worrisome for stroke, whereas the "abnormal" or "positive" HIT (eyes move with the head and then snap back in a corrective saccade to the examiner's nose) is reassuring for neuritis. Calling an HIT "normal," "abnormal," "negative," or "positive" is confusing (because the "negative" test is worrisome and the "positive" test is reassuring). It is preferable to report the presence or absence of a corrective saccade.[45,50] Approximately 10% of HITs with a "reassuring" corrective saccade are false positives due to strokes,[45] usually of the AICA or labyrinthine artery territories.[3]

The fourth component of the AVS evaluation is to look for any CNS findings due to posterior circulation ischemia. In addition to a general motor and sensory examination, a brief but systematic examination targeting the cranial nerves, cerebellar function, and visual fields should be done. Any (new) abnormality indicates a central finding and therefore would be inconsistent with neuritis. Anisocoria and ptosis (Horner syndrome) suggests a lateral medullary infarct. The unilateral facial sensory loss in lateral medullary stroke involves pain and temperature, not light touch, which is the usual

Table 2
Summary of useful physical examination findings in symptomatic patients with the acute vestibular syndrome

Examination Component	Peripheral (*All* Must be Present to Diagnose Vestibular Neuritis)	Central (Any *One* of These Findings Suggests Posterior Circulation Stroke)
Nystagmus (straight-ahead gaze and rightward & leftward gaze)	Dominantly horizontal, direction-fixed, beating away from the affected side[a]	Dominantly vertical and/or torsional or dominantly horizontal, direction-changing on left/right gaze[b]
Test of skew (alternate cover test)	Normal vertical eye alignment and no corrective vertical movement (ie, no skew deviation)	Skew deviation (small vertical correction on uncovering the eye)
Head impulse test (HIT)	Unilateral presence of a corrective refixation saccade (abnormal) when the is moved rapidly toward the affected side [c]	No corrective saccade (abnormal)
Targeted neurologic examination (see text)	No cranial neuropathy, brainstem, or cerebellar signs or field cut	Presence of limb ataxia, dysarthria, diplopia, ptosis, anisocoria, facial sensory loss (pain/temperature), unilateral decreased hearing, or field cut
Gait and truncal ataxia	Able to walk unassisted and to sit up in stretcher without holding on or leaning against bed or rails	Unable to walk unassisted or sit up in stretcher without holding on or leaning against bed or rails

[a] Inferior branch vestibular neuritis will present with downbeat-torsional nystagmus, but this is a rare disorder. From the emergency medicine perspective, vertical nystagmus in a patient with an AVS patient should be considered to be central (a stroke).
[b] More than half of posterior circulation strokes will have direction-fixed horizontal nystagmus that, alone, cannot be distinguished from that typically seen with vestibular neuritis.
[c] Some patients with strokes in the anterior inferior cerebellar artery (AICA) territory have a corrective saccade on head impulse testing that mimics vestibular neuritis, but hearing loss may be present and gait is severely altered. If a patient has bilaterally abnormal HIT, this is also suspicious for a central lesion if nystagmus is present (as may be seen in Wernicke syndrome).
From Gurley, K.L. and J.A. Edlow, *Acute Dizziness.* Semin Neurol, 2019. 39(1): p. 27-40; with permission.

modality tested by most nonneurologists. It is important to recognize that acute hearing loss, traditionally associated with a peripheral process, can also occur with an acute cerebrovascular event involving either the AICA or labyrinthine artery.[3]

Finally, the gait should be tested in patients with dizziness. Patients who are unsteady cannot be safely discharged from the ED. Furthermore, greater degrees of gait abnormality correlate with stroke. In a series of 114 patients with AVS (67% with neuritis and 33% with stroke), most neuritis patients could walk independently, whereas most patients with stroke could not.[51] In fact, two-thirds of the stroke

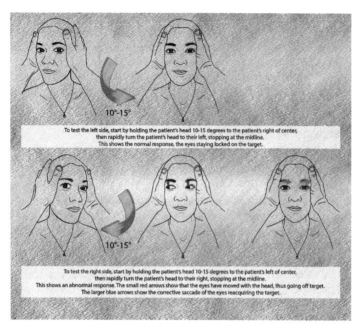

To test the left side, start by holding the patient's head 10-15 degrees to the patient's right of center, then rapidly turn the patient's head to their left, stopping at the midline. This shows the normal response, the eyes staying locked on the target.

To test the right side, start by holding the patient's head 10-15 degrees to the patient's left of center, then rapidly turn the patient's head to their right, stopping at the midline. This shows an abnormal response. The small red arrows show that the eyes have moved with the head, thus going off target. The larger blue arrows show the corrective saccade of the eyes reacquiring the target.

Fig. 7. Head impulse test. (*Courtesy of* Marie Rossettie.)

patients could not even stand up independently. All of the 10 patients with AICA stroke (whose HIT can be misleading) had severe gait instability.[51] **Table 2** summarizes these findings.

SPONTANEOUS EPISODIC VESTIBULAR SYNDROME

Patients with an s-EVS endorse one or more episodes of dizziness of variable duration not triggered by head or body position changes. Because, by definition, these patients are no longer symptomatic and are not triggerable, physical examination is not useful to distinguish the 2 most common diagnoses (vestibular migraine and posterior circulation TIA). Diagnosis relies on history and epidemiologic context.[6] If a patient with vestibular migraine or TIA were still symptomatic at the time of evaluation, one would proceed as if they had an AVS just as if a patient with an anterior circulation TIA still had symptoms at the time of presentation, they would be assumed to be having a stroke.

For vestibular migraine, there is a strong (5:1) female predominance.[52] Patients have multiple episodes of dizziness with or without headaches that may not occur with the dizziness.[53] When headaches do occur, they are usually (not always) similar to migraines that occur without the dizziness. The duration of the dizziness is variable lasting minutes to days.[54] Because migraine is a central phenomenon, the associated nystagmus can be of a central type.[55]

Half of patients who have posterior circulation TIAs have isolated transient dizziness.[39] Other symptoms include deficits involving the long tracts that pass through the brainstem, cranial nerve dysfunction, or visual field cuts. Contrary to conventional wisdom, short-term stroke risk may be higher with posterior circulation TIA than with anterior circulation TIA.[38,56]

Recognizing that none of these elements can be used in a binary yes/no fashion, factors that suggest vestibular migraine over TIA include younger age, more frequent attacks over a longer period of time, other migraine-related symptoms (such as headache, phonophobia, photophobia), and absent traditional vascular risk factors.

Patients with Menière disease (relatively uncommon in ED series of dizzy patients) also present with an s-EVS and will usually have ringing or buzzing in the ear and over time, progressive hearing loss.[57]

TRIGGERED EPISODIC VESTIBULAR SYNDROME

The physical examination is very helpful in patients with a t-EVS and will usually establish a specific diagnosis (**Table 3**). Although the utility of orthostatic vital signs has been downplayed in emergency medicine, patients with dizziness on standing up and orthostatic vital signs likely have orthostatic hypotension as a cause of the dizziness, and the evaluation should be directed at finding its underlying cause.

BPPV should be suspected in patients with very brief episodes of dizziness, generally lasting less than a minute. Episodes of dizziness that wakes a patient from sleep are nearly always due to BPPV.[58–61] In patients with suspected BPPV, bedside testing can confidently establish the diagnosis (see **Table 3**). The most commonly affected canal is the posterior (pc-BPPV), which is tested by the Dix-Hallpike maneuver. If this test is negative on both sides, then the horizontal canal (hc-BPPV) should be tested by the supine head roll test.

Patients with occasional BPPV have no nystagmus.[62–64] Possible causes are a small number of otoliths in the canal, use of vestibular suppressants at the time of diagnosis, or small amplitude nystagmus that the examiner is not perceiving due to visual fixation by the patient. In addition, some patients with hc-BPPV will have spontaneous (or more persistent) nystagmus, normally not seen with BPPV.[65,66] This occurs because, depending on the orientation of the patient's head, otoliths in the horizontal canal may be moving in a patient sitting up looking forward.

Finally, very rarely, patients with CPPV, caused by structural lesions (usually a tumor, multiple sclerosis plaque, or small brainstem stroke) adjacent to the fourth ventricle, will exhibit nystagmus or other features that are atypical for BPPV such as headache or diplopia, atypical nystagmus, or poor response to therapeutic maneuvers.[44,67]

IMAGING

Diagnostic studies in patients who are suspected of having some general medical (toxic, metabolic, infectious) condition causing their dizziness will depend on the suspected diagnosis, that is, blood glucose for suspected hypoglycemia, stool guaiac, and hematocrit for suspected gastrointestinal bleeding, etc.

In patients with an AVS, the physical examination should reliably distinguish between stroke (or other central causes) and vestibular neuritis or labyrinthitis. A key point is that not only is imaging not required but in fact, has serious limitations in patients with a posterior circulation stroke. The "reassurance" that an abnormal CT scan in dizzy patients excludes a central cause is false reassurance.[27] Unreliable for any acute ischemic stroke, CT performs even worse in the posterior circulation. An abnormal CT scan should never be relied on by itself to exclude posterior circulation ischemic stroke especially those presenting with an AVS.[68–73] In 2 large series of consecutive ED patients with dizziness who had CT, 0/344 (0%) and 7/448 (1.6%) had emergent findings on CT relevant to the dizziness.[72,73] Furthermore, intracranial hemorrhage (ICH) rarely presents as an isolated AVS. In one series of 595 cases of

Table 3
Benign paroxysmal positional vertigo physical examination, type of nystagmus, and therapeutic maneuvers

Canal Involved, Mechanism (Proportion of BPPV Cases)	Provocative Diagnostic Maneuver/Test	Expected Type of Nystagmus	Therapeutic Maneuver
pc-BPPV (80%–85%)	Dix-Hallpike	Up beating (from patient's perspective) and torsional	Epley maneuver Alternative: Semont maneuver
hc-BPPV (15%–20%) (sometimes called lateral canal)			
Canalolithiasis (most of the horizontal canal cases)	Supine head roll	Geotropic (beats toward the floor) horizontal that is transient Occurs on both sides, but is more intense on the *affected* side	Lempert log roll maneuver Alternative: Gufoni maneuver
Cupulolithiasis (minority of horizontal canal cases)	Supine head roll	Apogeotropic (beats toward the ceiling) horizontal, that is persistent Occurs on both sides but is more intense on the *healthy* unaffected side	Gufoni maneuver
sc-BPPV (~1%–2%) (sometimes called anterior canal)	Dix-Hallpike	Downbeating vertical nystagmus	Can use Epley but this form of BPPV usually resolves spontaneously

Abbreviation: pc-BPPV, posterior canal BPPV.
From Gurley, K.L. and J.A. Edlow, *Acute Dizziness.* Semin Neurol, 2019. **39**(1): p. 27-40; with permission.

ICH, the only patient who had an isolated AVS also had cerebellar dysmetria and rotatory nystagmus on examination.[74] Conversely, in the series of 448 patients presenting with dizziness, only 2 (0.5%) had an ICH. However, if associated headache is prominent or clinical findings that suggest CPPV, CT may be justified.

Less well known, early MRI, even diffusion-weighted MRI (DWI-MRI), can miss stroke in patients scanned in the first 48 hours. In a meta-analysis of 3236 patients with acute ischemic stroke, nearly 7% had an abnormal DWI-MRI, and this was strongly associated with a posterior circulation location.[75] The proportion of false-negative DWI-MRI when done in the first 72 hours in patients with the AVS ranges from 12% to 18%[45,46,76,77] and approaches 50% in small strokes (<10 mm in axial diameter)[46] Another large study found that number was 4% but it is not clear what percentage of the patients in the whole group had transient versus persistent symptoms.[78] Importantly, in all of these series, large vessel disease was common. Delayed MRI with DWI-MRI after 72 hours should reliably diagnose stroke and is considered the gold standard.

In patients with the s-EVS, there is no specific test that distinguishes vestibular migraine from posterior circulation TIA, and decision-making must be individualized based on history, epidemiology, and context. In patients with a t-EVS who likely have BPPV, no diagnostic testing beyond physical examination is needed. A therapeutic canalith repositioning maneuver might be considered a "diagnostic" test (see **Table 3**).

CONTROVERSIES

Use of the HINTS examination by emergency physicians in routine practice has never been validated. To learn and perform the HINTS examination requires time and commitment. If emergency physicians who use HINTS encounter ambiguous findings, one should probably err on the side of patient safety (overcalling something as possibly central rather than peripheral). The original HINTS study enrolled patients with stroke risk factors that do not mirror an unselected ED population of dizzy patients.[45] A recent meta-analysis of use of HINTS (N = 617 patients) concluded that the performance characteristics of HINTS testing by emergency physicians was inadequate to rule out stroke.[79]

Investigators are studying the use of a portable goggle device with an embedded infrared device to record the eye movements when the patient is being taken through each of the component movements of the HINTS examination. Proof of concept exists with results that then come out as worrisome for a central event or reassuring for a peripheral one.[80] Further studies are currently ongoing to investigate this approach.

Another recent study showed that perfusion-weighted MRI can help make a stroke diagnosis in 86 patients presenting with s-EVS.[81] Inclusion criteria were "rapid onset of vertigo/dizziness," "resolution of symptoms within 24 hours," and "no previous history of recurrent vertigo." Of the 86 patients, 23 were still symptomatic at the time of presentation so the HINTS testing was done and meaningful. Of the 63 asymptomatic patients, 32 had strokes, of which DWI-MRI was abnormal in half. In 9 of these 63 (14%), perfusion-weighted MRI showed cerebellar hypoperfusion as a cause of the event. The duration of the dizziness in these patients ranged from "several minutes" (50%) to "several hours" (50%).

SUMMARY

Using an algorithmic approach to acutely dizzy patients, physicians can often confidently make a specific diagnosis that leads to correct treatment and should reduce the misdiagnosis of cerebrovascular events. Emergency clinicians should try to become familiar with an approach that exploits timing and triggers as well as some basic "rules" of nystagmus. Emergency physicians should try to learn the HINTS examination although confirmation of accuracy in routine practice is currently lacking. The gait should always be tested in all patients who might be discharged. CT scans are unreliable to exclude posterior circulation stroke presenting as dizziness, and early MRI (within the first 72 hours) also misses 10% to 20% of these cases.

CLINICS CARE POINTS

- Use a "timing and triggers" (rather than a "symptom quality") approach to the diagnosis of patients with dizziness.
- Each acute timing and triggers category (AVS, s-EVS, and the t-EVS) is tightly associated with a specific differential diagnosis.
- Approximately 95% of patients with the AVS have either neuritis (vestibular neuritis or labyrinthitis) or posterior circulation stroke.
- In patients with the AVS presenting in the first 48 hours, bedside examination can help to distinguish between neuritis and stroke with greater sensitivity than MRI.
- The major differential diagnosis of patients with the s-EVS is vestibular migraine and posterior circulation TIA. Because these patients are asymptomatic and the dizziness cannot be triggered, physical examination is not helpful.
- Use physical examination to diagnose patients with the t-EVS.
- Because BPPV is so common and easily treatable, learn how to diagnose this condition by physical examination and treat with a bedside repositioning maneuver. A confident diagnosis of BPPV essentially excludes a central cause.
- CT scan is a poor test to exclude posterior circulation stroke and acutely should never be relied on in this setting.
- Approximately 10% to 20% of patients with the AVS who present within 48 hours of onset will have a false-negative MRI, even with DWI.

REFERENCES

1. Newman-Toker DE, Hsieh YH, Camargo CA, et al. Spectrum of dizziness visits to US emergency departments: cross-sectional analysis from a nationally representative sample. Mayo Clin Proc 2008;83(7):765–75.
2. Drachman DA, Hart CW. An approach to the dizzy patient. Neurology 1972;22(4):323–34.
3. Edlow JA. Diagnosing patients with acute-onset persistent dizziness. Ann Emerg Med 2018;71(5):625–31.
4. Gurley KL, Edlow JA. Missed stroke in acute vertigo and dizziness: It is time for action, not debate. Ann Neurol 2019;79(1):27–31.
5. Edlow JA. Diagnosing dizziness: we are teaching the wrong paradigm! Acad Emerg Med 2013;20(10):1064–6.
6. Edlow JA. Managing patients with acute episodic dizziness. Ann Emerg Med 2018;72(5):602–10.
7. Halmagyi GM, Curthoys IS. A clinical sign of canal paresis. Arch Neurol 1988;45(7):737–9.

8. Kerber KA, Fendrick AM. The evidence base for the evaluation and management of dizziness. J Eval Clin Pract 2010;16(1):186–91.
9. Gurley KL, Edlow JA. Avoiding misdiagnosis in patients with posterior circulation ischemia: a narrative review. Acad Emerg Med 2019;26(11):1273–84.
10. Royl G, Ploner CJ, Leithner C. Dizziness in the emergency room: diagnoses and misdiagnoses. Eur Neurol 2011;66(5):256–63.
11. Goldstein LB, Simel DL. Is this patient having a stroke? JAMA 2005;293(19): 2391–402.
12. Arch AE, Weisman DC, Coca S, et al. Missed ischemic stroke diagnosis in the emergency department by emergency medicine and neurology services. Stroke 2016;47(3):668–73.
13. Kerber KA, Brown DL, Lisabeth LD, et al. Stroke among patients with dizziness, vertigo, and imbalance in the emergency department: a population-based study. Stroke 2006;37(10):2484–7.
14. Lee CC, Ho HC, Su YC, et al. Increased risk of vascular events in emergency room patients discharged home with diagnosis of dizziness or vertigo: a 3-year follow-up study. PLoS One 2012;7(4):e35923.
15. Atzema CL, Grewal K, Lu H, et al. Outcomes among patients discharged from the emergency department with a diagnosis of peripheral vertigo. Ann Neurol 2015; 79(1):32–41.
16. Kerber KA, Meurer WJ, Brown DL, et al. Stroke risk stratification in acute dizziness presentations: A prospective imaging-based study. Neurology 2015; 85(21):1869–78.
17. Kim AS, Fullerton HJ, Johnston SC. Risk of vascular events in emergency department patients discharged home with diagnosis of dizziness or vertigo. Ann Emerg Med 2011;57(1):34–41.
18. Calic Z, Cappelen-Smith C, Anderson CS, et al. Cerebellar infarction and factors associated with delayed presentation and misdiagnosis. Cerebrovasc Dis 2016; 42(5–6):476–84.
19. Masuda Y, Tei H, Shimizu S, et al. Factors associated with the misdiagnosis of cerebellar infarction. J Stroke Cerebrovasc Dis 2013;22(7):1125–30.
20. Sangha N, Albright KC, Peng H, et al. Misdiagnosis of cerebellar infarctions. Can J Neurol Sci 2014;41(5):568–71.
21. Lee H, Sohn SI, Cho YW, et al. Cerebellar infarction presenting isolated vertigo: frequency and vascular topographical patterns. Neurology 2006;67(7):1178–83.
22. Dubosh NM, Edlow JA, Goto T, et al. Missed serious neurologic conditions in emergency department patients discharged with nonspecific diagnoses of headache or back pain. Ann Emerg Med 2019;74(4):549–61.
23. Kerber KA, Newman-Toker DE. Misdiagnosing dizzy patients: common pitfalls in clinical practice. Neurol Clin 2015;33(3):565–viii.
24. Nakajima M, Hirano T, Uchino M. Patients with acute stroke admitted on the second visit. J Stroke Cerebrovasc Dis 2008;17(6):382–7.
25. Tarnutzer AA, Lee SH, Robinson KA, et al. ED misdiagnosis of cerebrovascular events in the era of modern neuroimaging: A meta-analysis. Neurology 2017; 88(15):1468–77.
26. Kerber KA, Morgenstern LB, Meurer WJ, et al. Nystagmus assessments documented by emergency physicians in acute dizziness presentations: a target for decision support? Acad Emerg Med 2011;18(6):619–26.
27. Grewal K, Austin PC, Kapral MK, et al. Missed strokes using computed tomography imaging in patients with vertigo: population-based cohort study. Stroke 2015; 46(1):108–13.

28. Newman-Toker DE, Cannon LM, Stofferahn ME, et al. Imprecision in patient reports of dizziness symptom quality: a cross-sectional study conducted in an acute care setting. Mayo Clin Proc 2007;82(11):1329–40.
29. Lawson J, Johnson I, Bamiou DE, et al. Benign paroxysmal positional vertigo: clinical characteristics of dizzy patients referred to a Falls and Syncope Unit. QJM 2005;98(5):357–64.
30. Newman-Toker DE, Dy FJ, Stanton VA, et al. How often is dizziness from primary cardiovascular disease true vertigo? A systematic review. J Gen Intern Med 2008; 23(12):2087–94.
31. Edlow JA, Gurley KL, Newman-Toker DE. A new diagnostic approach to the adult patient with acute dizziness. J Emerg Med 2018;54(4):469–83.
32. Edlow JA, Newman-Toker D. Using the physical examination to diagnose patients with acute dizziness and vertigo. J Emerg Med 2016;50(4):617–28.
33. Kerber KA. Vertigo and dizziness in the emergency department. Emerg Med Clin North Am 2009;27(1):39–viii, viii.
34. Edlow JA. A new approach to the diagnosis of acute dizziness in adult patients. Emerg Med Clin North Am 2016;34(4):717–42.
35. Edlow JA, Newman-Toker DE. Medical and nonstroke neurologic causes of acute, continuous vestibular symptoms. Neurol Clin 2015;33(3):699, xi.
36. Pula JH, Newman-Toker DE, Kattah JC. Multiple sclerosis as a cause of the acute vestibular syndrome. J Neurol 2013;260(6):1649–54.
37. Kattah JC. The spectrum of vestibular and ocular motor abnormalities in thiamine deficiency. Curr Neurol Neurosci Rep 2017;17(5):40.
38. Gulli G, Marquardt L, Rothwell PM, et al. Stroke risk after posterior circulation stroke/transient ischemic attack and its relationship to site of vertebrobasilar stenosis: pooled data analysis from prospective studies. Stroke 2013;44(3): 598–604.
39. Paul NL, Simoni M, Rothwell PM. Transient isolated brainstem symptoms preceding posterior circulation stroke: a population-based study. Lancet Neurol 2013; 12(1):65–71.
40. Hoshino T, Nagao T, Mizuno S, et al. Transient neurological attack before vertebrobasilar stroke. J Neurol Sci 2013;325(1–2):39–42.
41. Lavallee PC, Sissani L, Labreuche J, et al. Clinical significance of isolated atypical transient symptoms in a cohort with transient ischemic attack. Stroke 2017; 48(6):1495–500.
42. Plas GJ, Booij HA, Brouwers PJ, et al. Nonfocal symptoms in patients with transient ischemic attack or ischemic stroke: occurrence, clinical determinants, and association with cardiac history. Cerebrovasc Dis 2016;42(5–6):439–45.
43. Dunniway HM, Welling DB. Intracranial tumors mimicking benign paroxysmal positional vertigo. Otolaryngol Head Neck Surg 1998;118(4):429–36.
44. Soto-Varela A, Rossi-Izquierdo M, Sánchez-Sellero I, et al. Revised criteria for suspicion of non-benign positional vertigo. QJM 2013;106(4):317–21.
45. Kattah JC, Talkad AV, Wang DZ, et al. HINTS to diagnose stroke in the acute vestibular syndrome: three-step bedside oculomotor examination more sensitive than early MRI diffusion-weighted imaging. Stroke 2009;40(11):3504–10.
46. Saber Tehrani AS, Kattah JC, Mantokoudis G, et al. Small strokes causing severe vertigo: frequency of false-negative MRIs and nonlacunar mechanisms. Neurology 2014;83(2):169–73.
47. Chen L, Lee W, Chambers BR, et al. Diagnostic accuracy of acute vestibular syndrome at the bedside in a stroke unit. J Neurol 2011;258(5):855–61.

48. Vanni S, Nazerian P, Casati C, et al. Can emergency physicians accurately and reliably assess acute vertigo in the emergency department? Emerg Med Australas 2015;27(2):126–31.

49. Vanni S, Pecci R, Edlow JA, et al. Differential diagnosis of vertigo in the emergency department: a prospective validation study of the STANDING algorithm. Front Neurol 2017;8:590.

50. Cnyrim CD, Newman-Toker D, Karch C, et al. Bedside differentiation of vestibular neuritis from central "vestibular pseudoneuritis. J Neurol Neurosurg Psychiatry 2008;79(4):458–60.

51. Carmona S, Martínez C, Zalazar G, et al. The diagnostic accuracy of truncal ataxia and HINTS as cardinal signs for acute vestibular syndrome. Front Neurol 2016;7:125.

52. Neuhauser H, Lempert T. Vestibular migraine. Neurol Clin 2009;27(2):379–91.

53. Furman JM, Marcus DA, Balaban CD. Vestibular migraine: clinical aspects and pathophysiology. Lancet Neurol 2013;12(7):706–15.

54. Dieterich M, Obermann M, Celebisoy N. Vestibular migraine: the most frequent entity of episodic vertigo. J Neurol 2016;263(Suppl 1):S82–9.

55. Polensek SH, Tusa RJ. Nystagmus during attacks of vestibular migraine: an aid in diagnosis. Audiol Neurootol 2010;15(4):241–6.

56. Flossmann E, Rothwell PM. Prognosis of vertebrobasilar transient ischaemic attack and minor stroke. Brain 2003;126(Pt 9):1940–54.

57. Sajjadi H, Paparella MM. Meniere's disease. Lancet 2008;372(9636):406–14.

58. Bisdorff A. Vestibular symptoms and history taking. Handb Clin Neurol 2016;137: 83–90.

59. Ichijo H. Onset time of benign paroxysmal positional vertigo. Acta Otolaryngol 2017;137(2):144–8.

60. Lindell E, Finizia C, Johansson M, et al. Asking about dizziness when turning in bed predicts examination findings for benign paroxysmal positional vertigo. J Vestib Res 2018;28(3–4):339–47.

61. Luscher M, Theilgaard S, Edholm B. Prevalence and characteristics of diagnostic groups amongst 1034 patients seen in ENT practices for dizziness. J Laryngol Otol 2014;128(2):128–33.

62. Balatsouras DG, Korres SG. Subjective benign paroxysmal positional vertigo. Otolaryngol Head Neck Surg 2012;146(1):98–103.

63. Huebner AC, Lytle SR, Doettl SM, et al. Treatment of objective and subjective benign paroxysmal positional vertigo. J Am Acad Audiol 2013;24(7):600–6.

64. Tirelli G, D'Orlando E, Giacomarra V, et al. Benign positional vertigo without detectable nystagmus. Laryngoscope 2001;111(6):1053–6.

65. De Stefano A, Kulamarva G, Citraro L, et al. Spontaneous nystagmus in benign paroxysmal positional vertigo. Am J Otolaryngol 2010;32(3):185–9.

66. Imai T, Takeda N, Sato G, et al. Differential diagnosis of true and pseudo-bilateral benign positional nystagmus. Acta Otolaryngol 2008;128(2):151–8.

67. Macdonald NK, Kaski D, Saman Y, et al. Central positional nystagmus: a systematic literature review. Front Neurol 2017;8:141.

68. Ahsan SF, Syamal MN, Yaremchuk K, et al. The costs and utility of imaging in evaluating dizzy patients in the emergency room. Laryngoscope 2013;123(9): 2250–3.

69. Hwang DY, Silva GS, Furie KL, et al. Comparative sensitivity of computed tomography vs. magnetic resonance imaging for detecting acute posterior fossa infarct. J Emerg Med 2012;42(5):559–65.

70. Kabra R, Robbie H, Connor SE. Diagnostic yield and impact of MRI for acute ischaemic stroke in patients presenting with dizziness and vertigo. Clin Radiol 2015;70(7):736–42.
71. Kerber KA, Schweigler L, West BT, et al. Value of computed tomography scans in ED dizziness visits: analysis from a nationally representative sample. Am J Emerg Med 2010;28(9):1030–6.
72. Lawhn-Heath C, Buckle C, Christoforidis G, et al. Utility of head CT in the evaluation of vertigo/dizziness in the emergency department. Emerg Radiol 2013; 20(1):45–9.
73. Wasay M, Dubey N, Bakshi R. Dizziness and yield of emergency head CT scan: is it cost effective? Emerg Med J 2005;22(4):312.
74. Kerber KA, Burke JF, Brown DL, et al. Does intracerebral haemorrhage mimic benign dizziness presentations? A population based study. Emerg Med J 2011;29(1):43–6.
75. Edlow BL, Hurwitz S, Edlow JA. Diagnosis of DWI-negative acute ischemic stroke: A meta-analysis. Neurology 2017;89(3):256–62.
76. Choi JH, Kim HW, Choi KD, et al. Isolated vestibular syndrome in posterior circulation stroke: frequency and involved structures. Neurol Clin Pract 2014;4(5): 410–8.
77. Akoglu EU, Akoglu H, Cimilli Ozturk T, et al. Predictors of false negative diffusion-weighted MRI in clinically suspected central cause of vertigo. Am J Emerg Med 2018;36(4):615–9.
78. Choi JH, Oh EH, Park MG, et al. Early MRI-negative posterior circulation stroke presenting as acute dizziness. J Neurol 2018;265(12):2993–3000.
79. Ohle R, Renee-Anne M, Virginie M, et al. Can emergency physicians accurately rule out a central cause of vertigo using the HINTS examination? a systematic review and meta-analysis. Acad Emerg Med 2020. https://doi.org/10.1111/acem.13960.
80. Newman-Toker DE, Saber Tehrani AS, Mantokoudis G, et al. Quantitative video-oculography to help diagnose stroke in acute vertigo and dizziness: toward an ECG for the eyes. Stroke 2013;44(4):1158–61.
81. Choi JH, Park MG, Choi SY, et al. Acute transient vestibular syndrome: prevalence of stroke and efficacy of bedside evaluation. Stroke 2017;48(3):556–62.

Sedation for Rapid Sequence Induction and Intubation of Neurologically Injured Patients

Jesse Shriki, DO, MS[a],*, Samuel M. Galvagno Jr, DO, PhD, FCCM[b]

KEYWORDS

- Traumatic brain injury • Rapid sequence intubation • Anesthesia • Sedation
- Neurologic disease

KEY POINTS

- Airway management should be carefully planned, reviewed, and executed.
- Traumatic brain injury (TBI) and a Glasgow Coma Scale less than 9 have an almost 50% higher mortality than patients without TBI.
- Normocarbia should be preserved with a goal $Paco_2$ between 35 and 45 mm Hg.
- Oxygen saturation less than 90% is associated with an increase in mortality in TBI.
- Hypotensive episodes can result in increased mortality even if short (<10 minutes).

INTRODUCTION

Patients with neurologic injury are prone to physiologic derangements, specifically during the period of initial stabilization, which includes establishing a definitive airway. In this article, the selection of sedatives that may help to optimize cerebral perfusion and ensure favorable outcomes is discussed. A focus on traumatic brain injury (TBI) is maintained throughout, but many of the principles discussed are applicable to any patient with a neurologic disease whereby cerebral or spinal cord perfusion may be compromised.

BACKGROUND/EPIDEMIOLOGY

TBI contributes to a growing and significant morbidity and mortality burden in the United States. In 2007, there were 1.9 million TBI-related emergency department visits, hospitalizations, and deaths; this increased almost 120% in 2013 to 2.4 million.[1]

[a] Surgical Critical Care, R Adams Cowley Shock Trauma Center, Program in Trauma, University of Maryland School of Medicine, 22 South Greene Street, Baltimore, MD 21201, USA; [b] Multi Trauma Critical Care Unit, R Adams Cowley Shock Trauma Center, Program in Trauma, University of Maryland School of Medicine, Baltimore, MD, USA
* Corresponding author.
E-mail address: Jesse.Shriki@umm.edu

Emerg Med Clin N Am 39 (2021) 203–216
https://doi.org/10.1016/j.emc.2020.09.012
0733-8627/21/© 2020 Elsevier Inc. All rights reserved.

In a study that examined TBI incidence and outcomes in California, a 57.7% increase in the number of TBI emergency department visits was observed, representing a 40.5% increase in visit rates over a 10-year period (346–487 per 100,000 residents) with 40.5% representing a revisit during the first year.[2] As the number of TBI-related deaths has continued to increase annually,[3] the epidemiology of various injury patterns has changed. Before 2006, most TBIs were associated with motor vehicle crashes (**Fig. 1**). Overall, TBI-related deaths make up 2.2% of all deaths in the United States. Mortality largely comprises patients with a low Glasgow Coma Scale (GCS), especially those with a GCS less than or equal to 6 (**Fig. 2**),[4] with some studies citing up to a 76% mortality in patients with GCS 3.[5]

Given the remarkable disease burden associated with TBI, prehospital, emergency, and critical care clinicians must understand the nuances of airway management. Appropriate selection of sedatives during airway management may help optimize physiology and prevent unfavorable outcomes.

PHYSIOLOGIC CONSIDERATIONS IN PATIENTS WITH TRAUMATIC BRAIN INJURY

The path to intubate a patient with TBI is fraught with peril and each step should not be undertaken without expert knowledge of the physiology. From the decision to intubate through the postintubation period, the airway management of the patients with TBI with TBI should be carefully planned and skillfully executed. Similar to TBI, patients with spinal cord injury are equally at risk for complications, and many of the same physiologic principles are applicable. The current literature suggests that the possibility for harm can occur when intubating patients with TBI. Denninghoff and colleagues[6] showed there was an increase in death in patients with TBI, with an odds ratio (OR) of 14 compared with nonintubated patients with TBI, and this increased OR persisted when adjusting for injury severity. It has also been shown that, of patients with a similar GCS, those who have a TBI and GCS less than 9 have an almost 50% higher mortality than those without TBI.[4] Underpinning the harm of intubation in this population is the concept of secondary injury. A secondary insult, initiated by the primary injury, occurs

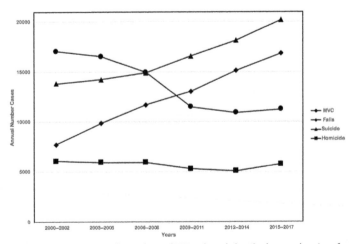

Fig. 1. Estimated average annual number of TBI-related deaths by mechanism from 2000 to 2017. MVC, motor vehicle crash. (*Data from* Taylor CA, Bell JM, Breiding MJ, L X. Traumatic Brain Injury-Related Emergency Department Visits, Hospitalizations, and Deaths - United States, 2007 and 2013. MMWR Surveill Summ 2017:1-1.)

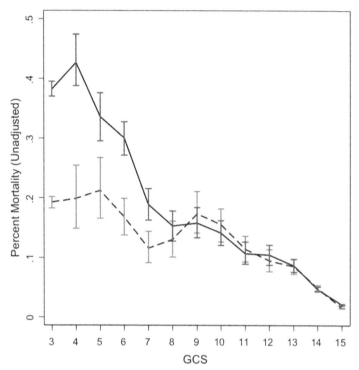

Fig. 2. Mortality percentage by GCS in patients with and without TBI.[4] Unadjusted proportion of deaths for each GCS level for TBI (*solid line*) and non-TBI (*dashed line*). (*From* Osler T CA, Glance LG. The differential mortality of Glasgow Coma Score in patients with and without head injury. Injury 2016;47:1879-85I with permission.)

and is characterized by a cascade of biochemical events responsible for clinical deterioration.[7] The pathophysiology from the primary insult induces an ischemic environment in the brain via microvascular and neuronal injury. This ischemic environment precipitates a vicious cycle characterized by an impaired cerebral metabolic rate, impaired cerebral perfusion and blood flow, increased cerebral edema, and increased intracranial pressure (ICP) (**Fig. 3**). Additional mechanisms resulting in injury include the initiation of glutamate-induced excitotoxicity and calcium channel injury leading to formation of free radicals.[8] Secondary clinical insults include hypotension, hypoxia, hyperoxia, hypocarbia, hypercarbia, and acidosis. Hence, when selecting sedatives to facilitate airway management, this pathophysiology must be understood.

Systemic hypotension, notorious for inciting secondary injury, has long been known to correlate with increased morbidity and mortality.[9] Hypotension can result in increased mortality even if these episodes are short (<10 minutes).[10] However, the numerical target for blood pressure control has been widely debated. Guidelines recommend maintaining a mean arterial pressure (MAP) greater than 80 mm Hg and a systolic blood pressure (SBP) greater than 100 mm Hg,[11] while not allowing the SBP to decrease to less than 90 mm Hg.[12] It is also recommended to increase the threshold to an SBP of 110 mm Hg for patients aged greater than 70 years.[12] Some investigators have argued that this target may still be too low and that an SBP closer 120 mm Hg is optimal.[13] What seems clear in the literature is that hypotension, whether occurring early or late in a patient's clinical course, is associated with

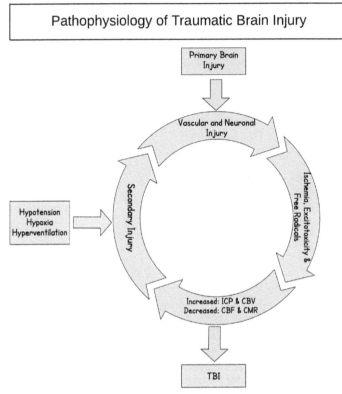

Fig. 3. Pathophysiology of TBI. CBF, cerebral blood flow; CBV, cerebral blood volume; CMR, cerebral metabolic rate.

increased mortality. In one of the most widely cited studies on this topic, by Chestnut and colleagues,[14] a 28% increase in mortality in early (within 8 hours) shock and a 49% increase in mortality in those with late (median 31 hours) shock was reported.

Low oxygen levels also may contribute to secondary brain injury. Hypoxemia (low Pao_2) leads to hypoxia (inadequate oxygen supply to neurologic structures). In the prehospital setting, 1 study showed that hypoxemia (defined as an oxygen saturation [Spo_2] of <90%) was associated with a 17% increase in mortality in patients with TBI.[15] Other reports have shown similar deleterious effects of hypoxemia.[9,16] A combination of hypoxemia and hypotension is at least additive, if not synergistic.[9,15,16] In contrast, hyperoxia, likely extreme hyperoxia (arterial oxygen pressure >300 mm Hg), may also be deleterious.[17]

Hypocapnia is well established to decrease cerebral blood volume, which decreases the intracranial volume and thus has been used to decrease ICP.[18] Arterial CO_2 pressure ($Paco_2$) is a potent vasoconstrictor of the cerebral arteries, causing cerebral blood flow (CBF) to decrease by about 3% per millimeter of mercury change in $Paco_2$, thus a decrease from 40 to 30 mm Hg represents a 33% decrease in brain volume.[19] Such a decrease can result in cerebral ischemia. It is now well accepted that hyperventilation to a $Paco_2$ less than 25 mm Hg is harmful,[20,21] and prolonged periods are not recommended. Thus, maintenance of normocarbia ($Paco_2$ between 35 and 45 mm Hg) is a primary goal during TBI management.[12] However, several studies have shown that this goal is infrequently attained in the prehospital and emergency settings.[22,23] Hyperventilation to a low $Paco_2$ should only be used for short periods of time in imminent brain herniation as a temporizing method while mobilizing neurosurgery for a possible decompressive craniectomy. Moreover, the effect of hypocarbia is short lived and the cerebrospinal fluid is able to normalize CBF quickly in the setting of hypocarbia, within about 4 hours.[19]

Protocolized care that allows for proper clinical decision making has been shown to improve outcomes. The EPIC (Excellence in Prehospital Injury Care) study was a statewide public health initiative in Arizona designed to implement Brain Trauma Foundation guidelines[12] into prehospital protocols to improve adherence and minimize causes of secondary brain injury.[24] Adjusted survival doubled in patients with severe TBI and tripled in the intubated cohort after statewide guidelines were effected. In addition, the incidence of hypoxemia and hypotension among patients with TBI was decreased.

ESTABLISHING AN AIRWAY

Understanding the deleterious consequences of altered oxygen, carbon dioxide, and blood pressure is fundamental when planning an approach for airway management of a patient with TBI. The goal of airway management is to establish a definitive airway while simultaneously optimizing physiologic parameters. Rapid sequence induction and intubation (RSII) is the technique of choice for TBI.[25–27] Once the decision is made to secure the airway with RSII, decisions regarding selection of induction and neuromuscular blocking agents are critical. Compounding the difficulty in selection of appropriate agents is the fact that neuronal injury is frequently associated with cardiac dysfunction. Although this is well known in nontraumatic aneurysmal subarachnoid hemorrhage, it has also been observed in cases of TBI where decompressive hemicraniectomy was required.[28] Both cardiac and neurologic function should be considered before the administration of induction agents. Although the usual reflex responses to stimulation by intubation include glottic closure, hypertension, tachycardia, and reflex bronchoconstriction,[29] any of a myriad of pathophysiologic derangements can occur, including hypoxia, hypotension, apnea with hypercarbia, bradycardia, and even cardiac arrest, with a nonnegligible incidence.[29]

ADJUNCTIVE MEDICATIONS

A variety of medications have historically been used to attenuate increases in ICP and to attenuate other effects associated with endotracheal intubation. However, the data to support the use of adjunctive medications are sparse and often extrapolated from small case series and heterogeneous patient populations.

Lidocaine has been used before RSII to prevent hypertension, tachycardia, and increased ICP based largely on data extrapolated from patients with hydrocephalus and brain tumors.[30] A Vaughan Williams class Ib antiarrhythmic, lidocaine, suppresses automaticity of conduction tissue and blocks both the initiation and conduction of nerve impulses by decreasing the neuronal membrane's permeability to sodium ions. At least 2 well-conducted reviews do not support the routine use of lidocaine as a pretreatment of RSII in patients with TBI.[31,32] If used, a dose of 1 to 2 mg/kg may be considered, but the drug must be given several minutes before RSII for maximal effect. Putative advantages include blunting of fasciculations associated with succinylcholine, a relatively safe side effect profile, and variable blockade of sympathetic response during RSII.[33,34] Disadvantages include the burden of drawing up an additional medication during an emergency airway scenario, arterial hypotension, minimal ICP protection, inconsistent protection against hypertension or tachycardia, and no direct evidence of benefit.[33,35]

A Cochrane Review examined the role of multiple different adjunctive medications, including lidocaine, β-blockers, calcium channel blockers, alpha-agonists, and opioids.[36] The review found a decrease in the OR of arrhythmias (OR, 0.1; 95% confidence interval [CI], 0.14–0.26) but a much larger OR of adverse events, including hypotension and bradycardia for local anesthetics (OR, 12.27; 95% CI, 4.03–37.36) and adrenergic blockers (OR, 24.17; 95% CI, 8.88–65.79).[36] For opiates, the adverse events OR was much higher (OR, 149.5; 95% CI, 35.07–637.65), including at least 1 case of chest rigidity (alfentanil).[36] Thus, the use of adjuncts should be considered on a case-by-case basis, balancing the harm and benefit.

INDUCTION AGENTS

There are no firm recommendations favoring one induction agent rather than another in terms of neuroprotective effects.[37] Ultimately, the ideal drug is the one with which the clinician is most comfortable. **Table 1** lists properties and doses of commonly used induction agents. For hemodynamically unstable patients, one technique that may help with dosing involves the use of the shock index (heart rate/blood pressure). As a composite measure for hemodynamic instability (ie, a shock index >0.9), shock index–based dosing may prevent the exacerbation of hypotension, including populations of patients at risk for this complication (**Table 2**). Midazolam has not been extensively studied as either a sole or adjunctive medication for RSII but, in a retrospective review of 219 patients who had prehospital RSII, use of this agent as an induction agent was associated with a dose-related incidence of hypotension.[38] Similarly, use of fentanyl as a single-drug induction agent in patients with trauma produced worse neurologic variables in a small retrospective study.[39] Hence, the use of opioids and benzodiazepines as sole induction agents is not discussed here; this article emphasizes the 3 principal sedative agents used for RSII in TBI and patients with neurologic injuries: propofol, etomidate, and ketamine.

Propofol

Propofol is a widely used intravenous anesthetic that works by increasing the gamma-aminobutyric acid (GABA)–mediated inhibitory tone within the central nervous system. Advantages include consistent decreases in ICP and cerebral metabolic rate (CMR), but at the cost of decreased CBF.[40,41] There are also some reports that propofol may decrease airway resistance postintubation.[42] Deleterious effects of propofol include a decrease in brain autoregulation; however, this is more likely to occur with

Table 1 Physiologic changes by pharmacologic interventions						
Agent	MAP	ICP	CBF	CPP	CMR	Dose (mg/kg)
Propofol	↓	↓	↓	↓	↓	1–2
Propofol (in shock)[a]	—	↓	↓	↓	↓	0.5–1
Etomidate	↔	↓	↓	↑/↓/↔	↓	0.15–0.3
Ketamine	↑	↓[b]	↑	↑	↑/↓[c]	1–2

Abbreviations: CMR, cerebral metabolic rate; CPP, cerebral perfusion pressure.
[a] Potency of propofol; likely increased in shock.
[b] See text for details; likely decreases or causes no change.
[c] Region-specific changes; increased in cingulate cortex, decreased elsewhere.

Table 2
Dosing considerations based on shock index

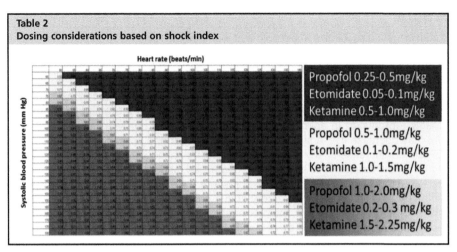

Shock index = heart rate/SBP. Dose reductions are also recommended for patients with heart failure, advanced age (>70 years), severe hypertension, high cervical spine injuries, history of β-blocker use, or amputated limbs (decreased volume of distribution).

higher doses.[43] Propofol seems to cause some degree of postintubation hypotension in up to 30% of patients, especially in hemodynamically unstable patients.[44–46] This systemic hypotension can produce a further decrease in cerebral perfusion pressure (CPP). Animal studies suggest that a dose reduction is required, at least in the swine model of hemorrhagic shock, with some investigators suggesting a concordant decrease in propofol dose by as much as 5-fold.[47,48] When dosed judiciously, propofol is a cheap, easily accessible agent for induction. At our institution, propofol is dosed according to shock index, with doses in the range of 0.25 to 1 mg/kg for patients with hypotension or deemed to be at risk for hypotension.[49] Allergic reactions to propofol are rare, and allergies to egg, soy, or peanuts should not be a deterrent to its use.[50]

Etomidate

Etomidate is an imidazole compound that, like propofol, stimulates GABA receptors to depress the reticular activating system. Like all sedative hypnotics, etomidate can decrease CBF and cerebral metabolic activity,[42,51] thereby decreasing ICP. Etomidate has been used extensively in neurosurgical patients.[49] In a study by Prior and colleagues,[52] CPP increased with a bolus of etomidate in 40 patients, decreased CPP in 19, and stayed the same in 2; the mean change in CPP was 5 mm Hg. Etomidate has a favorable hemodynamic profile overall, even when studied at full doses in porcine hemorrhagic shock models.[47] Nevertheless, although more hemodynamically bland than most other induction agents, etomidate can precipitate hypotension.[52,53] With even a single dose, etomidate can cause adrenal suppression, as shown by measurable suppression of cortisol levels; nonetheless, this seems to occur immediately after administration and dissipates in as little as 5 hours, although the effect could persist for up to 24 hours.[53,54] No statistically significant association with increased mortality has been consistently shown in patients with trauma[55] or critically ill patients.[56] Etomidate may cause hemolysis based on 1 animal study[57] and another human study showing increased transfusion requirements.[53] Other side effects seen with etomidate include myoclonus.[58]

Ketamine

Ketamine is a dissociative anesthetic that works at the N-methyl-ᴅ-aspartate (NMDA) receptor to cause region-specific changes in CMR. Ketamine causes increases in the CMR in the anterior cingulate cortex but decreases in CMR elsewhere throughout the brain. Ketamine is thought to have neuroprotective benefits, as shown by in vitro studies that have shown decreased excitotoxicity caused by antagonism of the NMDA receptor with resultant decreased calcium influx, but this effect has not been reliably reproduced in animal models.[51] Ketamine does not seem to increase ICP and may decrease it.[59] A systematic review by Zeiler and colleagues[60] showed that ICP did not increase in any of the studied patients, although the quality of evidence in that review was low. In 3 studies, ICP decreased, and, in 2 of the studies, ketamine increased CPP and mean arterial blood pressure.[60] Ketamine also has antiepileptic effects and may be useful in refractory status epilepticus.[61] Although known to be a direct myocardial depressant, the predominant effect of ketamine is indirect sympathomimetic activity mediated by catecholamine release with resultant increased cardiovascular tone.[49] Hence, ketamine preserves blood pressure and increases heart rate, but these effects may be diminished in patients who are catecholamine depleted (ie, patients in advanced stages of shock).

Given the theoretic benefits of ketamine and propofol, a mixture of the two has been suggested for induction. Given the portmanteau ketofol, this mixture has been studied and has been found to have a hemodynamic profile similar to etomidate.[46,53] Issues with ambiguous doses when the drugs are mixed together and the requirement for multiple medication administration are factors that may limit use in emergency settings.

Neuromuscular Blockers

The choice of neuromuscular blocker is a highly contentious area, with advocates on both sides. The 2 choices are rocuronium and succinylcholine. Succinylcholine has a short onset of action (30 seconds) and duration (8–10 minutes), allowing repeat neurologic examinations after RSII. This agent is associated with several adverse effects, including the possibility of increased ICP, hyperkalemia, and cardiovascular instability, which can increase exponentially in the setting of muscular disease and immobility in susceptible patients.[62] Succinylcholine must be avoided in patients with known preexisting neurologic disease (**Table 3**). Succinylcholine also causes muscle fasciculations, which was acknowledged in at least 1 study to be associated with more rapid desaturation.[63]

Rocuronium is an intermediate-acting aminosteroid analogue of vecuronium with an average onset of action of 60 seconds. In a 2019 multicenter, randomized controlled study that included 1248 patients requiring RSII, rocuronium was found to be noninferior to succinylcholine.[64] When used at a dose of 1.2 mg/kg, the onset of action and time to optimal intubating conditions is only slightly longer than those of succinylcholine. Although most trials have shown little difference between succinylcholine and rocuronium, 1 trial showed an increase in mortality. In a retrospective observation study of 233 patients undergoing paralysis with rocuronium or succinylcholine, the succinylcholine group had a higher mortality in patients with a critical head injury.[65] Rocuronium is associated with a longer duration of action (typically about 30 minutes, and prolonged with hypothermia) and thus early postintubation sedation is mandatory to prevent paralysis without sedation. The effects of rocuronium may be rapidly reversed with the gamma-cyclodextrin derivative sugammadex.

Table 3
Considerations for sedatives and adjunctive medications during airway management in patients with concomitant neurologic disease

Condition	Drugs to Avoid	Comment
Parkinson disease	Phenothiazines Metoclopramide	Dopamine antagonists can exacerbate parkinsonism
Multiple sclerosis Guillain-Barré syndrome (acute inflammatory demyelinating polyneuropathy)	Succinylcholine	Life-threatening hyperkalemia is possible with succinylcholine; patients may have an unpredictable response to nondepolarizing neuromuscular blockers Dysautonomia may lead to increased cardiovascular instability during induction
ALS	Succinylcholine	Life-threatening hyperkalemia is possible with succinylcholine; patients may have an unpredictable response to nondepolarizing neuromuscular blockers because of lower motor neurologic disorder associated with ALS
Myasthenic syndromes (ie, myasthenia gravis, Lambert-Eaton myasthenic syndrome)	Nondepolarizing neuromuscular blockers (lower doses required) Lidocaine	Exaggerated response to nondepolarizing neuromuscular blockers (increased blockade at lower doses); unpredictable response to succinylcholine Lidocaine may be associated with exacerbations in rare circumstances
Muscular dystrophy	Succinylcholine	Exaggerated response to nondepolarizing neuromuscular blockers (increased blockade at lower doses)
Patients with prolonged immobility (ie, spinal cord injuries)	Succinylcholine	Patients may require higher doses of nondepolarizing neuromuscular blockers

Abbreviation: ALS, amyotrophic lateral sclerosis.

HYPOXIA, HYPOVENTILATION, AND RAPID SEQUENCE INDUCTION AND INTUBATION: THE CHICKEN OR THE EGG?

Clinicians are confronted with a conundrum when a brain-injured patient presents with hypoxia before RSII. A typical response is to provide bag mask ventilation to correct hypoxemia. This technique may cause hyperventilation, which may induce cerebral vasoconstriction, which is a deleterious effect in patients with TBI. Poste and colleagues[66] studied prehospital intubations in patients with TBI and found that the lowest postintubation end-tidal CO_2 level was associated with higher OR for mortality (OR, 7.71; 95% CI, 1.03–58.03) as opposed to the lowest Spo_2 (OR, 1.39; 95% CI, 0.35–5.55). Only an Spo_2 less than 70% was associated with a statistically significant increase in mortality.[66] This study suggests that hyperventilation may be more deleterious than mild decreases in Spo_2 during RSII. The authors recommend appropriate oxygenation without aggressive hyperventilation when mild hypoxemia is encountered during RSII.

Table 4
Stepwise approach to the intubation of patients with brain injuries

Step/Pitfall	Critical Action
Preparation	• Prepare the team for patient arrival • Consider appropriate focal neurologic examination, including appropriate spinal reflexes as situation allows
Preoxygenation	• Ensure preoxygenation with as close to 90% Fio_2 as tolerated • Make every attempt to denitrogenate the patient to provide maximal oxygenation during apneic period
Positioning	• If possible, place the patient's head in a sniffing position (ear canal level with the anterior shoulder) to align the oral, pharyngeal, and laryngeal axes • Most brain-injured patients require cervical immobilization; the front aspect of the cervical collar may be removed while manual in-line stabilization is maintained
Induction	• Use the agent the clinician is most comfortable with (etomidate, propofol, ketamine). • Consider avoiding midazolam for induction
Hypotension	• Avoid SBP <90 mm Hg, maintain SBP >100–120 mm Hg using push-dose pressors as needed
Hypoxia	• Mild hypoxia during RSI may be tolerated in exchange to avoid reflexive hyperventilation • Maintain Spo_2 >92%
Hypocarbia	• Strict monitoring using calibrated continuous $ETco_2$ or frequent blood gas monitoring • Ensure normocarbia 35–45 mm Hg
Paralysis	• Use either rocuronium or succinylcholine • Be cognizant of paralysis without sedation
Intubation	• Most experienced clinician to get first pass • Avoid excessive manipulation of airway
Postintubation	• Use appropriate ventilator settings • Frequent vent checks with adjustment • Balance PEEP for lung protective settings; adjust RR if needed • Ensure adequate sedation
Monitoring	• Examine for seizures and need for prophylaxis • Possible need for intraventricular monitoring

Abbreviations: $ETco_2$, end-tidal CO_2; Fio_2, fraction of inspired oxygen; PEEP, positive end-expiratory pressure; RR, respiration rate; RSI, rapid sequence intubation; Spo_2, oxygen saturation.

SUMMARY

This article discusses the pathophysiology of TBI and its mortality. There are many layers to the data of RSII and TBI, and clinician should be well versed in them. Understanding the major concepts and key factors in morbidity and mortality are extremely important in the care of injured patients. Simplifying the steps, reviewing the literature, and practicing the principles is vital. This article elucidates those themes. Using the principles discussed, safe intubation strategies (**Table 4**) and thoughtful preparation are vital for the care of patients with TBI.

DISCLOSURE

The authors have no disclosures. This work was not funded.

REFERENCES

1. Taylor CA, Bell JM, Breiding MJ, et al. Traumatic Brain Injury-Related Emergency Department Visits, Hospitalizations, and Deaths - United States, 2007 and 2013. MMWR Surveill Summ 2017;66(9):1–16.
2. Xu RY, Markowitz AJ, Guo J, et al. Ten-year trends in traumatic brain injury: a retrospective cohort study of California emergency department and hospital revisits and readmissions. BMJ Open 2018;8(12):e022297.
3. Daugherty J, Waltzman D, Sarmiento K, et al. Traumatic Brain Injury-Related Deaths by Race/Ethnicity, Sex, Intent, and Mechanism of Injury - United States, 2000-2017. MMWR Morb Mortal Wkly Rep 2019;68(46):1050–6.
4. Osler T, Cook A, Lecky F, et al. The differential mortality of Glasgow Coma Score in patients with and without head injury. Injury 2016;47(9):1879–85.
5. Demetriades D, Kuncir E, Velmahos GC, et al. Outcome and prognostic factors in head injuries with an admission Glasgow Coma Scale score of 3. Arch Surg 2004; 139(10):1066–8.
6. Denninghoff KR, Griffin MJ, Bartolucci AA, et al. Emergent endotracheal intubation and mortality in traumatic brain injury. West J Emerg Med 2008;9(4):184–9.
7. Kochanek PM, Clark RS, Ruppel RA, et al. Biochemical, cellular, and molecular mechanisms in the evolution of secondary damage after severe traumatic brain injury in infants and children: Lessons learned from the bedside. Pediatr Crit Care Med 2000;1(1):4.
8. Kaur P, Sharma S. Recent Advances in Pathophysiology of Traumatic Brain Injury. Curr Neuropharmacol 2018;16(8):1224–38.
9. Chesnut RM, Marshall LF, Klauber MR, et al. The role of secondary brain injury in determining outcome from severe head injury. J Trauma 1993;34:216–22.
10. Manley G, Knudson MM, Morabito D, et al. Hypotension, hypoxia, and head injury: frequency, duration, and consequences. Arch Surg 2001;136(10): 1118–23.
11. Picetti E, Rossi S, Abu-Zidan FM, et al. WSES consensus conference guidelines: monitoring and management of severe adult traumatic brain injury patients with polytrauma in the first 24 hours. World J Emerg Surg 2019;14:53.
12. Carney N, Totten AM, O'Reilly C, et al. Guidelines for the Management of Severe Traumatic Brain Injury, Fourth Edition. Neurosurgery 2017;80(1):6–15.
13. Brenner M, Stein DM, Hu PF, et al. Traditional systolic blood pressure targets underestimate hypotension-induced secondary brain injury. J Trauma Acute Care Surg 2012;72(5):1135–9.
14. Chesnut RM, Marshall SB, Piek J, et al. Early and late systemic hypotension as a frequent and fundamental source of cerebral ischemia following severe brain injury in the Traumatic Coma Data Bank. Acta Neurochir Suppl (Wien) 1993;59: 121–5.
15. Chi JH, Knudson MM, Vassar MJ, et al. Prehospital hypoxia affects outcome in patients with traumatic brain injury: a prospective multicenter study. J Trauma 2006;61(5):1134–41.
16. Stocchetti N, Furlan A, Volta F. Hypoxemia and arterial hypotension at the accident scene in head injury. J Trauma 1996;40:764–7.
17. Davis DP, Meade W, Sise MJ, et al. Both hypoxemia and extreme hyperoxemia may be detrimental in patients with severe traumatic brain injury. J Neurotrauma 2009;26(12):2217–23.
18. Davis D. Early ventilation in traumatic brain injury. Resuscitation 2008;76(3): 333–40.

19. Curley G, Kavanagh BP, Laffey JG. Hypocapnia and the injured brain: more harm than benefit. Crit Care Med 2010;38:1348–59.
20. Muizelaar JP, Marmarou A, Ward JD, et al. Adverse effects of prolonged hyperventilation in patients with severe head injury: a randomized clinical trial. J Neurosurg 1991;75:731–9.
21. Caulfield EV, Dutton RP, Floccare DJ, et al. Prehospital hypocapnia and poor outcome after severe traumatic brain injury. J Trauma 2009;66(6):1577–83.
22. Thomas SH, Orf J, Wedel SK, et al. Hyperventilation in traumatic brain injury patients: inconsistency between consensus guidelines and clinical practice. J Trauma 2002;52(1):47–52.
23. Warner KJ, Cuschieri J, Copass MK, et al. The impact of prehospital ventilation on outcome after severe traumatic brain injury. J Trauma 2007;62(6):1330–6.
24. Spaite DW, Bobrow BJ, Keim SM, et al. Association of Statewide Implementation of the Prehospital Traumatic Brain Injury Treatment Guidelines With Patient Survival Following Traumatic Brain Injury: The Excellence in Prehospital Injury Care (EPIC) Study. JAMA Surg 2019;154:e191152.
25. Jung JY. Airway management of patients with traumatic brain injury/C-spine injury. Korean J Anesthesiol 2015;68:213–9.
26. Groth CM, Acquisto NM, Khadem T. Current practices and safety of medication use during rapid sequence intubation. J Crit Care 2018;45:65–70.
27. Bernard SA. Paramedic intubation of patients with severe head injury: a review of current Australian practice and recommendations for change. Emerg Med Australas 2006;18(3):221–8.
28. Krishnamoorthy V, Mackensen GB, Gibbons EF, et al. Cardiac Dysfunction After Neurologic Injury: What Do We Know and Where Are We Going. Chest 2016; 149(5):1325–31.
29. Mort T. The incidence and risk factors for cardiac arrest during emergency tracheal intubation: a justification for incorporating the ASA Guidelines in the remote location. J Clin Anesth 2004;16(7):508.
30. Donegan MF, Bedford RF. Intravenously administered lidocaine prevents intracranial hypertension during endotracheal suctioning. Anesthesiology 1980;52(6): 516–8.
31. Robinson N, Clancy M. In patients with head injury undergoing rapid sequence intubation, does pretreatment with intravenous lignocaine/lidocaine lead to an improved neurological outcome? A review of the literature. Emerg Med J 2001; 18:453–7.
32. Qi DY, Wang K, Zhang H, et al. Efficacy of intravenous lidocaine versus placebo on attenuating cardiovascular response to laryngoscopy and tracheal intubation: a systematic review of randomized controlled trials. Minerva Anestesiol 2013;79: 1423–35.
33. Lin CC, Yu JH, Lin CC, et al. Postintubation hemodynamic effects of intravenous lidocaine in severe traumatic brain injury. Am J Emerg Med 2012;30:1782–7.
34. Weingart S. Additional thoughts on the controversy of lidocaine administration before rapid sequence intubation in patients with traumatic brain injuries. Ann Emerg Med 2007;50:353.
35. Vaillancourt C, Kapur AK. Opposition to the use of lidocaine in rapid sequence intubation. Ann Emerg Med 2007;49:86–7.
36. Khan FA, Ullah H. Pharmacological agents for preventing morbidity associated with the haemodynamic response to tracheal intubation. Cochrane Database Syst Rev 2013;(7):CD004087.

37. Schifilliti D, Grasso G, Conti A, et al. Anaesthetic-related neuroprotection: intravenous or inhalational agents. CNS Drugs 2010;24(11):893–907.
38. Davis DP, Kimbro TA, Vilke GM. The use of midazolam for prehospital rapid-sequence intubation may be associated with a dose-related increase in hypotension. Prehosp Emerg Care 2001;5(2):163–8.
39. Michetti CP, Maguire JF, Kaushik A, et al. Single-drug sedation with fentanyl for prehospital postintubation sedation in trauma patients. J Trauma Acute Care Surg 2012;72:924–9.
40. Pinaud M, Lelausque JN, Chetanneau A, et al. Effects of propofol on cerebral hemodynamics and metabolism in patients with brain trauma. Anesthesiology 1990; 73(3):404–9.
41. Ravussin P, Guinard JP, Ralley F, et al. Effect of propofol on cerebrospinal fluid pressure and cerebral perfusion pressure in patients undergoing craniotomy. Anaesthesia 1988;43(Suppl):37–41.
42. Eames WO, Rooke GA, Wu RS, et al. Comparison of the effects of etomidate, propofol, and thiopental on respiratory resistance after tracheal intubation. Anesthesiology 1996;84(6):1307–11.
43. Steiner LA, Johnston AJ, Chatfield DA, et al. The effects of large-dose propofol on cerebrovascular pressure autoregulation in head-injured patients. Anesth Analg 2003;97(2):572–6.
44. Ishimaru T, Goto T, Takahashi J, et al. Association of ketamine use with lower risks of post-intubation hypotension in hemodynamically-unstable patients in the emergency department. Sci Rep 2019;9(1):17230.
45. Dietrich SK, Mixon MA, Rogoszewski RJ, et al. Hemodynamic Effects of Propofol for Induction of Rapid Sequence Intubation in Traumatically Injured Patients. Am Surg 2018;84(9):1504–8.
46. Smischney NJ, Beach ML, Loftus RW, et al. Ketamine/propofol admixture (ketofol) is associated with improved hemodynamics as an induction agent: a randomized, controlled trial. J Trauma Acute Care Surg 2012;73(1):94–101.
47. Johnson KB, Egan TD, Kern SE. The influence of hemorrhagic shock on propofol: a pharmacokinetic and pharmacodynamic analysis. Anesthesiology 2003;99(2): 409–20.
48. Shafer S. Shock values. Anesthesiology 2004;101(3):567–8.
49. Sikorski RA, Koerner AK, Fouche-Weber LY, et al. Choice of General Anesthetics for Trauma Patients. Curr Anesthesiol Rep 2014;4(3):225–32.
50. Asserhøj LL, Mosbech H, Krøigaard M, et al. No evidence for contraindications to the use of propofol in adults allergic to egg, soy or peanut. Br J Anaesth 2016; 116(1):77–82.
51. Hoffman WE, Charbel FT, Ausman JI. Cerebral blood flow and metabolic response to etomidate and ischemia. Neurol Res 1997;19(1):41–4.
52. Prior JG, Hinds CJ, Williams J, et al. The use of etomidate in the management of severe head injury. Intensive Care Med 1983;9(6):313–20.
53. Smischney NJ, Nicholson WT, Brown DR, et al. Ketamine/propofol admixture vs etomidate for intubation in the critically ill: KEEP PACE Randomized clinical trial. J Trauma Acute Care Surg 2019;87:883–9.
54. Archambault P, Dionne CE, Lortie G, et al. Adrenal inhibition following a single dose of etomidate in intubated traumatic brain injury victims. CJEM 2012;14: 270–82.
55. Hinkewich C, Green R. The impact of etomidate on mortality in trauma patients. Can J Anaesth 2014;61:650–5.

56. Alday NJ, Jones GM, Kimmons LA, et al. Effects of etomidate on vasopressor use in patients with sepsis or severe sepsis: a propensity-matched analysis. J Crit Care 2014;29:517–22.
57. Drummond JC, Patel DJ, Cole PM, et al. Focal cerebral ischemia during anesthesia with etomidate, isoflurane, or thiopental: a comparison of the extent of cerebral injury. Neurosurgery 1995;37:742–8.
58. Holdcroft A, Morgan M, Whitwam JG, et al. Effect of dose and premedication on induction complications with etomidate. Br J Anaesth 1976;48:199–205.
59. Filanovsky Y, Kao J. Myth: ketamine should not be used as an induction agent for intubation in patients with head injury. CJEM 2010;12:154–7.
60. Zeiler FA, Teitelbaum J, West M, et al. The ketamine effect on ICP in traumatic brain injury. Neurocrit Care 2014;21:163–73.
61. Zeiler FA, Teitelbaum J, Gillman LM, et al. NMDA antagonists for refractory seizures. Neurocrit Care 2014;20:502–13.
62. Martyn JA, Richtsfeld M. Succinylcholine-induced hyperkalemia in acquired pathologic states: etiologic factors and molecular mechanisms. Anesthesiology 2006;104:158–69.
63. Taha SK, El-Khatib MF, Baraka AS, et al. Effect of suxamethonium vs rocuronium on onset of oxygen desaturation during apnoea following rapid sequence induction. Anaesthesia 2010;65:358–61.
64. Guihard B, Chollet-Xémard P, Lakhnati P, et al. Effect of Rocuronium vs Succinylcholine on Endotracheal Intubation Success Rate Among Patients Undergoing Out-of-Hospital Rapid Sequence Intubation: A Randomized Clinical Trial. JAMA Surg 2019;322:2303–12.
65. Patanwala AE, Erstad BL, Roe DJ, et al. Succinylcholine Is Associated with Increased Mortality When Used for Rapid Sequence Intubation of Severely Brain Injured Patients in the Emergency Department. Pharmacotherapy 2016;36: 57–63.
66. Poste JC, Davis DP, Ochs M, et al. Air medical transport of severely head-injured patients undergoing paramedic rapid sequence intubation. Air Med J 2004;23: 36–40.

NeuroEthics and End of Life Care

Kelsey Cacic, MD[a],*, Jordan Bonomo, MD, FCCM, FNCS[b,c,d]

KEYWORDS

- Neuroethics • Devastating brain injury • Resource scarcity • Prognostication

KEY POINTS

- Neuroethics in the emergency department is part of daily practice and requires and understanding of the pillars of medical ethics and their application to the neurologically injured emergency department patient.
- Self-fulfilling prophesies inherently conflict with the traditional pillars of medical ethics and ultra-early prognostication in the neurologically injured is not morally sound.
- Resource limitations in neurologic therapeutics markedly alter the ethical framework of care, especially in the context of neurointerventional strategies for acute stroke management.
- True autonomy is rare in the neurologically injured patient; substituted consent and proxy autonomy are critical and susceptible to extreme bias.

INTRODUCTION

Ethics is an integral part of standard of care. In tort law, the standard of care is the degree of prudence and caution required of an individual providing the care who thereby has a legal obligation to adhere to certain standards while performing care that could cause foreseeable harm others, that is, maleficence. The requirements of this standard are closely dependent on circumstances; whether a standard of care has been breached is usually framed in terms of a "reasonable person" and if the intended beneficence outweighs any maleficence.[1]

Background

The emergency department (ED) is often the first point of hospital entry for patients with neurologic diseases and the location in which many ethical challenges related to care are initially identified. The emergency care ecosystem is a unique environment

[a] Department of Neurology and Rehabilitation Medicine, University of Cincinnati, Mail Location 0525, Stetson Building, 260 Stetson Street, Suite 2300, Cincinnati, OH 45267-0525, USA;
[b] Department of Emergency Medicine, University of Cincinnati, Cincinnati, OH, USA;
[c] Department of Neurology and Rehabilitation Medicine, University of Cincinnati, Cincinnati, OH, USA; [d] Department of Neurosurgery, University of Cincinnati, Cincinnati, OH, USA
* Corresponding author.
E-mail address: cacicky@ucmail.uc.edu

Emerg Med Clin N Am 39 (2021) 217–225
https://doi.org/10.1016/j.emc.2020.09.013
0733-8627/21/Published by Elsevier Inc.
emed.theclinics.com

and one in which complex decisions related to neurologic care and the attendant ethical issues must be made with limited information and under marked time constraints. Neuroethics as a discipline has recently been identified as its own entity, with subspecialty training now available as well. As a subdiscipline of biomedical ethics, neuroethics focuses on the unique disease states, prognostic challenges, and end of life care that often accompany neurologic illnesses. Both chronic and acute neurologic illness and injury share common features that are specific to this subdiscipline and the interface of neuroethics and emergency medicine has become more complex as treatments have become more advanced and the push for ultra-early prognostics has followed. Faced with decision making in real time that can have a profound impact on the likelihood of survival, and expected to make these decisions as a function of outcome prediction, the emergency care practitioner is placed in a very challenging position with these patients. As a result, a discussion of neuroethics in the emergency medicine environment is warranted and timely.

Definitions and Discussion

Generally speaking, the 4 most commonly accepted pillars of medical ethics are autonomy, beneficence, nonmaleficence, and justice. The application of these foundational underpinnings of bioethics to the practice of emergency medicine is not unfamiliar to most emergency physicians owing to the challenging ethical dilemmas faced by emergency physicians in everyday practice. However, there are nuanced differences inherent in the application of neuroethics to certain ED patients that warrants exploration. Specifically, there are 2 overarching realities of the care of the neurologically injured patient in the ED that challenge some of the more common understandings of the application of the pillars of medical ethics.

1. First, ultra-early prognostication in the neurologically injured is fraught with uncertainty, bias, and error.
2. Second, the true risks and benefits of many therapeutic interventions is not known with definitive certainty

Prognostication in the ultra-early phase is so challenging that the Neurocritical Care Society guidelines for the management of devastating brain injury specifically caution against limiting lifesaving care within the first 72 hours of injury in most neurologically injured patients.[2] The supposition is that self-fulfilling prophesies regarding devastating brain injury lead to early limitations in resuscitative care, yet data continue to demonstrate the inability of clinicians to accurately prognosticate in severely injured neurologic patients, even with the best of intentions and the best technology available. In 2009, a landmark investigation was published describing the outcomes of patients with blunt head trauma and Glasgow Coma Score of 3 at presentation. In this review of 189 patients, 13.2% of the cohort achieved good functional outcomes after 6 months.[3] In a similar style review of patients with intracerebral hemorrhage (ICH), the validity of the ICH score as a criterion standard for risk stratification and prediction of 30-day mortality was questioned. The authors found that the ICH score does not accurately predict the mortality rate regardless of surgical intervention and that survival exceeded the index assessment of outcome from the baseline ICH score.[4] These examples clearly underscore the challenges faced by emergency physicians when attempting to align clinical decision making with time-sensitive prognostic models that are likely to induce mortality bias, the end result of which is loss of therapeutic opportunity for the patient.

When the challenges noted are applied to the pillars of medical ethics, certain critical assessments must be addressed. With respect to autonomy, it is required that the patient be able to make an informed decision, with the necessary facts, risks, and benefits clearly delineated and the likelihood of success reasonably estimated. In the case of acute, severe neurologic injury, the information regarding treatment and prognosis is highly technical and it is nearly impossible for those patients to operate with fully informed consent when making decisions about their health, even in the rare circumstances when they can participate. The very nature of the injuries themselves renders these patients' capacity for expression of autonomy incomplete. When unable to participate in those discussions, proxy expressions of consent and autonomy are sought from those with close relationships to the patients under the pretext that those identified as such will have particular insights into the goals of care wishes of the patient and express them accordingly. However, it is again important to note that the expression of proxy decision making as a substitute for autonomy is held to the same technical standards regarding the possession of a reasonable understanding of risks and benefits and prognosis. In the acutely neurologically injured patient, the veracity of autonomous decision making, even when expressed via proxy, is subject to much disagreement and warrants careful scrutiny to ensure internal consistency and the absence of bias.

Beneficence (the requirement that care be provided with the intent of doing good for the patient) is a more straightforward principle, even in the care of the neurologically injured patient. Neurotherapeutics are developed and deployed for the benefit of the patient. Although all therapeutics carry a risk of side effects, the overall intent is the good of the patient and the risk of the side effects is balanced against the absence of therapeutic intervention. Nonmaleficence (requiring that the care rendered does not harm the patient or society at large) is less straightforward in neuroethics discussions in the emergency setting. Despite the intent to do good for the patient, many neurotherapeutics carry high risks of rare but devastating complications. The treatment of acute ischemic stroke with intravenous tissue plasminogen activator carries a risk of symptomatic ICH of 6.4% and the use of endovascular therapy for mechanical thrombectomy in stroke carries an aggregate risk of symptomatic ICH of 4.4% in the largest 5 trials of endovascular therapy.[5,6] When attempting to provide these life-saving therapies to acute stroke patients, a consideration of the risk of intervention is critical in assessing the ethical underpinnings of the treatment. Only patients with acute, disabling strokes are eligible for treatment, but many of those patients would survive without the interventions. And some, although mildly disabled at time of treatment, are infrequently worsened by attempts at therapeutic intervention. The weighing of neurologic disability against the risk of intervention-associated morbidity and mortality requires a nuanced understanding of the belief system of the patient and an expression of societal norms that would support the view that, in fact, some disabilities are worse than death.

The fourth pillar of medical ethics, justice, has particular applicability to the emergency medicine ecosystem, and has been applied during times of scarcity and widespread disease. Most recently, the global severe acute respiratory disease coronavirus-2 (coronavirus disease-19) pandemic has brought the discussion of justice to the modern practitioner in a way that many have not seen before. Specifically, justice requires the fair and equitable distribution of care and resources, and attention to competing needs, rights and obligations. It is important to make the distinction between equal distribution and equitable distribution in emergency medicine. Fairness, as applied to need, defines equitable care, but not necessarily equal care.[7] These competing claims have been illuminated in times of scarcity; as an example, when neurointensive care unit beds are used for surge capacity during pandemics, the specialized neurologic care that would otherwise be available to the patients being admitted through the ED may not be available. Neurointerventional procedures, including endovascular therapy, may also not be available as a result of resource scarcity including a lack of appropriately trained proceduralists as a result of staff illness and quarantine requirements. However, assigning resources to those with the most need respects the principle of distributive justice, even in times of scarcity. Broadly speaking, justice in emergency medicine requires the fair and impartial treatment of patients in the ED; however, issues related to treatment and prognostic bias in neurologically injured patients are potentially in conflict with justice and must be recognized and mitigated thoughtfully.

THE ETHICS OF ENDOVASCULAR STROKE THERAPY FOR PATIENTS IN THE EMERGENCY DEPARTMENT

In acute stroke care, tissue plasminogen activator has been an accepted standard of care treatment for decades with endovascular treatment (EVT) via mechanical thrombectomy more recently introduced. Per the American Heart Sacculation/American Stroke Association stroke guidelines, mechanical thrombectomy is the standard of care for patients with low premorbid modified Rankin scale (mRS), significant disability, causative proximal occlusion, and early treatment initiation; class of recommendations I, level of evidence A.[8] The latest guidelines have even expanded the time window for EVT up to 24 hours (and beyond in clinical trials) in cases of mismatch between clinical deficit and volume of infarct, effectively evaluating salvageable tissue, based on imaging criteria.[9]

A standard of care, however, is not without its ethical dilemmas, as has been highlighted by the coronavirus disease-19 pandemic. In times of scarcity, whether owing to limited providers or facilities, the standard of care may informally shift as increased emphasis is placed on justice, both in terms of distribution and rationing. For EVT, scarcity may be in the form of limited expert physicians to perform the procedure, limited availability of transport to capable facilities, or limited intensive care beds in which to take care of postprocedural patients.

As a standard of care treatment, there is already a degree of explicit rationing of EVT based on clearly defined and well-accepted criteria for patient appropriateness for therapy.[1] But for those who do not clearly meet class of recommendations I, level of evidence A criteria, the guidelines are less defined and at higher risk of implicit rationing based on subjective usefulness. Per the American Heart Sacculation/American Stroke Association Guidelines, patients with a premorbid mRS of greater than 1 who do not meet other criteria have a class of recommendations IIB, level of evidence B-R for thrombectomy (ie, more randomized data is needed), but may be reasonable candidates. It can be reasonably assessed that there is decreasing marginal benefit relative to increasing baseline mRS, but where is the threshold of futility?

Patient autonomy, insofar as definition of quality of life, should be a primary consideration when considering interventions, even in the acute setting. Intensive care unit-level interventions should generally be considered inappropriate when there is no reasonable expectation that the patient will improve significantly enough to allow him or her to perceive the benefits of the treatment.[10] But if marginal improvement can be obtained, even in the face of severe remaining deficits, that may be acceptable to some.[11] For patients not capable of autonomous consent, a proxy decision maker is asked to express what that patient would have wanted, which can be fraught with bias and difficult decision making. Although these conversations around quality of life and goals of care are challenging owing to time and resource limitations, it remains very reasonable to expect that they be done in the ED when time allows.

BRAIN DEATH IN THE EMERGENCY DEPARTMENT

Unlike prognostication in early catastrophic brain injury where various prediction models and shared decision making factor significantly, a declaration of death by neurologic criteria is decided by clear-cut legally and morally binding criteria.

The first criteria for brain death determination were created in 1968 with multiple similar, although not identical, guidelines created by various societies since that time, all based fundamentally on the Uniformed Determination of Death Act of 1981.[12] The American Academy of Neurology published brain death criteria for adults in 1995, revised in 2010, and clarified in 2019, which are considered the primary guidelines throughout the United States for death by neurologic criteria, although practices vary widely. Using these criteria for diagnosis, no case of recovery of neurologic function has been observed after determination of brain death.[13]

The diagnosis of brain death requires multiple components including exclusion of confounders, clearance of sedating and paralytic agents, clear causative and irreversible etiology, correlative neuroimaging, and an examination consistent with cessation of whole brain function. Although the mechanics of the examination itself may be accomplished in the acute period, the other components are not as easily achieved. To ensure clearance, waiting at least 5 half-lives for any central nervous system depressants that are present may require days based on pharmacokinetics and pharmacodynamics in critically ill patients. The addition of therapeutic hypothermia after cardiac arrest specifically alters both the pharmacokinetics and pharmacodynamics of sedatives and requires cautious analysis to exclude residual effects that can obfuscate the neurologic examination. Although this factor is less likely to be a confounder in the ED, hypothermia on arrival may have similar effects on drug clearance. Equally important, early neuroimaging can be falsely reassuring, leaving prerequisites for brain death unfulfilled.

Although it may be tempting to declare brain death in the acute phase to spare the patient's family the agony of waiting, to limit potentially futile interventions, or to preserve intensive care unit capacity during times of scarcity, an early diagnosis of brain death should rarely, if ever, occur in the clinical course of devastating neurologic injury.

The Neurocritical Care Society published recommendations that specifically caution against early prognostication in devastating brain injury, recommending a 72-hour window immediately after the injury during which withdrawal from life-sustaining treatment should be delayed and maximal resuscitative efforts should be pursued to avoid a self-fulfilling prophecy.[2] Although there is no minimally acceptable period of observation before a diagnosis of brain death after a devastating brain injury, it is reasonable to follow similar guidelines for a minimum of a 72-hour window, effectively excluding the diagnosis of brain death in the ED setting.[14]

If brain death were to be inappropriately declared too early, at worst it becomes a self-fulfilling prophecy and at best that patient disproves the diagnosis and the trust between the physician and family is damaged. At the base of the diagnosis is nonmaleficence; give a patient time to declare themselves and ensure criteria are met to ensure you inflict no harm. It is not ethically justified, therefore, to declare brain death early in the acute phase when harm outweighs beneficence.

If death by neurologic criteria is not to be declared in the acute period, is there then a limit to interventions, specifically resuscitation? With advancement of resuscitative technology such as extracorporeal membrane oxygenation, the continuum between life and death has become increasingly complicated. Mired in this controversy is organ donation and the potential for competing interests between resuscitative efforts and potential donation. Ethically, the physician's responsibility lies in the patient in front of them rather than a potential transplant candidate elsewhere; therefore, all resuscitative efforts should continue when futility is not yet established, as is often the case in the acute phase before death by neurologic criteria. If the patient becomes hemodynamically unstable, Dalle Ave and colleagues[15] concluded in their work that organ preserving cardiopulmonary resuscitation ought to be performed only when specific consent is obtained from the patient's family.

AIRWAY MANAGEMENT IN DEVASTATING NEUROLOGIC CONDITIONS

The astute physician knows the airways, breathing, and circulation take precedence over diagnosis and prognosis, but in devastating neurologic conditions, prognosis may be key to medical decision making before even the basic airways, breathing, and circulations are considered.

If an evidence-based prognosis offers reasonable hope for improvement, many patients and their surrogates opt for aggressive therapies for maximal benefit. When the prognosis for neurologic recovery is poor; however, it is reasonable to opt for more palliative goals. In the case of airway management, the case is fairly straightforward for a compromised airway in time-limited acute conditions because, once a treatment is instituted, there is reasonable hope for not only improvement, but likely return to baseline in the near future. The situation becomes complex when the timeline is extended or the prognosis is less clear; when offering therapy may equate to prolonged suffering the decision to proceed bears significant moral consequence.

Stroke is a common diagnosis for ethics consults in neurocritical care patients, with a majority of the consults for withdrawal of life support or futility.[16] In large territory infarcts or hemorrhages, ventilatory support may be required to sustain life while the stroke evolves, and potentially longer if the patient survives the acute phase with significant continued deficits. Interventions may be possible during this phase that will prolong quantity with an unknown effect on quality of life, potentially prolonging suffering. Does the beneficence of potential therapy outweigh the potential maleficence of associated complications? The patient's wishes and prognosis will often tip the scale, although research has shown significant variability in physician prognosis, particularly in the early phases.[17] It is key to strike a balance between careful optimism and nihilism because at one end of the spectrum is the self-fulfilling prophecy of a dismal prognosis and at the other is prolonged suffering without additional gain.[18–20]

The situation is similar for neuromuscular respiratory failure. A patient with Guillain-Barre syndrome requiring early intubation may eventually wean from mechanical ventilation after weeks or months with unknown residual deficits or he or she may require mechanical ventilation indefinitely. The same is true of acute high thoracic spinal cord injuries; a ventilator may be needed initially and possibly indefinitely, although it is often too early to know in the acute phase of injury. The acute phase will be difficult, but is the suffering worth the unknown end result? Only the patient can truly make that decision with input from the critical care team. Again, prognosis and autonomy are cornerstones of this dilemma with careful avoidance of clinical nihilism in self-fulfilling prophecies.[21]

CONSENT IN CRITICAL NEUROLOGIC PATIENTS

All the tenets of medical ethics stand alone, but beneficence and autonomy are linked in that it is reasonable for individuals to want the best for themselves and others. This tenet comes under scrutiny in the form of consent in incapacitated critical neurologic patients. Consent is rooted in respect, dignity, and autonomy with 2 prerequisites: disclosure, capacity, and voluntariness.[1] Ideally, when a patient is incapacitated, the legal proxy would be present and well-informed of the wishes of the patient but in time-sensitive cases, the proxy may be unknown or unreachable in the acute phase. Is it ethically justifiable to make educated guesses based on mRS and prognosis?

A common example is a patient presenting with a stroke—perhaps with aphasia or otherwise altered—who is unable to provide consent for tPA or EVT. Without therapy, the deficits will likely remain, whereas with therapy, there is a potential for significant recovery. Is it ethically justifiable to assume what a patient would want? Per American Heart Sacculation/American Stroke Association Stroke Guidelines (2018), when a patient cannot provide consent and a legally authorized representative is not immediately available, it is justified to proceed with IV thrombosis in an otherwise eligible adult patient with a disabling acute ischemic stroke.[2] Although not explicitly stated, it can be extrapolated that the same holds true of EVT as treatment for the same etiology so long as eligibility criteria are met. To withhold these treatments owing to lack of consent would be to deny the patient their right to therapeutic opportunity.

A more complicated case exists in the encephalopathic patient. There are no clear guidelines for a standard of care in undiagnosed encephalopathy, particularly for diagnostic testing.

When there is no clear prognosis, it is uncertain if any risk is worth the reward, and the "reasonable person" standard becomes nebulous. This situation brings into question whether assumed consent can be decoupled from prognosis. Failure to obtain informed consent is a basis for medical malpractice but, in practice, few medical malpractice suits are predicated on the basis of absent informed consent; rather it serves to undermine cases where it is absent.[1]

Retrospectively, aggressive treatment will be looked upon more favorably in those with a good outcome than those with a poor outcome. For those physicians not fortunate enough to have a crystal ball, the "reasonable person" must remain the guiding standard—would most people, given the known facts, accept the known risks to gain the possible rewards—with any nonurgent procedures delayed until clear informed consent can be properly obtained.

ORGAN DONATION IN EMERGENCY MEDICINE

The respect for autonomy may, at times, require that care be rendered for those who would otherwise be limited from receiving aggressive care and resuscitation. Specifically, when it is known that a patient with a neurologically devastating injury has a first-person consent for organ donation, either through his or her own communication or that of a proxy, it is reasonable to consider that the preservation of their opportunity for donation respects their autonomy, beneficence and nonmaleficence, as well as simultaneously paying deference to justice. In general, discussions related to organ donation are not had with patients and their families in the ED by emergency medicine providers. Instead, those discussions are left for the so-called effective requestors, specially trained staff of the organ procurement organizations or nonphysician staff at the hospitals with unique skills to facilitate the necessary discussions about organ donation, donor status, and consent for donation. Even though discussions regarding organ donation generally do not occur in the ED, the care rendered in the ED may dramatically affect the opportunity for organ donation after admission. Resuscitative efforts aimed at hemodynamic stabilization preserve organ function and the potential for delayed decision making regarding donor suitability. These opportunities are often seen as beneficial to the surviving families and should be preserved whenever possible. Often described in terms of duty, efforts to preserve organ donation possibilities are generally consistent with justice and should be the default action unless specifically understood, a priori, to be contrary to the wishes of the patient expressed via legal documentation or proxy.

SUMMARY

The application of traditional pillars of medical ethics to the care of the neurologically injured patient in the emergency setting requires attention to the risks of bias, errors in prognostication, and a lack of evidence-based therapeutics. The unique environmental conditions of emergency medicine require rapid assessment and application of nuanced ethical principles, often under the shroud of stress and emotional shock. It is precisely these challenges that necessitate an a priori understanding of the limitations of both prognosis and autonomy in many of these situations. Generally speaking, when moral conflict arises in the emergency setting, erring on the side of preserving life and allowing time to observe the trajectory of prognosis is ethically sound and may eliminate moral distress in caregivers, patients, and surrogates.

CLINICS CARE POINTS

- Ultra-early prognosis in neurologic injury is fraught with bias, error and a lack of compelling data. Even patient with an initial Glasgow Coma Score of 3 after blunt trauma may have the potential to recover.
- Neurologic injury renders traditional assessments of autonomy impossible in many situations. Care must be taken when using proxy expressions of patient's wishes after neurologic injury.
- Many interventions in neurologic injury carry a risk of rare but devastating consequences; understanding the belief system of the patient is crucial to know if these risks are acceptable.
- Scarcity may shift the standard of care; be aware of resource limitations that may affect patient care.

DISCLOSURE

The authors attest that they have no relevant disclosures for this work. Dr J. Bonomo has served as a speaker and consultant for the Portola and Genentech companies.

REFERENCES

1. Szalados JE. Ethics and law for neurosciences clinicians: foundations and evolving challenges. New Brunswick, NJ: Rutgers University Press; 2019.
2. Souter MJ, Blissitt PA, Blosser S, et al. Recommendations for the critical care management of devastating brain injury: prognostication, psychosocial, and ethical management. Neurocrit Care 2015;23(1):4–13.
3. Chamoun RB, Robertson CS, Gopinath SP. Outcome in patients with blunt head trauma and a Glasgow Coma Scale score of 3 at presentation. J Neurosurg 2009; 111(4):683–7.
4. McCracken DJ, Lovasik BP, McCracken CE, et al. The intracerebral hemorrhage score: a self-fulfilling prophecy? Neurosurgery 2019;84(3):741–8.
5. National Institute of Neurological Disorders and Stroke rt-PA Stroke Study Group. Tissue plasminogen activator for acute ischemic stroke. N Engl J Med 1995; 333(24):1581–8.

6. Meinel TR, Kniepert JU, Seiffge DJ, et al. Endovascular Stroke Treatment and Risk of Intracranial Hemorrhage in Anticoagulated Patients. Stroke 2020;51(3): 892–8.
7. Jacobus C. 10 Issues Related to Justice. 2012 SAEM Ethics Curriculum. 2012. Available at: https://www.saem.org/docs/default-source/saem-documents/ education/module-10-issues-related-to-justice.pdf?sfvrsn=653624fd_2. Accessed July 20, 2020.
8. Powers WJ, Rabinstein AA, Ackerson T, et al. 2018 Guidelines for the Early Management of Patients With Acute Ischemic Stroke: a guideline for healthcare professionals from the American Heart Association/American Stroke Association. Stroke 2018;49:e46–99.
9. Nogueira RG, Jadhav AP, Haussen DC, et al. Thrombectomy 6 to 24 hours after stroke with a mismatch between deficit and infarct. N Engl J Med 2018;378(1): 11–21.
10. Kon AA, Shepard EK, Sederstrom NO, et al. Defining futile and potentially inappropriate interventions: a policy statement from the Society of Critical Care Medicine Ethics Committee. Crit Care Med 2016;44(9):1769–74.
11. Nakagawa K, Bianchi MT, Nakagawa SS, et al. Aggressive care after a massive stroke in young patients: is that what they want? Neurocrit Care 2010;13(1): 118–22.
12. Rubin M, Bonomo J, Hemphill JC III. Intersection of prognosis and palliation in neurocritical care. Curr Opin Crit Care 2017;23(2):134–9.
13. Lewis A, Greer D. Current controversies in brain death determination. Nat Rev Neurol 2017;13(8):505.
14. Machado C, Jeret JS, Shewmon DA, et al. Evidence-based guideline update: determining brain death in adults: report of the Quality Standards Subcommittee of the American Academy of Neurology. Neurology 2011;76(3):307–9.
15. Dalle Ave AL, Shaw DM, Gardiner D. Extracorporeal membrane oxygenation (ECMO) assisted cardiopulmonary resuscitation or uncontrolled donation after the circulatory determination of death following out-of-hospital refractory cardiac arrest—An ethical analysis of an unresolved clinical dilemma. Resuscitation 2016; 108:87–94.
16. Boissy AR, Ford PJ, Edgell RC, et al. Ethics consultations in stroke and neurological disease: a 7-year retrospective review. Neurocrit Care 2008;9(3):394.
17. Zahuranec DB, Fagerlin A, Sánchez BN, et al. Variability in physician prognosis and recommendations after intracerebral hemorrhage. Neurology 2016;86(20): 1864–71.
18. Hemphill JC III, Newman J, Zhao S, et al. Hospital usage of early do-not-resuscitate orders and outcome after intracerebral hemorrhage. Stroke 2004; 35(5):1130–4.
19. Morgenstern LB, Zahuranec DB, Sánchez BN, et al. Full medical support for intracerebral hemorrhage. Neurology 2015;84(17):1739–44.
20. Hoogmoed J, Van den Berg R, Coert BA, et al. A strategy to expeditious invasive treatment improves clinical outcome in comatose patients with aneurysmal subarachnoid haemorrhage. Eur J Neurol 2017;24(1):82–9.
21. Hemphill JC III, White DB. Clinical nihilism in neuroemergencies. Emerg Med Clin North Am 2009;27(1):27–37.

Novel Treatments for Transient Ischemic Attack and Acute Ischemic Stroke

Matthew S. Siket, MD, MSc[a,b,*], Rhonda Cadena, MD[c,d,e]

KEYWORDS

- Acute ischemic stroke • Intravenous alteplase • Endovascular thrombectomy

KEY POINTS

- Nearly 700,000 people experience a stroke every year and 240,000 experience a transient ischemic attack.
- Primary prevention is important in stroke prevention and includes controlling hypertension, diabetes, cholesterol, weight, and cardiac risk factors, and getting plenty of physical activity, abstaining from cigarette smoking and alcohol, and eating a nutritious diet.
- In patients who are not candidates for reperfusion therapy, treatment involves perfusing the ischemic penumbra to prevent worsening of the infarcted region.

INTRODUCTION

Each year, nearly 700,000 people will suffer an acute ischemic stroke (AIS)[1] and an additional 240,000 people will experience a transient ischemic attack (TIA).[2] Before the coronavirus disease-19 outbreak, stroke was the fifth leading cause of death in the United States and remains a leading cause of long-term disability. Over the last 25 years, researchers have been searching for novel ways of treating TIA and AIS that are both effective and safe. Although researchers have yet to identify better treatments, recent trials have shown better patient selection to extend the time window for some beyond the standard 3-hour window.

[a] Division of Emergency Medicine, Department of Surgery, Larner College of Medicine at the University of Vermont, 111 Colchester Avenue, EC2-216, Burlington, VT 05401, USA; [b] Department of Neurological Sciences, Larner College of Medicine at the University of Vermont, 111 Colchester Avenue, EC2-216, Burlington, VT 05401, USA; [c] Division of Neurocritical Care, Department of Neurology, University of North Carolina, 170 Manning Drive, CB#7025, Chapel Hill, NC 27517, USA; [d] Department of Neurosurgery, University of North Carolina, 170 Manning Drive, CB#7025, Chapel Hill, NC 27517, USA; [e] Department of Emergency Medicine, University of North Carolina, 170 Manning Drive, CB#7025, Chapel Hill, NC 27517, USA
* Corresponding author. Department of Neurological Sciences, Larner College of Medicine at the University of Vermont, 111 Colchester Avenue, EC2-216, Burlington, VT 05401.
E-mail address: Matthew.Siket@med.uvm.edu

Emerg Med Clin N Am 39 (2021) 227–242
https://doi.org/10.1016/j.emc.2020.09.014
0733-8627/21/© 2020 Elsevier Inc. All rights reserved.

EVALUATION

Any patient with suspected AIS should have a focused assessment aimed at identifying ongoing, functionally disabling focal neurologic deficits. Prehospital and emergency department professionals may use any number of validated stroke screening and severity grading tools (discussed elsewhere in this article) to aid in efficient stroke detection.[3] The use of prehospital stroke screens have been linked with improved thrombolytic treatment rates and faster door-to-needle times, whereas severity scales aid in the identification of patients with large vessel occlusion (LVO) stroke for faster door-to-groin times for endovascular candidates. The National Institutes of Health Stroke Scale (NIHSS) is a standardized and commonly used assessment of neurologic deficits intended to be easily reproducible, using 11 items to produce a score of 0 to 42. Generally speaking, the higher the NIHSS, the larger the area of infarction and the worse the outcome for patients. Documentation of the NIHSS at the time of the initial evaluation and before stroke treatment is a quality performance metric. NIHSS training and certification is available to EM clinicians and is encouraged, particularly where neurologic expertise is unavailable.

Establishing the time that the patient was "last known well" (LKW), that is, without symptoms, is of paramount importance. It is distinct from the time of symptom discovery and should be used as the presumed time of stroke onset in all cases when the patient cannot clearly recall the precise time symptoms began. The patient's premorbid functional status (level of independence immediately before the stroke) should also be assessed. The modified Rankin Scale (mRS) is a 6-point ordinal measurement of functional disability and is commonly used as an outcome measure in stroke treatment trials (**Table 1**).[4]

Early Stabilization and Resuscitation

All emergency department patients should first have their airway, breathing, and circulation assessed and standard resuscitative measures enacted to ensure hemodynamic stability. The role of the emergency clinician in immediate assessment of suspected stroke patients upon arrival is key, because a minority may lose protective airway reflexes and require emergent endotracheal intubation before ascertaining diagnostic imaging. Hypotension should be avoided and corrected immediately if present. Unless the patient is to receive intravenous (IV) thrombolysis, permissive

Table 1 The mRS	
Score	Description
0	No symptoms at all
1	No significant disability despite symptoms; able to carry out all usual duties and activities
2	Slight disability; unable to carry out all previous activities, but able to look after own affairs without assistance
3	Moderate disability; requiring some help, but able to walk without assistance
4	Moderately severe disability; unable to walk without assistance, unable to attend to needs without assistance
5	Severe disability; bedridden, incontinent, and requiring constant nursing care and attention
6	Dead

hypertension (up to 220 mm Hg systolic) should be allowed. Patients receiving thrombolytics should have their blood pressure maintained at or below 185/110 mm Hg in accordance with the American Heart Association/American Stroke Association (AHA/ASA) recommendations.[5]

Primary Stroke Prevention

Because 76% of patients with stroke are experiencing this for the first time,[1] primary prevention is an important factor in treatment. The top 10 modifiable risk factors for strokes include[6]:

- Hypertension
- Diabetes
- Dyslipidemia
- Cigarette smoking
- Obesity
- Poor diet
- Physical inactivity
- Stress or depression
- Alcohol intake
- Cardiac causes such as atrial fibrillation and valvular disease

Controlling these risk factors reduces the risk of first stroke. **Table 2** shows the current recommendations for primary prevention of stroke based on the AHA/ASA guidelines for primary prevention of stroke.[7]

Non–stroke-related visits to the emergency department are important opportunities for screening, counseling, and referring patients with conditions such as asymptomatic hypertension, undiagnosed or uncontrolled diabetes, obesity, and cigarette smoking.

INTRAVENOUS THROMBOLYSIS
History

Thrombolytic therapies for AIS have been under investigation since the 1950s, preceding computed tomography (CT) technology. The predominant risk of treatment is hemorrhagic conversion of the area of infarction leading to intracerebral hemorrhage (ICH) and high rates of mortality. Early studies predominantly used streptokinase and urokinase, which shifted to recombinant tissue plasminogen activator (rt-PA) in the 1990s. In 1995, the European Cooperative Acute Stroke Study (ECASS)-I was the first randomized trial of alteplase (an rt-PA) for AIS patients within 6 hours of LKW and enrolled 620 patients throughout Europe. No difference in outcomes (disability or mortality) were found in the intention-to-treat population, but after accounting for protocol violations in more than 17% of the study population, rt-PA treatment showed an overall benefit.[14] Later the same year, the National Institute of Neurological Disorders and Stroke (NINDS)-II trial of 624 stroke patients showed a significant improvement in clinical outcome at 3 months for AIS patients treated with t-PA within 3 hours, despite an increased risk of symptomatic ICH of 6.4%.[15] Overall, the NINDS trial found that t-PA treated patients were 30% more likely to have minimal or no disability at 3 months. One year later, the US Food and Drug Administration approved t-PA for the treatment of AIS up to 3 hours after symptom onset.

ECASS III, published in 2008, was the next trial to show clinical efficacy of patients receiving rt-PA up to 4.5 hours of LKW. This study randomized 821 patients to treatment between 3.0 and 4.5 hours from LKW (as treatment within 3 hours had become

Table 2
Recommendations for primary stroke prevention based on the 2014 AHA/ASA guidelines[7]

	Recommendation for Primary Stroke Prevention
Physical inactivity	Moderate-intense aerobic physical activity 3–4 times/wk for 40 min/d[8]
Dyslipidemia	Treatment with a statin medication in patients for a goal LDL $\leq$70 or a high 10-y risk for cardiovascular events[9,10]
Diet and nutrition	Reduced intake of sodium and saturated fat Increased intake of potassium, fruits, vegetables, and low-fat dairy products
Hypertension	Regular blood pressure screening, diet modification for patients with prehypertension (120–139/80–89 mm Hg), and medical treatment of patients with hypertension for a goal BP of <140/90 mm Hg[11]
Obesity	Weight reduction for overweight (BMI = 25–29 kg/m²) and obese (BMI >30 kg/m²) patients[12]
Diabetes	In addition to controlling diabetes, patients with type I or type II diabetes should have control of hypertension to a goal of <140/90 mm Hg and treated with a statin medication for a goal LDL $\leq$70[13]
Cigarette smoking	Smoking cessation with the use of drug therapy or nicotine replacement[10]
Atrial fibrillation	Long-term anticoagulation in patients without hemorrhagic risk factors for patients with a high risk for stroke, defined as a CHA2DS2-VASc score of $\geq$2
Other cardiac conditions	
Valvular disease	Long term aspirin therapy for patients with bioprosthetic valves and long term anticoagulation in patients with mitral stenosis, left atrial thrombus, and after mechanical valve replacement therapy
CHF	Aspirin or anticoagulation can be used if no previous thromboembolic events.
MI	Anticoagulation can be considered in patients with asymptomatic left ventricular mural thrombi and for patients with STEMI and anterior apical akinesis or dyskinesis if no contraindications.
PFO	Antithrombotic treatment and catheter-based closure are not recommended in patients with PFO if no history of thromboembolic events

Abbreviations: BMI, body mass index; BP, blood pressure; CHF, congestive heart failure; LDL, low-density lipoprotein cholesterol; MI, myocardial infarction; PFO, patent foramen ovale; STEMI, ST-elevation myocardial infarction.

standard of care) and a favorable outcome was observed in 52.4% of treated patients versus 45.2% of controls.[16]

The International Stroke Trial-3 trial enrolled a total of 3035 out of an intended 6000 patients in a 1:1 open controlled design and is the largest clinical trial to date investigating rt-PA efficacy. This study was conducted after thrombolysis had become the standard of care for patients up to 4.5 hours from LKW, so only patients meeting the "uncertainty principle" for whom clinical equipoise remained were enrolled (e.g., 53% of patients treated with rt-PA were >80 years old). Although this trial did not achieve its primary outcome measure (proportion alive and independent at 6 months), there was a significant ordinal decrease in disability at 6 months, and those treated within 3 hours of onset showed significant benefit. Overall, this trial further reinforced the use of rt-PA.

In the subsequent 25 years since the NINDS publication, the debate regarding the clinical efficacy of fibrinolysis in stroke has continued.[17] Some trials following NINDS, including ECASS II (0–3 hours and 3–6 hours from LKW)[18] and Alteplase Thrombolysis for Acute Noninterventional Therapy in Ischemic Stroke (ATLANTIS) B (3–5 hours from LKW)[19] did not demonstrate a similar benefit of rt-PA therapy. In addition, other trials have shown higher percentages of hemorrhages, but these are likely due to a large number of protocol deviations including treatment beyond the 3-hour time window, administration of antiplatelets or anticoagulants in the first 24 hours, or uncontrolled blood pressures, all of which have been shown to increase the risk of ICH.[20–22]

Several pooled analyses have explored the overall efficacy of rt-PA[23] and, although subject to methodologic heterogeneity, the collective evidence from these analyses supports a time-dependent treatment effect of rt-PA.[24]

Current Recommendations

Although the US Food and Drug Administration has approved the use of rt-PA for AIS only up to 3 hours from LKW, multiple organizations including the AHA/ASA, American College of Emergency Physicians, American College of Cardiology, European Stroke Organization, National Stroke Foundation, and National Institute for Health and Care Excellence have endorsed its use up to 4.5 hours of LKW, which is widely considered the international standard of care. Of note, some groups including the Canadian Association of Emergency Physicians and Australasian College for Emergency Medicine have called for more research before considering rt-PA standard of care based on conflicting available evidence, and it is anticipated that the recent reanalysis of ECASS-III may lead to others following suit.[25]

Although the lack of consensus regarding the use of rt-PA in AIS may leave the emergency clinician hesitant to administer and/or recommend it, it is clear that rt-PA should not be considered life saving, but rather autonomy preserving. The decision to pursue thrombolysis should be based on individual patient wishes, and made using shared decision making after a brief discussion of risks and benefits (American College of Emergency Physicians Level C recommendation).[26] Written informed consent is generally not required, but documentation of a discussion of risks and benefits with the patient and/or health care proxy should be reflected in the medical record.

Thrombolytic treatment should be reserved for only those patients with ongoing, disabling, focal neurologic deficits not meeting any exclusion criteria.[27] Treatment of minor and nondisabling symptoms has been a source of debate, but the Phase IIIB, Double-Blind, Multicenter Study to Evaluate the Efficacy and Safety of Alteplase in Patients With Mild Stroke: Rapidly Improving Symptoms and Minor Neurologic Deficits (PRISMS) trial recently explored this and was halted after enrollment of only 313 of an intended 948 subjects. In this study, patient with an NIHSS of 0 to 5 with symptoms described as "not clearly disabling" were randomized to rt-PA versus control. Although halted prematurely, there was no significant difference in 90-day mRS between groups, yet the treated group had a much higher rate of symptomatic ICH (3.2% vs 0%).[28]

Recent Advances

In an effort to maximize the likelihood of a good patient outcome, significant effort has been made to expedite door-to-needle times for AIS patients receiving rt-PA.

One such initiative has been to bring stroke reperfusion therapies to the scene, bypassing the emergency department all together. Mobile stroke units have emerged in many metropolitan areas as an innovative way to improve stroke treatment efficiency. Patients are met on scene by an ambulance equipped with a portable CT scanner, many of which have full CT angiography capabilities to detect LVO stroke. To date, approximately 20 locations around the world deploy mobile stroke units, despite their high initial investment and operating costs.[29] The overall clinical benefits and broader generalizability of mobile stroke units are undetermined, but likely dependent on individual geographic and treatment factors.[30]

Telestroke has emerged as a practical way to bring cerebrovascular neurologic expertise to rural and resource-conservative settings in an effort to improve acute stroke treatment, and small hospitals using telestroke have been associated with reduced door-to-needle times.[31] Regardless of the technology used, a coordinated stroke system of care that emphasizes efficient diagnosis to minimize onset-to-treatment time is encouraged (AHA/ASA Class I, Level A recommendation).[32]

Extended window thrombolysis has been demonstrated with some success, despite the ongoing debate about the efficacy of rt-PA in the currently endorsed time window (0–4.5 hours from LKW). The Efficacy and Safety of MRI-Based Thrombolysis in Wake-Up Stroke (WAKE-UP) trial enrolled 503 of an intended 800 acute stroke patients in whom the time LKW could not be determined. Patients were randomized to receive rt-PA or not if MRI showed an area of restricted diffusion without changes on T2 fluid attenuated inversion recovery imaging. Patients treated with rt-PA were more likely to have a favorable outcome (mRS of 0–2 at 90 days), despite a trend toward increased risk of symptomatic ICH (2.0% vs 0.4%; $P = .15$).[33] The Extending the Time for Thrombolysis in Emergency Neurological Deficits (EXTEND) trial randomized 225 of a planned 310 subjects between 4.5 and 9.0 hours from LKW with a mismatch on CT scan or MR perfusion imaging and also favored rt-PA treatment despite increased symptomatic ICH.[34] The cautious selective use of rt-PA in patients with a favorable imaging pattern with LKW beyond 4.5 hours has been given a weak level of recommendation by the AHA/ASA, and further studies are warranted.

Alternative fibrinolytic agents have been explored to improve the safety and efficacy of thrombolysis in AIS. Although alteplase remains the treatment standard, its short half-life and need for continuous infusion over 1 hour after an initial bolus make it less ideal. Other agents such as tenecteplase have been shown to be more fibrin-specific and have a longer half-life after a bolus-only dose. Because tenecteplase causes less hypofibrinogenemia than alteplase, it is thought to cause less hemorrhagic transformation, which was demonstrated in a recent meta-analysis.[35] Tenecteplase has demonstrated noninferiority to alteplase in AIS and LVO patients undergoing endovascular treatment.[36,37] It is currently being investigated in multiple extended window trials.[38]

Sonothrombolysis is the concept of augmenting clot-dissolving capabilities of systemic fibrinolysis through ultrasound-induced mechanical agitation. Continuous transcranial Doppler examinations performed concurrently with t-PA administration seems to be a noninvasive way to promote fluid motion around a thrombus and increase rt-PA concentration within the clot.[39] Studies have been mixed in terms of clinical benefit, although most have shown an increased rate of vessel recanalization without an increased risk of mortality or symptomatic ICH.[40] The greatest potential benefit seems to be in proximal LVO stroke of the middle cerebral artery, where rt-PA alone is unlikely to be efficacious.[41]

ENDOVASCULAR STROKE CARE

A revolution in interventional stroke treatment occurred in 2015 with the publication of 5 prospective, randomized, multicenter trials that enrolled patients from around the world using confirmed LVO stroke. Each showed overwhelming benefit of mechanical thrombectomy with modern generation stent retrieval devices.[42–46] The Multicenter Randomized Clinical Trial of Endovascular Treatment for Acute. Ischemic Stroke in the Netherlands (MR CLEAN) trial was the first of this group to report its results and the other trials were subsequently closed prematurely citing lack of equipoise in light of other positive trials. Using pooled data from the Highly Effective Reperfusion Evaluated in Multiple Endovascular Stroke Trials (HERMES) collaboration of endovascular trials, the number needed to treat to decrease 90-day functional disability by 1 point on the mRS is 2.6,[47] and mechanical thrombectomy is now considered the standard of care for eligible patients with LVO stroke of less than 6 hours duration.[5]

It should be noted that the majority of patients in all 5 of the landmark endovascular trials also received IV rt-PA, wherein mechanical thrombectomy was an adjuvant therapy used in conjunction with systemic thrombolysis. Although this remains the current treatment standard, 1 head-to-head trial comparing combination therapy (IV rt-PA + thrombectomy) with thrombectomy alone reported noninferiority of endovascular treatment alone,[48] and multiple additional studies are currently underway.

Although the efficacy of endovascular reperfusion decreases over time, some patients have been shown to benefit from mechanical thrombectomy as far out as 24 hours from LKW. Careful selection of patients using advanced neuroimaging is key for patients in an LVO and LKW greater than 6 hours. The Endovascular Therapy Following Imaging Evaluation for Ischemic Stroke 3 (DEFUSE 3) trial identified patients 6 to 16 hours from LKW with an LVO and a diffusion/perfusion mismatch using CT- or MR-based perfusion imaging. A computer algorithm generated mismatch ratio (core/penumbra) of greater than 1.8 was needed for eligibility. Patients receiving endovascular therapy were much more likely than those who did not to have a mRS of −2 at 90 days (45% vs 17%).[49] The Diffusion Weighted Imaging (DWI) or Computerized Tomography Perfusion (CTP) Assessment With Clinical Mismatch in the Triage of Wake Up and Late Presenting Strokes Undergoing Neurointervention (DAWN) trial selected patients 6 to 24 hours from stroke onset using a mismatch of infarct volume on MRI to severity of clinical deficit. The likelihood of having a mRS of 0 to 2 at 90 days was 49% in those receiving thrombectomy and 13% in those who did not.[50] Collectively, the number needed to treat to restore 1 patient with LVO with a favorable imaging pattern presenting beyond 6 hours from LKW to functional independence at 90 days is between 3 and 4.

NEUROPROTECTIVE THERAPY

The ischemic cascade progresses from initially oligemic tissue to irreversible infarction, but increasing evidence suggests this sequence occurs at different rates among individuals experiencing a stroke. Strategies to slow and disrupt this progression have been the subject of numerous investigational studies. Apoptotic and excitatory pathway inhibitors, anti-inflammatory agents and free radical scavengers are among the most studied candidate agents, but to date none has demonstrated clear benefit. The subset of stroke patients that seems to be most likely to benefit includes those with large penumbral areas of tissue at risk, such as LVO patients awaiting thrombectomy. The recently published Efficacy and Safety of Nerinetide for the Treatment of Acute Ischaemic Stroke (ESCAPE-NA1) trial of IV nerinetide in patients with LVO within 12 hours of onset did not show any significant difference in clinical outcomes between treatment groups, but did not find an improved outcome in patients who did not receive rt-PA.[51] The Field Administration of Stroke Therapy–Magnesium (FASTMAG) trial of early IV magnesium administration was also negative in improving functional outcomes, but did pave the way for prehospital neuroprotective studies.[52] Adjuvant neuroprotective strategies are likely to remain an appealing and exciting area of acute stroke research for the foreseeable future.

CONTRAINDICATIONS TO REPERFUSION STRATEGIES

Whereas the primary goal in AIS is reperfusion of the occluded vessel, there are patients in whom IV thrombolytics and endovascular thrombectomy is contraindicated. For these patients, the goal must be focused on saving the at-risk surrounding ischemic region via improving cerebral perfusion, antiplatelet medications, and preventing cerebral hypoxia.

Blood Pressure

When blood flow is cut off from a region of the brain, there is infarcted tissue immediately downstream to the occluded vessel causing a core infarct area. Surrounding that region is an area of at-risk brain in which there is low blood flow and hypoxia, resulting in an ischemic penumbra (**Fig. 1**). This tissue is perfused by collateral vessels from other nonoccluded branches and, given these are smaller vessels and circumvent the standard flow, hypotension and hypovolemia should be avoided.[53–55] Given the paucity of data to determine the optimal blood pressure, the goal is not known and may be different for every patient. Therefore, in patients who did not receive IV alteplase or mechanical thrombectomy and have no comorbid conditions requiring urgent

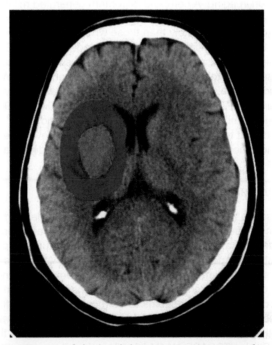

Fig. 1. A noncontrast CT scan of the head showing representation of a core infarct (*blue*) and surrounding ischemic penumbra (*red*). (Image source: Rhonda Cadena, MD)

antihypertensive treatment, allowing the blood pressure to rise up to 220/120 mm Hg might be reasonable. If there are signs of end-organ damage that need emergent treatment such as acute myocardial infarct, heart failure, aortic dissection, or eclampsia, a decrease of 15% of initial pressure is warranted.[34]

Twenty-fourhour blood pressure goals include:
- Before IV alteplase: less than 185/110 mm Hg
- After IV alteplase: ≤180/105 mm Hg
- After mechanical thrombectomy (0–6 h): ≤180/105 mm Hg
- After mechanical thrombectomy (6–24 h): ≤140/90 mm Hg
- No IV alteplase or mechanical thrombectomy: ≤220/120 mm Hg

Antiplatelet Therapy

In patients without contraindications, aspirin should be given within 24 hours of symptom onset. The initial dose should be at least 160 mg, because doses of 160 to 300 mg have been shown to be effective in decreasing the recurrence of stroke.[56,57] In patients who are deemed unsafe to swallow or who have not yet passed a dysphagia screening, rectal or nasogastric aspirin can be given. In patients with small strokes (NIHSS ≤3) who did not receive IV alteplase or mechanical thrombectomy, treatment with dual antiplatelet therapy (aspirin and clopidogrel) started within 24 hours of stroke may be effective in decreasing recurrent ischemic stroke.[58,59]

Cerebral Edema

The most life-threatening complication of large cerebral and cerebellar strokes is malignant cerebral edema and herniation (**Fig. 2**). Studies have shown a reduction in mortality if a decompressive hemicraniectomy is performed within 48 hours in patients 60 years of age or younger who experience neurologic decline.[60] Therefore, for patients with large strokes, intensive care unit admission in a facility with neurosurgery consultation should be considered.[61]

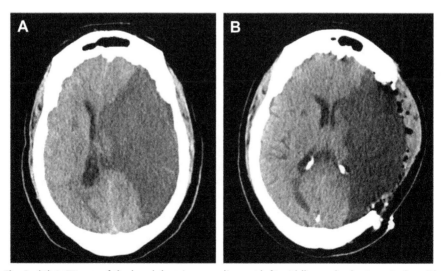

Fig. 2. (A) A CT scan of the head showing a malignant left middle cerebral artery stroke with cerebral edema and midline shift and (B) The same patient after a decompressive hemicraniectomy. (Images: Rhonda Cadena, MD.)

In patients with intracranial hypertension and clinical signs of herniation, hyperventilation (goal P_{CO_2} 30–34 mm Hg) or hyperosmolar therapy can be used to temporarily reduce intracranial pressures as a bridge to surgical intervention. Hypothermia or barbiturates in the setting of malignant cerebral or cerebellar edema are not recommended owing to limited data supporting benefit.[62] Corticosteroids have not been shown to be beneficial in the treatment of cerebral edema owing to AIS and may be associated with increased risk of infection; therefore, they are not currently recommended.[63]

Cerebellar infarction with brain stem compression and fourth ventricle effacement can lead to obstructive hydrocephalus. In these patients, ventriculostomy is recommended and suboccipital decompressive craniectomy may or may not be necessary on the basis of factors such as the size of the infarction, neurologic condition, degree of brainstem compression, and effectiveness of medical management.[63]

SPECIAL CIRCUMSTANCES
Cervical Artery Dissection

Stroke prevention with antithrombotic therapy remains the mainstay of treatment for patients with cervical artery dissections. Although there has not been a randomized trial of antithrombotic therapy versus placebo in patients with acute cervical artery dissection, observational studies and expert opinion suggest that it is reasonable to initiate antithrombotic therapy in the acute setting to prevent early thromboembolic events.[64] The ideal antithrombotic agent has not yet been determined but an antiplatelet agent is reasonable over anticoagulation if there are no contraindications.

In patients who present to the emergency department with an AIS owing to an extracranial or intracranial dissection without rupture, despite limited evidence on this specific population with regard to IV alteplase, a subgroup analysis in this population indicates it as effective and safe in patients without dissection.[65,66] Therefore, in a patient with neurologic deficits concerning for stroke, after an initial CT scan of the head without contrast is performed to rule out hemorrhage, IV alteplase is recommended in accordance with published guidelines if there are no contraindications, followed by endovascular treatment, if indicated. After treatment, further testing with CT angiography of the head and neck could be performed for evaluation of a dissection if suspicion exists.

Posterior Circulation Strokes

Posterior circulation strokes account for up to 19% of all strokes treated with IV alteplase,[67–69] but have been excluded from recent studies regarding treatment beyond the standard time windows owing to the risk of hemorrhage. A recent retrospective review of an ongoing prospective database of strokes reported that in the 14.6% of posterior circulation strokes that received IV alteplase, their bleeding risk was one-half of what was seen in anterior circulation strokes.[70] Current stroke guidelines suggest that mechanical thrombectomy is reasonable for posterior circulation occlusions up to 6 hours but do not guide further recommendations.[63] Currently there is a paucity of data guiding treatment outside of the 6-hour time window.

Small Strokes

The benefits of IV alteplase in patients with mild stroke (NIHSS 0–5) are unclear given various analyses of the data showing benefit in some and no benefit in others.[19,26,71] A recent randomized controlled trial looked at the efficacy of IV alteplase in patients with and NIHSS 0 to 5 with nondisabling symptoms.[30] In those patients, there was no benefit of treatment when given within 3 hours of onset because the risk of the IV alteplase may be more than the benefit. However, in patients with disabling mild strokes, such that would affect the ability to talk or perform activities of daily living, IV alteplase is recommended.[63]

TRANSIENT ISCHEMIC ATTACK

Much like AIS, the mainstay of treatment of TIA is to identify the underlying etiologic trigger and prevent a recurrent event. Both stroke and TIA should be regarded as cerebrovascular emergencies, warranting an early and frontloaded diagnostic evaluation. A TIA warns of impending stroke in 12% to 30% of patients experiencing a stroke and the risk is highest within the first 24 to 48 hours of the sentinel event.[72,73] When presenting to the emergency department, patients should undergo brain and cervicocephalic vascular imaging to differentiate stroke and nonstroke mimics and to identify high-risk vascular lesions (such as severe stenosis or dissection), and be assessed for common causes of cardiac embolism.[74]

Differentiating true ischemic events from mimics can prove diagnostically challenging because patients most often have a normal neurologic examination at the time of their index visit. A careful history focusing on the differentiation of symptoms that suggest irritative phenomenon like seizure or complex migraine can be helpful. A noncontrast CT scan is of low yield in patients with TIA and diffusion-weighted MRI is strongly preferred, but oftentimes logistically not feasible in the emergency department setting given the majority of US emergency departments do not have 24/7 access to MRI.[75] Perfusion imaging modalities (both CT scans and MRI) have been shown to identify patients with focal perfusion abnormalities in 30% to 42% of patients after a TIA, some of whom had no abnormalities detected on diffusion-weighted MRI.[76–78] Although this strategy may identify an additional subset of patients at risk of early progression to infarct, it is not commonly performed on patients with TIA on the whole.

Clinical risk prediction scores such as the ABCD2 score[79] have been shown to estimate short-term stroke risk after TIA with moderate accuracy, but should not alone drive disposition decisions from the emergency department. Imaging-enhanced tools such as the ABCD3-I score[80] have superior predictive ability compared with clinical tools, but add advanced diagnostic testing (such as diffusion-weighted MRI and vessel imaging), which make them less useful as clinical decision aids in the emergency department. The Canadian TIA Score provides a practical alternative, showing good discriminative capability in differentiating low, moderate and high-risk TIA patients in terms of 7-day subsequent stroke risk after emergency department presentation.[81] This score was recently validated in 14 emergency departments across Canada, with findings supporting the early discharge of patients deemed low risk, additional testing and secondary prevention initiation with close follow-up for those of moderate risk, and specialist consultation for those of high risk.[82]

If a cardioembolic source is identified, then patients should generally be started on anticoagulation unless contraindicated. For most other patients, antiplatelet therapy is recommended. Dual antiplatelet therapy with aspirin and clopidogrel (300 mg loading dose followed by 75 mg/d) for a total of 21 days is currently recommended by the AHA/ASA for high-risk patients with an ABCD2 score of greater than 4. Otherwise, the same secondary prevention strategies used in AIS are applicable to TIA with a focus on mitigating risk factors and adopting a healthy lifestyle.

DISCLOSURE

I have no commercial or financial conflicts.

REFERENCES

1. Benjamin EJ, Blaha MJ, Chiuve SE, et al. Heart disease and stroke statistics-2017 update: a report from the American Heart Association. Circulation 2017;135(10): e146–603.
2. Kleindorfer D, Panagos P, Pancioli A, et al. Incidence and short-term prognosis of transient ischemic attack in a population based study. Stroke 2005;36(4):720–3.
3. Nentwich LM. Diagnosis of Acute Ischemic Stoke. Emerg Med Clin North Am 2016;34(4):837–59.
4. van Swieten JC, Koudstaal PJ, Visser MC, et al. Interobserver agreement for the assessment of handicap in stroke patients. Stroke 1988;19(5):604–7.
5. Powers WJ, Rabinstein AA, Ackerson T, et al. 2018 Guidelines for the Early management of Patients with acute ischemic stroke: a guideline for healthcare professionals from the American Heart Association/American Stroke Association. Stroke 2018;49(3):e46–110.
6. O'Donnell MJ, Xavier D, Liu L, et al. Risk factors for ischaemic and intracerebral haemorrhagic stroke in 22 countries (the INTERSTROKE study): a case-control study. Lancet 2010;376(9735):112–23.
7. Meschia JF, Bushnell C, Boden-Albala B, et al. Guidelines for the primary prevention of stroke: a statement for healthcare professionals from the American Heart Association/American Stroke Association. Stroke 2014;45(12):3754–832.
8. Eckel RH, Jakicic JM, Ard JD, et al. 2013 AHA/ACC guideline on lifestyle management to reduce cardiovascular risk: a report of the American College of Cardiology/American Heart Association Task Force on Practice Guidelines. J Am Coll Cardiol 2014;63(25 Pt B):2960–84.
9. Grundy SM, Stone NJ, Bailey AL, et al. 2018 Guideline on the management of blood cholesterol: a report of the American College of Cardiology/American Heart Association Task Force on Clinical Practice Guidelines. Circulation 2019;139(25): e1082–143.
10. Wolf PA, D'Agostino RB, Belanger AJ, et al. Probability of stroke: a risk profile from the Framingham Study. Stroke 1991;22(3):312–8.
11. Sipahi I, Swaminathan A, Natesan V, et al. Effect of antihypertensive therapy on incident stroke in cohorts with prehypertensive blood pressure levels: a meta-analysis of randomized controlled trials. Stroke 2012;43(2):432–40.
12. Caterson ID, Finer N, Coutinho W, et al. Maintained intentional weight loss reduces cardiovascular outcomes: results from the Sibutramine Cardiovascular OUTcomes (SCOUT) trial. Diabetes Obes Metab 2012;14(6):523–30.
13. Nathan DM, Cleary PA, Backlund JY, et al. Intensive diabetes treatment and cardiovascular disease in patients with type 1 diabetes. N Engl J Med 2005;353(25): 2643–53.
14. Hacke W, Kaste M, Fieschi C, et al. Intravenous thrombolysis with recombinant tissue plasminogen activator for acute hemispheric stroke. The European Cooperative Acute Stroke Study (ECASS). JAMA 1995;274(13):1017–25.
15. National Institute of Neurological Disorders and Stroke rt-PA Stroke Study Group. Tissue plasminogen activator for acute ischemic stroke. N Engl J Med 1995; 333(24):1581–7.
16. Hacke W, Kaste M, Bluhmki E, et al. Thrombolysis with alteplase 3 to 4.5 hours after acute ischemic stroke. N Engl J Med 2008;359(13):1317–29.
17. Ingall TJ, O'Fallon WM, Asplund K, et al. Findings from the reanalysis of the NINDS tissue plasminogen activator for acute ischemic stroke treatment trial. Stroke 2004;35(10):2418–24.

18. Hacke W, Brott T, Caplan L, et al. Thrombolysis in acute ischemic stroke: controlled trials and clinical experience. Neurology 1999;53(7 Suppl 4):S3–14.

19. Clark WM, Wissman S, Albers GW, et al. Recombinant tissue-type plasminogen activator (Alteplase) for ischemic stroke 3 to 5 hours after symptom onset. The ATLANTIS Study: a randomized controlled trial. Alteplase Thrombolysis for Acute Noninterventional Therapy in Ischemic Stroke. JAMA 1999;282(21):2019–26.

20. Katzan IL, Furlan AJ, Lloyd LE, et al. Use of tissue-type plasminogen activator for acute ischemic stroke, The Cleveland area experience. JAMA 2000;283(9):1151–8.

21. Bravata DM, Kim N, Concato J, et al. Thrombolysis for Acute Stroke in Routine Clinical Practice. Arch Intern Med 2002;162:1994–2001.

22. Lopez-Yunez AM, Bruno A, Williams LS, et al. Protocol violations in community-based rTPA stroke treatment are associated with symptomatic intracerebral hemorrhage. Stroke 2001;32:12–6.

23. Wardlaw JM, Murray V, Berge E, et al. Thrombolysis for acute ischaemic stroke. Cochrane Database Syst Rev 2014;(7):CD000213.

24. Emberson J, Lees KR, Lyden P, et al. Effect of treatment delay, age, and stroke severity on the effects of intravenous thrombolysis with alteplase for acute ischaemic stroke: a meta-analysis of individual patient data from randomised trials. Lancet 2014;384(9958):1929–35.

25. Australasian College of Emergency Medicine. Statement on intravenous thrombolysis for ischaemic stroke. Available at: https://acem.org.au/getmedia/8dca8e1f-4de3-4c28-a2aa-a61400c02650/S129_Statement_on_IV_Thrombolysis_for_Ischaemic_Stroke_v4.aspx. Accessed July 23rd, 2020.

26. Brown MD, Burton JH, Nazarian DJ, et al. Clinical policy: use of intravenous tissue plasminogen activator for the management of acute ischemic stroke in the Emergency Department. Ann Emerg Med 2015;66(3):322–33.

27. The Brain Attack Coalition. TPA Stroke Study Group Guidelines. Available at: https://www.stroke-site.org/guidelines/tpa_guidelines/. Accessed on July 23rd, 2020.

28. Khatri P, Kleindorfer DO, Devlin T, et al. Effect of alteplase vs aspirin on functional outcome for patients with acute ischemic stroke and minor nondisabling neurologic deficits: the PRISMS Randomized Clinical Trial. JAMA 2018;320(2):156–66.

29. Liaw N, Liebeskind D. Emerging therapies in acute ischemic stroke. F1000Res 2020;9. F1000 Faculty Rev-546.

30. Holodinsky JK, Kamal N, Zerna C, et al. In what scenarios does a mobile stroke unit predict better patient outcomes? A modeling study. Stroke 2020;51(6):1805–12.

31. Heffner DL, Thirumala PD, Pokharna P, et al. Outcomes of spoke-retained telestroke patients versus hub-treated patients after intravenous thrombolysis: telestroke patient outcomes after thrombolysis. Stroke 2015;46(11):3161–7.

32. Powers WJ, Rabinstein AA, Ackerson T, et al. Guidelines for the early management of patients with acute ischemic stroke: 2019 update to the 2018 guidelines for the early management of acute ischemic stroke. Stroke 2019;50(12):e344–418.

33. Thomalla G, Simonsen CZ, Boutitie F, et al. MRI-guided thrombolysis for stroke with unknown time of onset. N Engl J Med 2018;379(7):611–22.

34. Ma H, Campbell BCV, Parsons MW, et al. Thrombolysis guided by perfusion imaging up to 9 hours after onset of stroke. N Engl J Med 2019;380(19):1795–803.

35. Xu N, Chen Z, Zhao C, et al. Different doses of tenecteplase vs alteplase in thrombolysis therapy of acute ischemic stroke: evidence from randomized controlled trials. Drug Des Devel Ther 2018;12:2071–84.

36. Logallo N, Novotny V, Assmus J, et al. Tenecteplase versus alteplase for management of acute ischaemic stroke (NOR-TEST): a phase 3, randomised, open-label, blinded endpoint trial. Lancet Neurol 2017;16(10):781–8.

37. Campbell BCV, Mitchell PJ, Churilov L, et al. Tenecteplase versus alteplase before thrombectomy for ischemic stroke. N Engl J Med 2018;378(17):1573–82.

38. Nelson A, Kelly G, Byyny R, et al. Tenecteplase utility in acute ischemic stroke patients: a clinical review of current evidence. Am J Emerg Med 2019;37(2):344–8.

39. Tsivgoulis G, Katsanos AH, Alexandrov AV. Reperfusion therapies of acute ischemic stroke: potentials and failures. Front Neurol 2014;5:215.

40. Li X, Du H, Song Z, et al. Efficacy and safety of sonothrombolysis in patients with acute ischemic stroke: a systematic review and meta-analysis. J Neurol Sci 2020;416:116998.

41. del Zoppo GJ, Poeck K, Pessin MS, et al. Recombinant tissue plasminogen activator in acute thrombotic and embolic stroke. Ann Neurol 1992;32(1):78–86.

42. Goyal M, Demchuk AM, Menon BK, et al. Randomized assessment of rapid endovascular treatment of ischemic stroke. N Engl J Med 2015;372(11):1019–30.

43. Berkhemer OA, Fransen PS, Beumer D, et al. A randomized trial of intraarterial treatment for acute ischemic stroke. N Engl J Med 2015;372(1):11–20.

44. Campbell BC, Mitchell PJ, Kleinig TJ, et al. Endovascular therapy for ischemic stroke with perfusion-imaging selection. N Engl J Med 2015;372(11):1009–18.

45. Saver JL, Goyal M, Bonafe A, et al. Stent-retriever thrombectomy after intravenous t-PA vs. t-PA alone in stroke. N Engl J Med 2015;372(24):2285–95.

46. Jovin TG, Chamorro A, Cobo E, et al. Thrombectomy within 8 hours after symptom onset in ischemic stroke. N Engl J Med 2015;372(24):2296–306.

47. Siket MS. Treatment of Acute Ischemic Stroke. Emerg Med Clin North Am 2016;34(4):861–82.

48. Goyal M, Menon BK, van Zwam WH, et al. Endovascular thrombectomy after large-vessel ischaemic stroke: a meta-analysis of individual patient data from five randomised trials. Lancet 2016;387(10029):1723–31.

49. Albers GW, Marks MP, Kemp S, et al. Thrombectomy for stroke at 6 to 16 hours with selection by perfusion imaging. N Engl J Med 2018;378(8):708–18.

50. Nogueira RG, Jadhav AP, Haussen DC, et al. Thrombectomy 6 to 24 hours after stroke with a mismatch between deficit and infarct. N Engl J Med 2018;378(1):11–21.

51. Hill MD, Goyal M, Menon BK, et al. Efficacy and safety of nerinetide for the treatment of acute ischaemic stroke (ESCAPE-NA1): a multicentre, double-blind, randomised controlled trial. Lancet 2020;395(10227):878–87.

52. Saver JL, Starkman S, Eckstein M, et al. Prehospital use of magnesium sulfate as neuroprotection in acute stroke. N Engl J Med 2015;372(6):528–36.

53. Castillo J, Leira R, García MM, et al. Blood pressure decrease during the acute phase of ischemic stroke is associated with brain injury and poor stroke outcome. Stroke 2004;35(2):520–6.

54. Manning LS, Mistri AK, Potter J, et al. Short-term blood pressure variability in acute stroke: post hoc analysis of the controlling hypertension and hypotension immediately post stroke and continue or stop post-stroke antihypertensives collaborative study trials. Stroke 2015;46(6):1518–24.

55. Wohlfahrt P, Krajcoviechova A, Jozifova M, et al. Low blood pressure during the acute period of ischemic stroke is associated with decreased survival. J Hypertens 2015;33(2):339–45.
56. International Stroke Trial Collaborative Group. The International Stroke Trial (IST): a randomised trial of aspirin, subcutaneous heparin, both, or neither among 19435 patients with acute ischaemic stroke. Lancet 1997;349(9065):1569–81.
57. CAST (Chinese Acute Stroke Trial) Collaborative Group CAST: randomised placebo-controlled trial of early aspirin use in 20,000 patients with acute ischaemic stroke. Lancet 1997;349(9066):1641–9.
58. Wang Y, Wang Y, Zhao X, et al. Clopidogrel with aspirin in acute minor stroke or transient ischemic attack. N Engl J Med 2013;369(1):11–9.
59. Johnston SC, Easton JD, Farrant M, et al. Clopidogrel and aspirin in acute ischemic stroke and high-risk TIA. N Engl J Med 2018;379(3):215–25.
60. Vahedi K, Hofmeijer J, Juettler E, et al. Early decompressive surgery in malignant infarction of the middle cerebral artery: a pooled analysis of three randomised controlled trials. Lancet Neurol 2007;6(3):215–22.
61. Wijdicks EF, Sheth KN, Carter BS, et al. Recommendations for the management of cerebral and cerebellar infarction with swelling: a statement for healthcare professionals from the American Heart Association/American Stroke Association. Stroke 2014;45(4):1222–38.
62. Wan YH, Nie C, Wang HL, et al. Therapeutic hypothermia (different depths, durations, and rewarming speeds) for acute ischemic stroke: a meta-analysis. J Stroke Cerebrovasc Dis 2014;23(10):2736–47.
63. Mostofi K. Neurosurgical management of massive cerebellar infarct outcome in 53 patients. Surg Neurol Int 2013;4:28.
64. Markus HS, Hayter E, Levi C, et al. Antiplatelet treatment compared with anticoagulation treatment for cervical artery dissection (CADISS): a randomised trial. Lancet Neurol 2015;14(4):361–7.
65. Tsivgoulis G, Zand R, Katsanos AH, et al. Safety and outcomes of intravenous thrombolysis in dissection-related ischemic stroke: an international multicenter study and comprehensive meta-analysis of reported case series. J Neurol 2015;262(9):2135–43.
66. Lin J, Sun Y, Zhao S, et al. Safety and efficacy of thrombolysis in cervical artery dissection-related ischemic stroke: a meta-analysis of observational studies. Cerebrovasc Dis 2016;42(3–4):272–9.
67. Förster A, Gass A, Kern R, et al. Thrombolysis in posterior circulation stroke: stroke subtypes and patterns, complications and outcome. Cerebrovasc Dis 2011;32(4):349–53.
68. Dorňák T, Král M, Hazlinger M, et al. Posterior vs. anterior circulation infarction: demography, outcomes, and frequency of hemorrhage after thrombolysis. Int J Stroke 2015;10(8):1224–8.
69. Breuer L, Huttner HB, Jentsch K, et al. Intravenous thrombolysis in posterior cerebral artery infarctions. Cerebrovasc Dis 2011;31(5):448–54.
70. Keselman B, Gdovinová Z, Jatuzis D, et al. Safety and outcomes of intravenous thrombolysis in posterior versus anterior circulation stroke: results from the safe implementation of treatments in stroke registry and meta-analysis. Stroke 2020; 51(3):876–82.
71. Wahlgren N, Ahmed N, Dávalos A, et al. Thrombolysis with alteplase 3-4.5 h after acute ischaemic stroke (SITS-ISTR): an observational study. Lancet 2008; 372(9646):1303–9.

72. Johnston SC, Gress DR, Browner WS, et al. Short-term prognosis after emergency department diagnosis of TIA. JAMA 2000;284(22):2901–6.
73. Chandratheva A, Mehta Z, Geraghty OC, et al. Population-based study of risk and predictors of stroke in the first few hours after a TIA. Neurology 2009; 72(22):1941–7.
74. Lo BM, Carpenter CR, Hatten BW, et al. Clinical policy: critical issues in the evaluation of adult patients with suspected transient ischemic attack in the emergency department. Ann Emerg Med 2016;68(3):354–70.e29.
75. Siket MS, Edlow JA. Transient ischemic attack: reviewing the evolution of the definition, diagnosis, risk stratification, and management for the emergency physician. Emerg Med Clin North Am 2012;30(3):745–70.
76. Grams RW, Kidwell CS, Doshi AH, et al. Tissue-negative transient ischemic attack: is there a role for perfusion MRI? AJR Am J Roentgenol 2016;207(1): 157–62.
77. Meyer IA, Cereda CW, Correia PN, et al. Factors Associated With Focal Computed Tomographic Perfusion Abnormalities in Supratentorial Transient Ischemic Attacks. Stroke 2018;49(1):68–75.
78. Lee J, Inoue M, Mlynash M, et al. MR perfusion lesions after TIA or minor stroke are associated with new infarction at 7 days. Neurology 2017;88(24):2254–9.
79. Johnston SC, Rothwell PM, Nguyen-Huynh MN, et al. Validation and refinement of scores to predict very early stroke risk after transient ischaemic attack. Lancet 2007;369(9558):283–92.
80. Merwick A, Albers GW, Amarenco P, et al. Addition of brain and carotid imaging to the $ABCD^2$ score to identify patients at early risk of stroke after transient ischaemic attack: a multicentre observational study. Lancet Neurol 2010;9(11): 1060–9.
81. Perry JJ, Sharma M, Sivilotti ML, et al. A prospective cohort study of patients with transient ischemic attack to identify high-risk clinical characteristics. Stroke 2014; 45(1):92–100.
82. Available at: https://www.cambridge.org/core/journals/canadian-journal-of-emergency-medicine/article/pl01-prospective-multicenter-validation-of-the-canadian-tia-score-for-predicting-subsequent-stroke-within-seven-days/DB9CA99BE32B22C83AEE9EA21386174BAccessed September 9th, 2020.

Moving?

Make sure your subscription moves with you!

To notify us of your new address, find your **Clinics Account Number** (located on your mailing label above your name), and contact customer service at:

Email: journalscustomerservice-usa@elsevier.com

800-654-2452 (subscribers in the U.S. & Canada)
314-447-8871 (subscribers outside of the U.S. & Canada)

Fax number: 314-447-8029

Elsevier Health Sciences Division
Subscription Customer Service
3251 Riverport Lane
Maryland Heights, MO 63043

*To ensure uninterrupted delivery of your subscription, please notify us at least 4 weeks in advance of move.

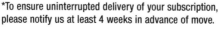